THE MYCELIAL HEALER

*A Comprehensive Guide to the
Cultivation and Traditional Uses
of Medicinal Mushrooms*

Christopher Parker and
Katherine Parker, PhD

Chelsea Green Publishing
White River Junction, Vermont
London, UK

First published in 2025 by Chelsea Green Publishing | PO Box 4529 | White River Junction, VT 05001
| West Wing, Somerset House, Strand | London, WC2R 1LA, UK | www.chelseagreen.com
A Division of Rizzoli International Publications, Inc. | 49 West 27th Street | New York, NY 10001
| www.rizzoliusa.com

Unless otherwise noted, all photographs copyright © 2025 by Christopher and Katherine Parker.
All illustrations copyright © 2025 by Naomi Gill.
Photo on page 266 by hilko_mari / iStock.

The information we present in this book is provided as an information resource only and is not to be used or relied
on for any diagnostic or treatment purposes. Please consult your health care team before implementing any
strategies we outline herein.

Publisher: Charles Miers
Deputy Publisher: Matthew Derr
Project Manager: Natalie Wallace
Developmental Editor: Fern Marshall Bradley
Copy Editor: Ashley Davila
Proofreader: Angela Boyle
Indexer: Shana Milkie
Designer: Melissa Jacobson
Page Layout: Abrah Griggs

ISBN 978-1-64502-281-7 (paperback) | ISBN 978-1-64502-282-4 (ebook)
Library of Congress Control Number: 2025026338 (print) | 2025026339 (ebook)

Our Commitment to Green Publishing
Chelsea Green sees publishing as a tool for cultural change and ecological stewardship. We strive to align our
book manufacturing practices with our editorial mission and to reduce the impact of our business enterprise in
the environment. We print our books using vegetable-based inks whenever possible. This book may cost slightly
more because it was printed on paper supplied by Versa from well-managed, FSC®-certified forests and other
controlled sources.

Authorized EU representative for product safety and compliance
Mondadori Libri S.p.A. | www.mondadori.it
via Gian Battista Vico 42 | Milan, Italy 20123

Printed in the United States of America.
10 9 8 7 6 5 4 3 2 1   25 26 27 28 29

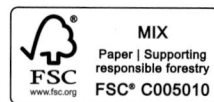

MIX
Paper | Supporting
responsible forestry
FSC
www.fsc.org   FSC® C005010

Praise for *The Mycelial Healer*

"*The Mycelial Healer* is a fantastic addition to the library shelf for growers and health-conscious consumers alike. The Parkers bring a wealth of information and expertise to this beautifully designed contribution. Well done!"

—ROBERT DALE ROGERS, author of *The Fungal Pharmacy*

"*The Mycelial Healer* is a profound journey into the fungal world—blending Indigenous wisdom, hands-on cultivation, and scientific insight. Parker and Parker invite us to reconnect with the unseen networks that sustain life. As an edible landscape enthusiast, I find this book an outstanding resource for optimizing all that shady space—transforming understory into abundance. More than just a guide for growers, it's also a profound meditation on the idea that true restoration and reconnection with the natural world begin beneath our feet, radiating outward from the soil."

—MICHAEL JUDD, author of *Edible Landscaping with a Permaculture Twist* and *For the Love of Pawpaws*

"In your hands is a comprehensive and immensely personal resource celebrating the power and provision of the fungal world. At once a moving exposition and a highly approachable technical compendium, *The Mycelial Healer* inspires, empowers, and nurtures by weaving together worldview and application rooted in deep tradition and experience. Your mycelial journey will certainly benefit from exploring the insights and methods shared within its pages."

—JOHN MUNSELL, professor and forest management extension specialist, Virginia Polytechnic Institute and State University; coauthor of *The Community Food Forest Handbook*

"*The Mycelial Healer* deserves a spot on every mushroom enthusiast's bookshelf. Chris and Katherine Parker set the stage for a fresh look at mushrooms as food and medicine. Their detailed, practical descriptions of how to set up a lab, grow mushrooms outdoors or indoors, and ethically wild-harvest are supported by dozens of photos and diagrams."

—JEANINE DAVIS, professor, North Carolina State University; very small farmer; author of *Growing and Marketing Ginseng, Goldenseal and Other Woodland Medicinals*

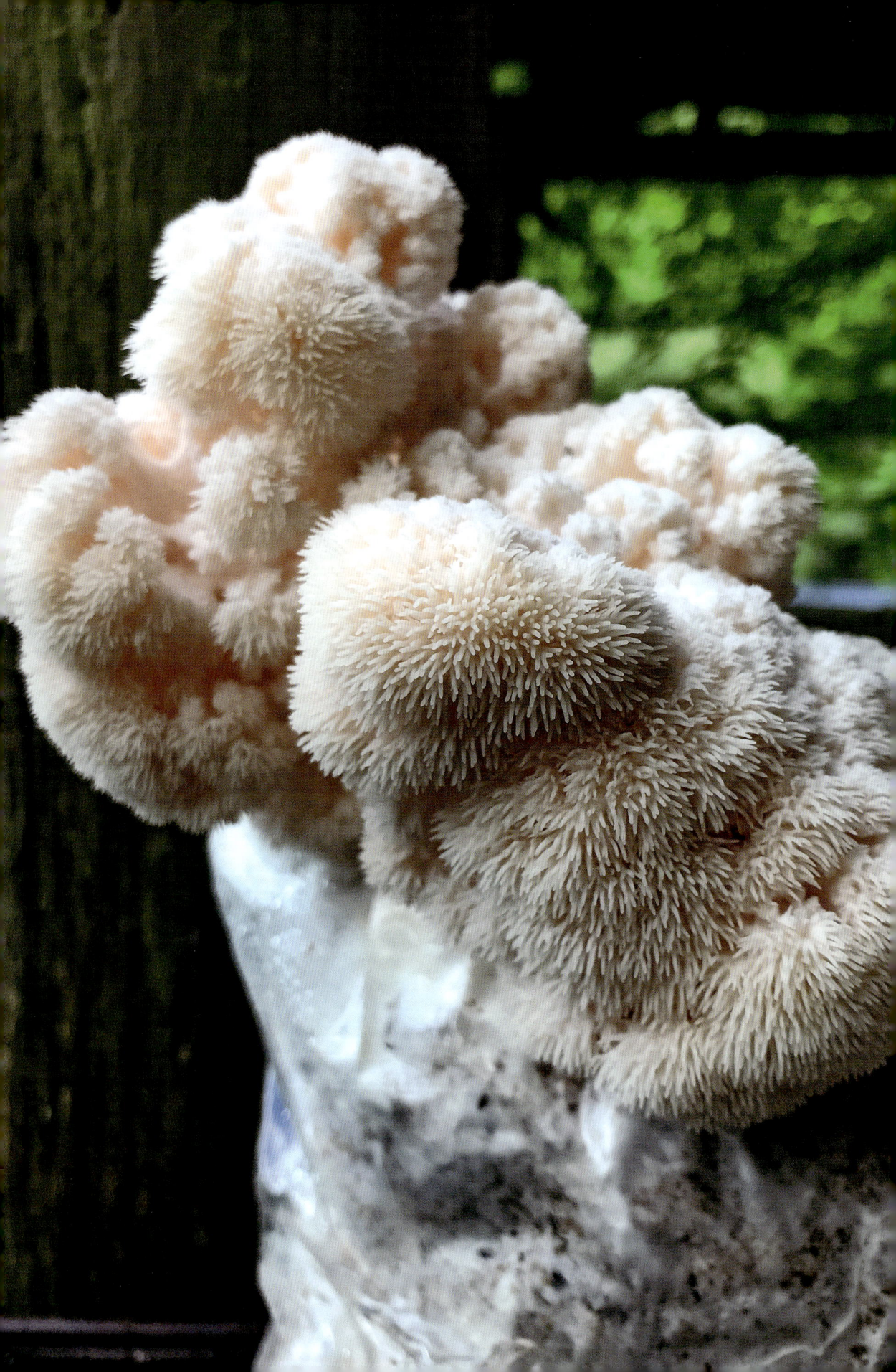

For our ancestors and the past generations.

For the future generations,
Adawehi and Sunalei Parker, Christopher's daughters, and
Leo and Heather Kelly, Katherine's nephew and niece.

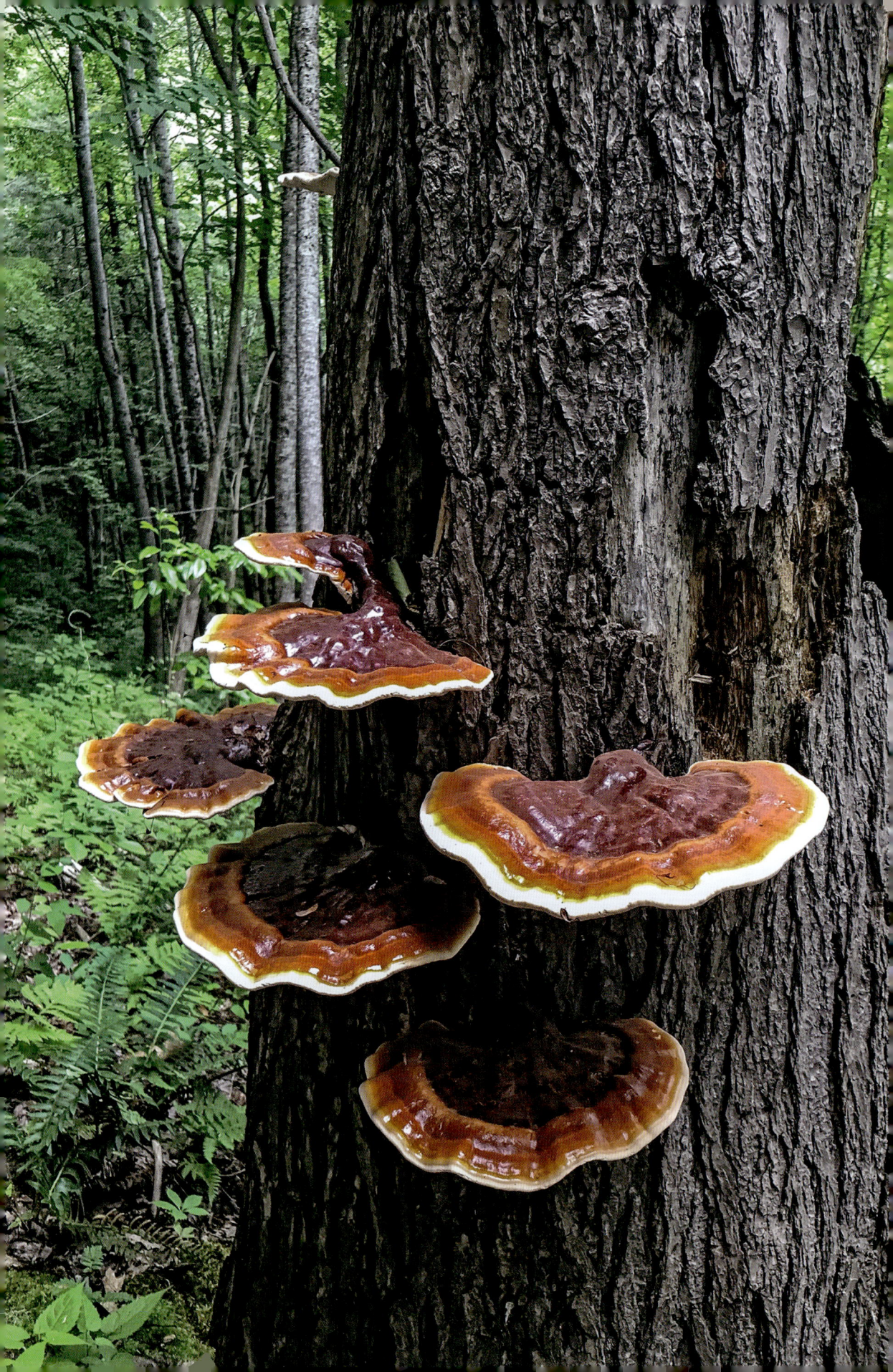

Contents

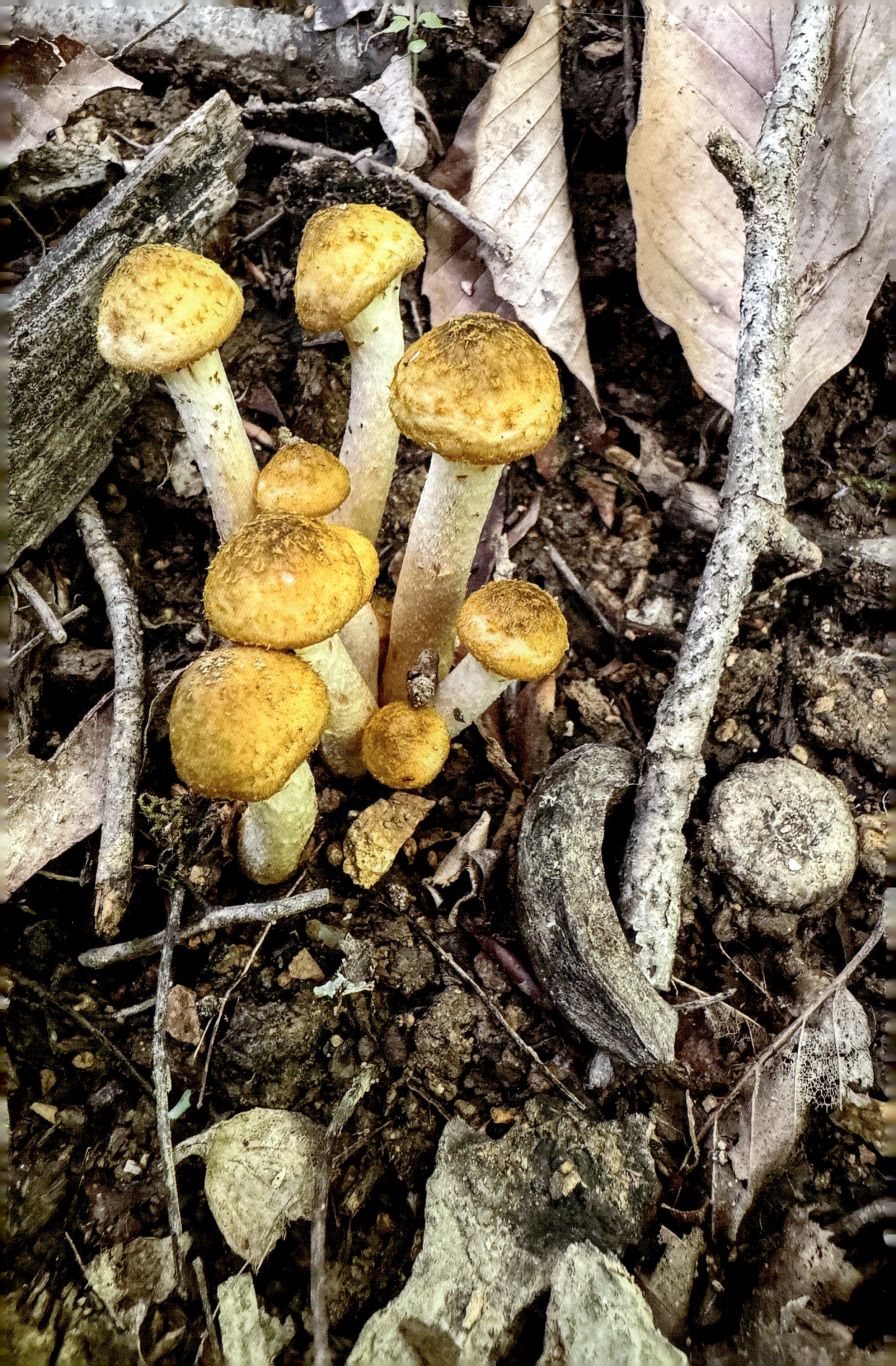

Introduction

The majority of my childhood was spent outdoors in the forests of the southeast parts of the oldest chain of mountains in the world. In one of my very first memories as a little boy, I am in the forest by a creek with my father. I'm looking under rocks for crawdads; climbing trees to their tops and riding them down to the ground. In one of the pine thickets where I used to climb trees, I came upon a huge mushroom. I was instantly captivated. It was the summer between kindergarten and first grade, so I may have only been six years old, but that mushroom is seared into memory. It was only later that I understood which mushroom I had encountered. It was an *Amanita*, beautiful but deadly poisonous. To this day it is one of those up-close memories of exquisite clarity where everything else fades into the background.

The *Amanita* was half as tall as six-year-old me, which meant it must have been around two feet tall. It is not out of the ordinary for certain mushroom species to reach such a height. The "warty" cap, straight stem, and bulbous base are still clear in my mind's eye over forty years later. Its pure whiteness against the backdrop of green pine needles, tree bark, and the brown needle–laden forest floor gave this mushroom a luminous quality. Little did I know how dangerous this mushroom was if consumed, a mushroom that would have likely killed me if I had eaten it. But all I did was touch it. Squeezing the stem; touching the cap in awe.

I frequented this part of the woods often, but I do not remember the mushroom being there the day before. It had popped up seemingly overnight.

A short period later, after the *Amanita* had come and gone, I had another memorable encounter in that same area of the forest. My parents had gotten me a puppy, but it had died of parvovirus, and I was sad about this loss. One of my parents—I don't remember which one—told me to bury the dog. Gathering a shovel and my pup, we went into that same patch of forest. I dug a hole to bury him, close to the spot where I had seen the mushroom. It was not intentional, but at some level, I felt drawn to bury him there. Some twenty years later, with a deepening understanding of how fungi and death are intertwined, these

1

incidents came rushing back to me. In hindsight, I understand now that my interaction with the mushroom in that part of the forest and the death of my puppy are all linked together. The transformational power of fungi to give life, take life, and take death and transmute it into life are now in my full view. Fungi are the great recyclers that hold the circle of space, time, and transformation.

Before I came to this realization of how fungi connect all of life and death on planet Earth, I started my journey to mushroom cultivation as a freshman in high school. Finding myself in a Future Farmers of America (FFA) program, I signed up for a class called "Introduction to Agriculture and Natural Resources." In this class we studied everything from soil and water conservation to forestry. The forestry end of the program was the most enjoyable for me. We participated in tree identification and tree judging (I had grown up with my father and both my grandfathers teaching me about the natural world, so tree identification was easy for me), and learned about the cultivation of Shiitake on small logs—the kind that would usually end up left behind, as waste, in slash piles after logging operations. It was wood that my instructors called a non-timber forest product. Slash piles are sometimes burned or just left to sit. It was fascinating to me that a log could be inoculated with spawn and produce mushrooms that people could eat or could sell to others, and that the logs would keep producing a new yearly harvest for five to seven years, according to the size of the log. I was hooked. This was in the early 1990s, and that operation was at a scale of about one thousand logs.

Shiitakes are the gateway mushroom for many people. The simplicity of Shiitake cultivation was inspiring, and I quickly wanted to know more about growing mushrooms. I started studying more about mycology with field guides and books on cultivation. Only a few were available. *Growing Gourmet and Medicinal Mushrooms* by Paul Stamets was one of the books I picked up in 1993. I learned a lot. The field guides were my favorite reference for a number of years because I could identify different mushrooms when out hunting or fishing. This passion kept moving, morphing and branching, just like mycelium.

After harvesting my first flush of Shiitakes, I found the confidence to start learning techniques for the earlier stages in the cultivation process. Once I had some success growing on logs, I embarked on the journey to learn the sterile techniques needed to produce sawdust spawn, a common starting material for mushroom cultivation. After I gained skill in that, I set my sights on grain spawn. That led to growing mycelium on petri plates and eventually to cloning mushrooms from the wild. I had very little equipment at first, and lots of failures helped me develop the skills I have today. Failure is one of the best teachers.

INTRODUCTION

Mycology is a field still in its infancy, but more and more people are undertaking different disciplines nested within the greater field of mycology. Some people are interested in growing mushrooms, some are interested in mycoremediation, some are interested in medicinal mushrooms, others are interested in the role of fungi in regenerative agriculture. We have branches that are looking for structural and industrial applications. The world of mycology is wide open. There are so many things to discover, learn about, and teach to others. This field of study has identified less than an estimated 10 percent of the species of fungi present on our planet—we have a lot more to learn. What we have learned so far has been fascinating, enchanting, and frightening.

Katherine (my wife and coauthor) and I steward a forest farm in the Southern Appalachian Mountains where we grow mushrooms under the canopy and in our indoor cultivation operation. We are slowly repopulating the forest with native species of plants and fungi while doing what we can to redress the balance by removing invasive species. We share the farm with an enthusiastic band of four-legged beings—goats, sheep, horse, donkey, cats, and dogs—and an orchestra of wild ones too. We keep experimenting with ways to grow mushrooms, and we offer this book as an invitation for you to join the adventure.

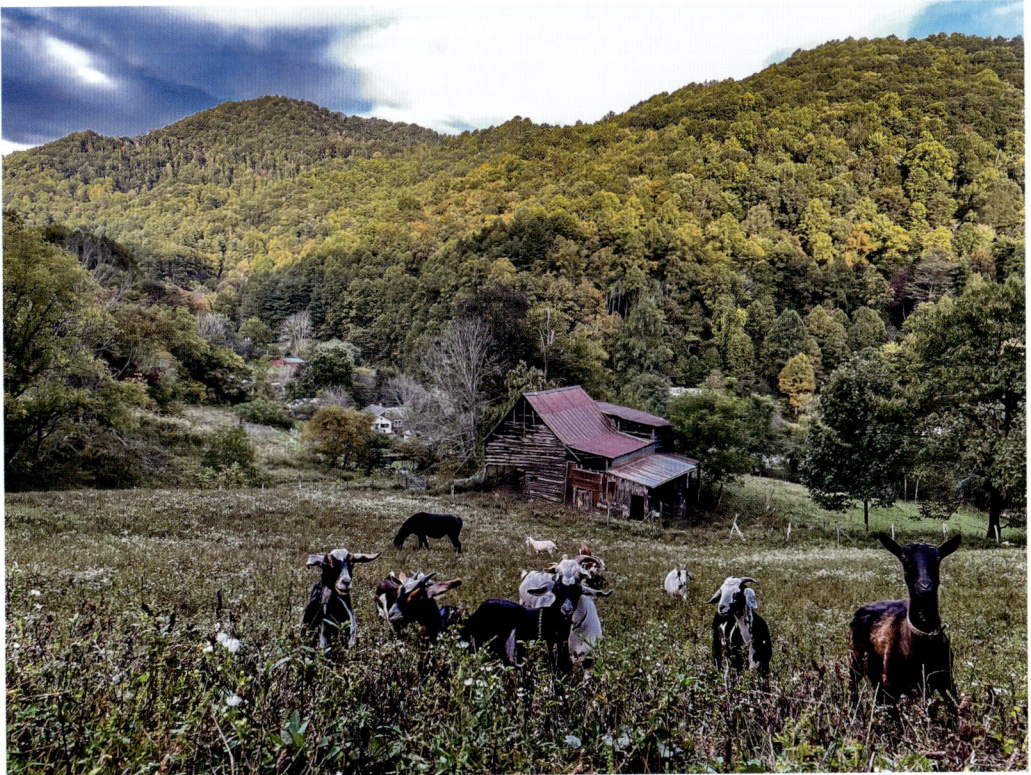

Figure 0.1. View of our forest farm.

One thing that keeps me excited about this journey is that mycologists have realized that we've been wrong about quite a few past assumptions. But we are also discovering that we had figured out some things about mushrooms before research confirmed them, and that there are more learning opportunities for everyone. Many generations of my ancestors have tended the forests in these mountains. Some of my ancestors are Cherokee. We have a long, deep relationship with the land here that changes as we all continue to evolve. As we learn more about mushrooms, we learn more about the forest and about what it means to be human. Some of my ancestors are from Scotland, England, and Ireland. Katherine was born and raised in the British Isles, where people have also had a long relationship with fungi. Traditional cultures from all over the world have been closely connected to fungi. Each mushroom cultivator brings their unique experience and fresh ways of thinking to this exploratory journey, braiding our histories together with new experiences. We are certain that the more we continue to experiment with farming medicinal and culinary mushrooms in the forest, the more will be revealed to us, all in fungal time.

About This Book

This book begins with a deep-time look at fungi and how they shaped our planet and all of life. Katherine and I explore the essence of their medicine and their ability to transform life and to build vast, multi-species collaborative networks. We look at how the blueprint they laid down in the early stages of life on Earth reflects throughout so much of the natural world, from the forest to our guts. Fungi are part of us, just as we are all part of the world. We also address ethical ways to harvest mushrooms from the wild that situate us humans as participants in a much wider web of life. We explore ways to be in relationship with the fungi as we wild-harvest and cultivate them and what they have to teach us about being a collaborative member of a thriving ecosystem.

In chapters 2 through 5, we provide you with the tools you need to start growing medicinal mushrooms for your own benefit and perhaps also to

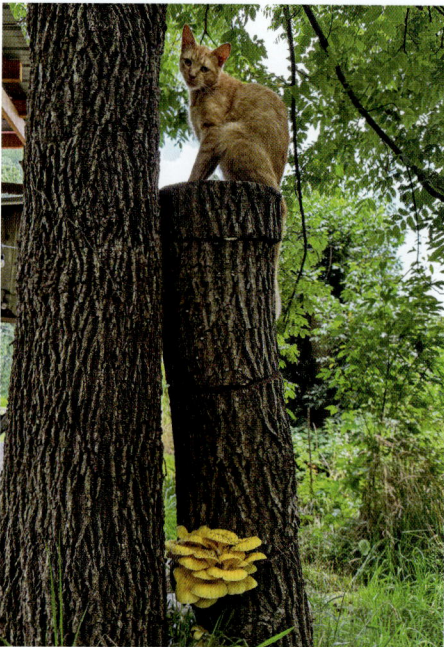

Figure 0.2. Mr. Butters the cat atop a totem fruiting Golden Oysters.

supply your community. We lead you through the entire process from finding mushrooms out in the wild to maintaining your own climate-controlled grow room. We include low-tech outdoor methods and beginner-level indoor methods in addition to more advanced, sterile lab techniques. It's a choose-your-own adventure, whether you envision a semi-automated indoor operation or simply a low-tech, hands off approach in the forest.

These chapters are not all-encompassing. It's beyond the scope of this book to provide full lessons on breeding mushroom varieties or naturalizing fungi. But we do provide a solid base of how-to-grow information for mushroom growers, market farmers, forest farmers, healers, herbalists, mycologists, or anyone along a journey of reconnection with their food and medicine. We hope this information will help you start, or deepen, your own cultivation journey.

We do not claim to have any new fundamental insights in the world of mycology. However, over the last thirty years, we have pushed the edge on mushroom cultivation techniques to see what we can discover. We encourage you to do the same. Feedback from new mushroom growers is invaluable to us because it opens our eyes to new ways of doing things and opens our minds to aspects that we otherwise would have never thought of. There are aspects of mycology so complicated that we could study fungi for multiple lifetimes and never cover it all. This is what keeps us excited about our work as producers and teachers.

How deeply you dive into cultivating culinary and medicinal mushrooms is up to you, and you'll need to balance your time and monetary means with your immediate or long-term goals. Our intention is to help you find where you would like to dive first. Your initial experiences will then guide you into the areas that most resonate for you.

In chapter 6 we describe some of the biochemical compounds that make mushrooms potent medicines and explain how to prepare mushrooms as medicine and as food, including a few of our favorite recipes.

Many species of mushrooms are medicinal; only a few are deadly like that Amanita I encountered as a child. We chose to focus on fourteen genera for *The Mycelial Healer*. Some of these are quite popular, including Chaga, Lion's Mane, Maitake, medicinal molds, Oyster, psychoactive mushrooms, Reishi, Shiitake, and Turkey Tail. Others you may never have heard of: Amadou, Birch Polypore, Cordyceps, Milky Caps, and Split Gill. We chose these fourteen mushrooms because they are the most widely used as medicinals around the world and have been the subjects of the most scientific research. Chapter 7 presents a profile of each of these mushrooms. We begin each profile with an overview of the characteristics of the mushrooms and where you might find them, and how they have been used traditionally across the world. A section on scientific research focuses on the more recent science that supports the use of these mushrooms as medicine. We also discuss ethical wild harvesting of these mushrooms and summarize the main cultivation methods.

In the chapters on cultivating mushrooms, we mention some species of culinary mushrooms that are not covered in the mushroom profiles in this book. There are good reasons to grow mushrooms apart from their specific medicinal properties. The real medicine is the journey with fungi and remembering our deep relationships with them.

Looking at the world in fungal time might start with slowing down and paying attention. Why the hurry? Do we know what we are missing? Often modern people do not. It takes time to see these things and understand them. That is what this book is about. A different perspective. A perspective that is older than me. A perspective of slowing down, looking with respect and curiosity, to see how these things work together. This is where culture comes from. Thousands of years of careful observations and working with the land, incorporating ourselves into the landscape.

Are you ready? We are excited to show you around the world of fungi.

CHAPTER ONE

The World According to Fungi

We modern humans like to view ourselves as being independent. We like to imagine that we have complete control over our lives and make all of our own decisions. Some of us even try to become as separate from nature as possible. However, as clever as we are, we still depend on the systems that tie all life on Earth together. We do not and cannot exist without the complex network of biological and geological relationships that birthed us and continue to feed us. Some people have big plans, like colonizing Mars or discovering the next subatomic particle, but it would be great if we could focus first on cleaning up the mess we have made here on Earth. The mess will clean itself up in the future, after humans go extinct, but wouldn't it be nice to leave the place better than how we found it? We are acting like teenagers; it is time to step into a more

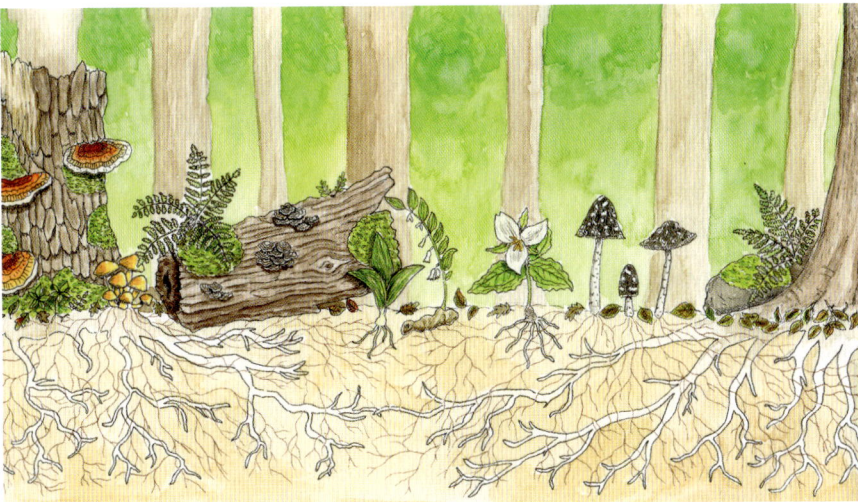

Figure 1.1. Fungal mycelium connects the forest community.

mature relationship with the planet. Fungi have been around a lot longer than we have—they are our Elders, and they carry wisdom we would do well to hear.

What we tend to think of as mushrooms are only a small part of any fungus. The part sticking up above the ground, that we pick and eat, is called the *fruiting body*. It is formed out of the underground (or within-tree) mycelium, a vast net made up of hyphae, which are thread-like tubes of protoplasm. Mycelium can be thought of as fungal "roots," and mycelial networks work their way through whatever substrate they are in, consuming anything edible and exuding metabolites (see figure 1.1). The fruiting body, which pops up periodically above the surface, essentially exists to produce spores. These spores are similar to seeds; they are distributed by wind, insects, or animals to spread fungi to new areas.

Over the 900 million years or so since fungi diverged from protists (unicellular, microscopic organisms), they have diversified into somewhere between 2 and 11 million species today, of which we have only identified and named around 150,000.[1] Many species of fungi that we will never know about have already flourished and gone extinct. As opposed to animals with skeletons, scales, or exoskeletons, many fungi are difficult to fossilize because of their soft nature and the rapid decomposition of mycelium and fruiting bodies. This makes studying their history difficult. Fungi that contain cells that are less easily broken down—such as Amadou (*Fomes fomentarius*) and Reishi (*Ganoderma* spp.)—are more likely to fossilize.

We do know that fungi are one of the most successful groups of organisms that this planet has ever seen. When an organism has been around in many shapes and forms for 900 million years, then other organisms will evolve to have similar structures. Spores from fungi, which have a very durable coating, have shown up in the fossil record around 715 to 800 million years ago.[2] Spores appear in the fossil record from early plants around 470 million years ago.[3] Fungi were pioneers in genetic reproduction and dispersal strategies around 330 million years before plants showed up to the party. Similarly, the branching structure in mycelium is replicated over and over in the plant and animal worlds.

Building Soils and Sharing Resources

For much of their early existence, fungi worked in collaboration with bacteria and algae to create the first soils, around 500 million years ago.[4] (Fungi continue to be exquisite collaborators, as we describe throughout this book.) This planet-wide, massive effort that resulted in soil formation likely started in tidepools and then moved to the terrestrial surface of the planet as organisms developed adaptations and strategies to begin to degrade stone. At this time, the Earth's crust was, well, a crust, and a stoney one at that. It was an extremely uninhabitable place.

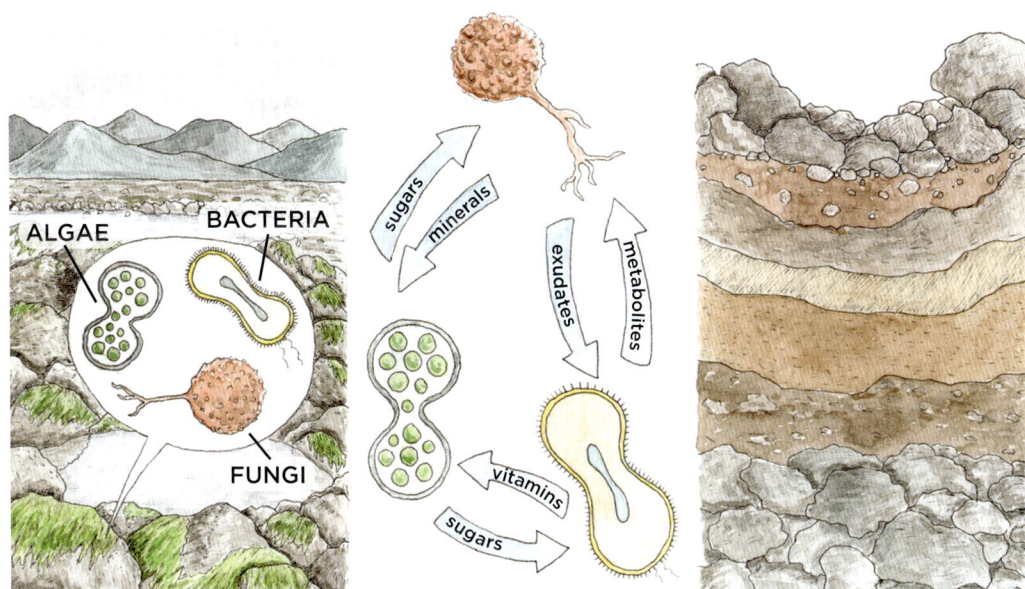

Figure 1.2. Fungi, algae, and bacteria collaborate to develop primitive soils that become the basis for all land-based life on Earth.

The degradation of stone through the symbiosis of algae, fungi, and bacteria was the beginning of soil formation, as shown in figure 1.2. Fungi are able to exude acids that break down rock, extracting essential minerals. Algae have the ability to photosynthesize, using solar energy to make sugars, which fungi use as fuel. Bacteria also exude rock-dissolving acids. Fungi likely fed on the bacteria and played the unique role of feeding the bacteria a carbon-rich diet, sourced from the algae. The metabolites from all three of these organisms, in combination with their decaying bodies, contributed to the first primitive soils. Together they transformed the hard crust of the planet into a fertile substrate that would eventually be able to support complex life, including us humans.

Death is transformational: it turns something that otherwise is unusable into something new and beautiful. Over countless generations, fungi, algae, and bacteria harvested rock, sunlight, and each other to create life. These tiny beings were able to lay the groundwork that gives Earth-based life sustenance. And they didn't stop there. To this day, fungi, bacteria, and algae continue to form a biological bedrock for plants, insects, and animals. As decomposers, they have transformed all the bodies of all biological beings since life began on this planet into nutrients that can be used by subsequent generations. They are our oldest ancestors.

The first living structures that stretched from the Earth's surface up toward the sky were not plants or trees—they likely were fungi called *prototaxites* (see figure 1.3), which may have reached over 26 feet (8 m) tall.[5] They existed between 420 and 350 million years ago, along with early types of plants, long

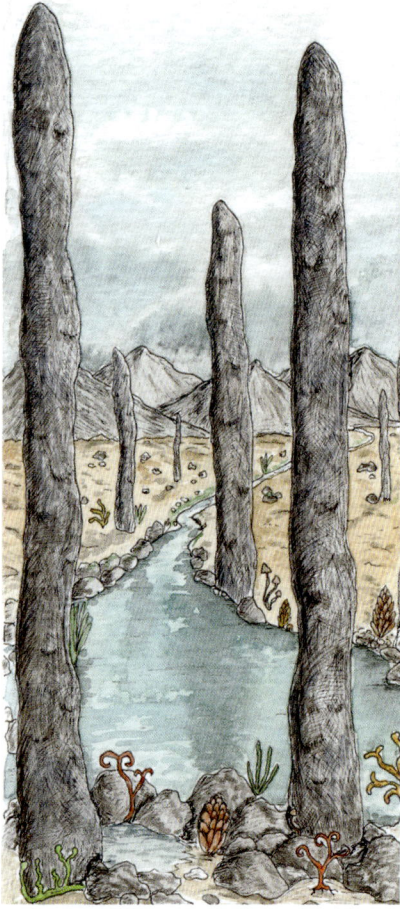

Figure 1.3. Possible view of *Prototaxites*.

before trees evolved. Scientists believe that these mammoths of the fungal world were responsible for the redistribution of water and nutrients through the soil to support the expansion of early plant life. This ancient sharing of resources is the basis of all life and can be seen as a foreshadowing of things that would come with mycorrhizal fungi—those that collaborate closely with plants.

Mycorrhizal Communities

Fungi gave rise to our first vascular plants. These early plants relied on a type of fungi called *arbuscular mycorrhizal fungi* (AMF), beginning at least 500 million years ago.[6] The word *arbuscular* has its roots in the word *arbor*, which means "tree" in Latin. This is in reference to the tree-like structures (arbuscules) incorporated into the root cells of plants (see figure 1.4). AMF are in a category we refer to as *endomycorrhizal*, with *endo-* meaning "in," *myco-* meaning "mushroom," and *-rhizal* referencing "root." These fascinating fungi incorporated themselves into the root structures of early vascular plants from the beginning, which allowed plants to begin to diversify into the complicated species of towering giants on Earth today.

This deep intertwining of mycelium and plant roots forms a foundational network on which global ecosystems are built. As plants evolved, their root structures became more developed, and some fungi evolved to connect on the outside of plant roots. These are *ectomycorrhizal*: *ecto-* meaning "outside." A great example of this type of collaboration are some bog and heathland ecosystems. Ericoid mycorrhizal fungi (EMF) are important drivers of these ecosystems. They are fungi that have evolved to collaborate with plants in the order Ericales, which includes rhododendrons, cranberries, and heather. EMF have retained their ability to decompose lignocellulose (the main components of woody plants), while other types of ectomycorrhizae have lost this characteristic. This allows EMF to decompose a wider range of substrates. These bogs and heathlands are acidic, and without these fungal partners, plants would not be able to extract the nutrients needed from these extreme environments.

When plants die the EMF breaks down the plant material and passes the nutrients on to the plants with which it has mycorrhizal association. The tight-knit recycling of carbon and nutrients in acidic ecosystems is important. These highly acidic bogs are well known for their ability to preserve plant material and animals for hundreds and sometimes thousands of years. Irish and Scottish bogs often turn up amazing artifacts, including 2,325-year-old "bog butter"![7] EMF seem to be the main drivers of these systems, and without them, the bogs could collapse.

The invisible microorganisms that exist in soils around the world live in such a complex manner that we have barely scratched the surface of understanding them. The jury is still out on the total number of species on planet Earth, but we know that our soils are the most diverse ecosystems, with estimates of up to 100 billion species living in Earth's soils. When working in concert with each other, soil microorganisms create a balance of harmony and resilience.

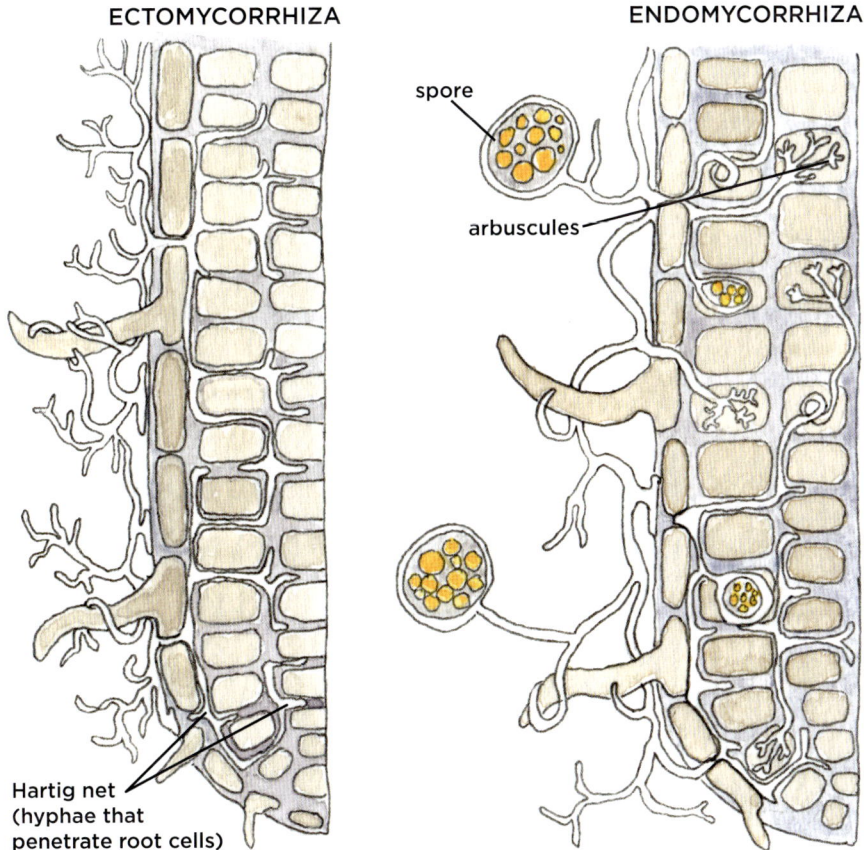

Figure 1.4. Ectomycorrhizal fungi connect to plants mostly on the outside of the roots, whereas endomycorrhizal fungi are deeply embedded within the structure of the plant root.

Our Microbiome

This tendency of deep collaboration between fungi and other microorganisms that build the foundations of all life on the planet is reflected in the microbiome of animals, including humans. *I Contain Multitudes* by science journalist Ed Yong is an eye-opening read for those of us culturally conditioned to think of ourselves as individuals. Our bodies are more "other" cells than human cells. We are dependent on this humming, multispecies orchestra of cells to maintain stability for this bipedal being we call *Homo sapiens*.

The number of human cells in our bodies is somewhere around 37 trillion, and 100 trillion other organisms—mostly fungi, bacteria, viruses, and protists—coinhabit us. Yes, we are composed of *three times* more nonhuman than human cells. The gut microbiome alone can weigh between 2 and 5 pounds, about the same weight as the human brain! A healthy gut microbiome supports our immune system, facilitates nutrient absorption, keeps the heart healthy, and works with our brain to ensure efficient cognitive processing. Disruptions of the microbiome can lead to weight gain, inflammatory bowel syndrome, and digestive issues, as well as increased harmful cholesterol and heart disease, out of control blood sugar levels, and increased risk of asthma, depression and anxiety, and cognitive decline. In short, the gut microbiome is essential for all aspects of keeping us healthy, just as the microorganisms in the soil play a massive role in keeping a forest functioning optimally.

Scientists still have much to discover about the human microbiome. We have learned that some medicinal mushrooms seem to work through interacting with bacteria or other fungi in our gut. Fungi from the forest are in conversation with those that inhabit our digestive system.

Human Roots in the Forest

We are forest creatures. Forests gave birth to us. The forest is where we belong, and it is where we return to find medicine. The forest is the medicine. Humans evolved from tree-dwelling apes and have been eating mushrooms for millions of years.[8] All of the plants, fungi, and animals that make the forest are greater than the sum of their parts. Just one example—more than twenty-two species of primates eat fungi, and Goeldi's Monkeys (*Callimico goeldii*), which live in Amazonian forests, spend over half of their feeding hours during the dry season consuming only four species of mushrooms.[9]

In the 1990s, Terence McKenna proposed that approximately 100,000 years ago humans encountered psychoactive mushrooms, and continuing encounters shaped human evolution.[10] This idea is sometimes called the stoned ape theory. Its merit is debated, and with good reason for both sides. The theory states that human consumption of psychoactive fungi was responsible for the cognitive revolution: our rapid increase in intelligence, language, and culture. More recent theorists additionally propose that our ancestors used psychoactive fungi to manage psychological distress, treat health problems, enhance social relations, and facilitate collective ritual and shared decision making.[11] Psychoactive fungi heighten the senses, possibly allowing for more astute observations of the world, leading to our ancestors securing more food, sensing the presence of predatory animals more keenly, or becoming more attuned predators themselves. Psychoactive fungi change our perceptions, conceivably leading to better problem-solving skills. (We discuss this in more detail in the psychoactive mushrooms profile on page 230.)

Regardless of how this all happened, trees, nuts, roots, fruits, mushrooms, and other foods from the forest have always supported us. Not only did the forests shape us, but we shaped them alongside other organisms big and small. How we continue this relationship with the forest is crucial to the ongoing flourishing of life on Earth. Learning how to responsibly gather and grow medicinal mushrooms is part of strengthening the forest–human relationship.

Hunting Mushrooms

Some people talk about "foraging" for mushrooms. This to me sounds as if they are stumbling through the forest, randomly looking around, without direction; it has never sat right for me. The word *forage* has its roots in the word *fodder*. Fodder is grass, silage or hay. The word *hunting* instead became my term of choice. The roots of *hunt* are something along the lines of "to seize, capture," "to stalk" or "to search until found." Why does this choice of words matter? Because our words allow others to understand our intentions and therefore what we focus on.

When we walk in the forest, or in our modern urban terrain, we are completely unaware of most of what surrounds us, even though human eyesight is among the best of all creatures on Earth. We can see only a shimmer of the band of light in the middle of the spectrum. Low-energy radio waves are invisible to us, as are the upper end of the high-energy gamma rays.

When out hunting mushrooms in the forests, it is important to soften our gaze and slow down, letting our senses become more attuned to the forest around us. If we do not, then the mushrooms beside our feet and on the trees around us may be invisible too.

We don't take hunting for morel mushrooms very seriously, but many people do. Over the years, a lot of people have asked me to take them out to look for these prized and elusive fungi. After a persistent friend asked many times, I agreed to go with him. I did not want to reveal my usual morel spots, so we went to other parts of the forest.

As we were driving, I suddenly told him to stop on the side of the road. He pulled over, and I led him down an embankment through some trees. In the Southern Appalachians, morels come out in successions. Black Morels show up first, then Half-Free Morels, White Morels, Tulip Poplar Morels, and finally, the big Yellow Morels. It was halfway through morel season on this day. Dogwoods were blooming, as were bloodroot. Jewelweed's fat dicot seed leaves were showing themselves. I started allowing my gaze to soften and traveled slowly across the forest floor. Two minutes into my calm, deliberate walk, the first morel came into view. Approaching it, I sat down close by, with the intention of just being with that mushroom. Again, I slowed the pace of my gaze and tried my best to align myself with the mushrooms. As I sat there, several more morels started to show up in the vicinity. I called my unsuccessful friend over. He came crashing through the undergrowth, striding right past several morels. I asked him to slow down. He still could not see them. After I pointed out several mushrooms, he saw them, but he did not find any for himself that day. He was amazed that I had known where to stop and had found our first morel of the day within minutes. But moving fast and crashing through the forest, it was impossible for him to find mushrooms. He had to slow down first.

When people first try hunting mushrooms, many have the city walk, moving as quickly as possible from one place to another. People who did not grow up hunting, fishing, picking wild foods, or spending time in the forest may have to relearn how to be in tune with natural spaces. This starts by simply slowing down, letting go of the idea of reaching a destination or a goal. Walk at a relaxed pace. Smell the air, listen to the sounds, feel the textures around you. This way you will start to recognize which microhabitats certain trees, plants, animals, and fungi tend to gravitate toward. You will begin to recognize forest communities—who hangs out with whom, in which degrees of light and moisture.

Out in the forest, walking for hours without finding any mushrooms, I can become tired. This kind of tired state is the perfect opportunity to allow your mind to "lift." I'm not sure how to fully explain this, but you let the thinking part of your mind drift up and slightly away. This allows you to follow your intuition; it is somewhat of an altered state. This state will allow you to find what you are seeking. It is what I imagine our ancestors experienced out hunting. Low blood sugar levels and their fuel source switching over to ketones. This changes many things with your experience in the forest. It may sound fantastical, but our nervous systems are sensitive, and you will be pulled in a direction if you can quiet your mind and pick up on the energies that flow in the forest. These heightened senses are what often kept our ancestors out of harm's way.

Regardless of what continent your ancestors lived on, they picked, ate, and used mushrooms as medicine. That medicine is still there if you allow it to come through you. Practice letting go of needing to achieve the goal and allow the mushrooms to show themselves to you. If you are directionally challenged, you may want to hunt with a friend or download a map of the area in advance to help you get back to your starting point after following your intuition in the forest.

When picking mushrooms to eat as food or medicine, paying close attention to the polycultures, or communities, of the forest is essential. This way when you pick the mushrooms you want to take, you will also be able to give back. We never take anything without giving back. One of many ways we give back on every hunt is to return some of the fungi to areas that are similar to the ones where we harvested. Or we return spores or spore solutions (a mixture of spores suspended in water) back to other areas that have the right environmental conditions. For example, when we harvest Chanterelle mushrooms, we pull them fully from the ground, with soil clinging to the butt of the stem. Some people advise against harvesting mushrooms this way. They will tell you that you are damaging the mycelium. This is not true. In fact, we find that if Chanterelles are harvested by cutting the stems and leaving a "stump" behind, molds may take hold in the stump cells that were damaged by the cutting knife. These dead cells are opportunities for other fungi to colonize. Pulling the stems rather than cutting them allows for the stems to separate from the rest of the mycelial bed without inviting such contamination.

This is one way to expand wild mushrooms and show respect to the fungi at the same time. Harvest the full mushroom, and then when you trim off the stem, place the stem with soil still attached into a bag dedicated to that species, or at least the same genus. As you continue hunting, you will probably walk through parts of the forest that have the same habitat as the site where you collected. Stop there, and use your foot to move the leaves back, plus a bit of soil. Drop a few stem butts onto the cleared spot, then use your foot to cover the stem butts with the leaves. This is especially effective if done right before a rain, or close to water sources. By doing this you are increasing the range of this mushroom, making it easier for it to increase the population in this part of the forest. If you are picking saprotrophic (wood-eating) fungi, you can spread them to new potential habitats by simply lifting the bark of dead or dying trees and placing the stem butts between the bark and sapwood.

When harvesting, we pick only the mushrooms that are vibrant and in their prime. The ones that are too young we leave. We pick in one cove or section of our forest one week and then the parallel section the next, the third section the week after that, and finally, after the fourth section of forest, we circle back to the first. With this cycle, we observe that some of the mushrooms are again perfect to pick, and some will be too old to harvest because they have already released their spores. The release of spores is essential to regenerate the genetics of the area. This method is highly recommended with any terrestrial fungi including morels, Milky mushrooms, lobsters, corals, boletes, and so on. We describe techniques in following chapters on how to encourage naturally simulated production of saprotrophic fungi. These harvesting techniques, along with expanding techniques, have sustained nations for thousands of years and will ensure resilient ecosystems and bountiful harvests for generations to come.

The Fungal Blueprint

Fungi have been on the planet for so long, and are foundational to so much other life, that their adaptive characteristics show up in a wide variety of other beings. As mentioned earlier in this chapter, arbuscular mycorrhizal fungi are named after the structure characteristic of trees. However, we have this backward. It is this microscopic fungal structure that gave rise to the trees in the first place. Without these fungi, trees would have never had the ability to evolve as they have. We can see trees as an amplification, a fractal, of the tiny pattern of foundational fungal structures, rising hundreds of feet into the air. Up in these heights, the trees produce leaves that serve the same function as the arbuscules, exchanging carbon dioxide and oxygen while releasing purified water back into the atmosphere. This mirrors what occurs in the underground arbuscules in the roots, where carbon exchange occurs in both directions. In this collaborative relationship, the plant receives nutrients and water from the fungi while the fungi receive sugars from their photosynthesizing friends.

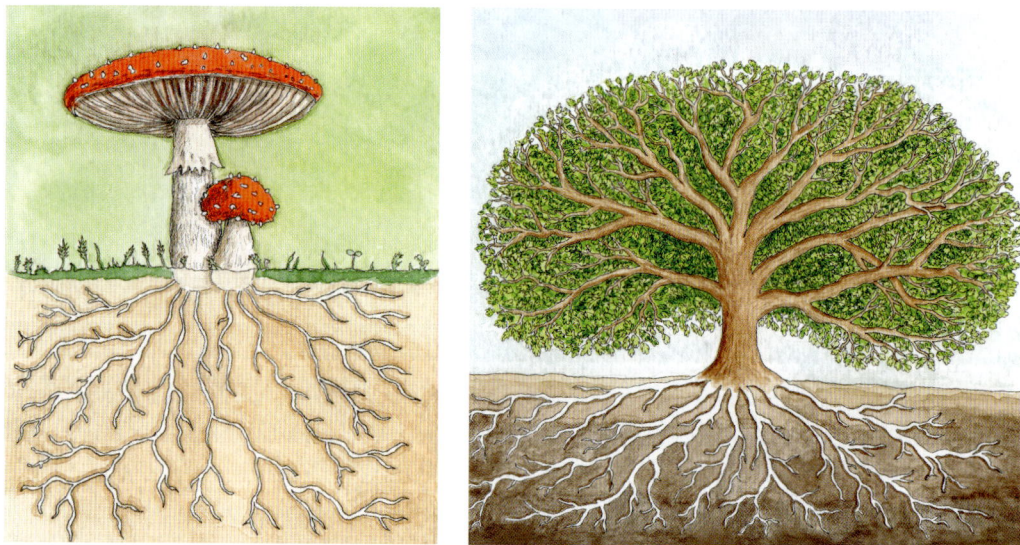

Figure 1.5. The branching pattern found in mycelium is reflected throughout the living world.

Fungi use hydraulic pressure for many operations. The growth of fungal hyphae is dependent on hydrostatic pressure inside the cells. Driven by this pressure, the hyphal tips expand outward to find food, deliver nutrients, and create fruitbodies. When droughts occur, fungi are able to direct water into dry areas by using hydraulic redistribution to deliver moisture to the community partners that they depend on. It has been found that mycorrhizal mycelium can increase the root surface area of plants, according to species, ten to one hundred times. That is a significant advantage to plants and trees. Obviously, trees have their cellular structure and are capable of hydraulic redistribution, but without their mycorrhizal partnerships water availability would be severely limited. The mycelial branching pattern allows them to most efficiently distribute water across wide areas.

Neurons in the nervous system of animals have a very similar branching pattern to mycelium and a similar exploratory nature as well. Mycelium will expand hyphae until it reaches the edge of its substrate. This is exactly what happens to a log that has been inoculated with mushroom spawn (this is shown in figure 2.8). The mycelium branches and explores until it reaches the bark layer, and then it knows it has reached the potential. The same happens with nerve cells in our bodies, so that we have full sensory experience. Right under our skin, which is just like the bark on a log, are nerve endings, which form one of our major senses—touch. The sense of touch keeps us from destroying our skin and bodies while it feeds back information about the world we are exploring. Some fungal hyphae transmit electrical pulses as a way to communicate across the large body of underground mycelium.[12] One section of hyphae can detect a food source and send electrical signals across the entire network in response. Our nervous system is a branching information highway that is constantly firing off electrical signals, just like mycelia do.

Fungi developed the ability to form chitin in their cell walls to give themselves structure and protection. Chitin is a structural polysaccharide, made of long chains of carbohydrates. We see chitin employed as a protective structure in the animal kingdom as well. Insects and ocean crustaceans, which share an ancestor with fungi (the ancient protists), have chitin in their exoskeletons. Crab shells can be up to 40 percent chitin, which, along with other minerals, forms their tough exterior, important for a crab's survival in their environment. Spider exoskeletons are mostly a rigid "skin" of protein and chitin. We explore more about fungal chitin and methods for breaking it down in "Making Mushroom Double Extractions" on page 129.

These are but a few examples of how modern plants and animals show the patterns of ancient fungi and their successes through the long history of planet Earth. It is estimated that 95 percent of the world's plant species belong to families that form mycorrhizal associations.[13] As the science progresses, more and more fungal collaborations are uncovered each year. Without their fungal partners, plants would not be able to function, and we see their foundational structures ripple through time as in these evolutionary patterns in the plant and animal kingdoms.

Fungi Shape Their Environments

We humans are interesting creatures, to say the least. Fungi are every bit as fascinating. It may come as a surprise that we share a common ancestor, even though this ancestor is nearly a billion years in the past. Our evolution together has left us with approximately 50 percent of our DNA shared with fungi. The divergence of humans and fungi is now a great chasm. We are very different on many levels, but we retain some similarities. It is hard to say what other similarities will be uncovered as research progresses. One fascinating similarity is that both fungi and humans have a tendency to shape their environment.

Like fungi, we cannot produce our own sugars. Neither humans nor fungi were blessed with the gift of photosynthesis, so we have both developed other strategies to ensure a supply of essential carbohydrates. What have we done? We have created huge disturbances in the landscape so that we can grow plants that produce a large amount of carbohydrates, or plants that are used for simple sugars. We farm the landscape, and so do fungi.

A fascinating study (published in 2013) shows that mycelium of the Thick-Footed Morel (*Morchella crassipes*) farms the bacteria *Pseudomonas putida*.[14] The research team was not using the word *farm* as a metaphor: they found evidence that the fungus was planting, cultivating, and harvesting the bacteria. Working with petri plates inoculated with both organisms, they saw quickly that the fungus was moving the bacteria around the plate. It was already known that fungi will allow, or encourage, certain bacteria to hitch a ride on growing hyphae so they can be propelled through the soil. (Bacteria cannot move with the efficiency that elongating fungal hyphae can.) As the mycelium grows, it exudes various metabolites that are generally a good source of sugars, aminos, and other nutrients. In this study the researchers saw that the fungal metabolites were a preferable food source for the bacteria *P. putida*. The fungus fed the bacteria so the bacteria grew bigger before the fungi harvested carbon from them. Just like human farmers.

Morels are known for creating sclerotia (see figure 1.6). A *sclerotium* is a hardened mass of mycelium that acts as a nutrient reserve. In this study the researchers found that hundreds of thousands of bacteria were incorporated into the sclerotia to form carbon reserves. These sclerotia were created away

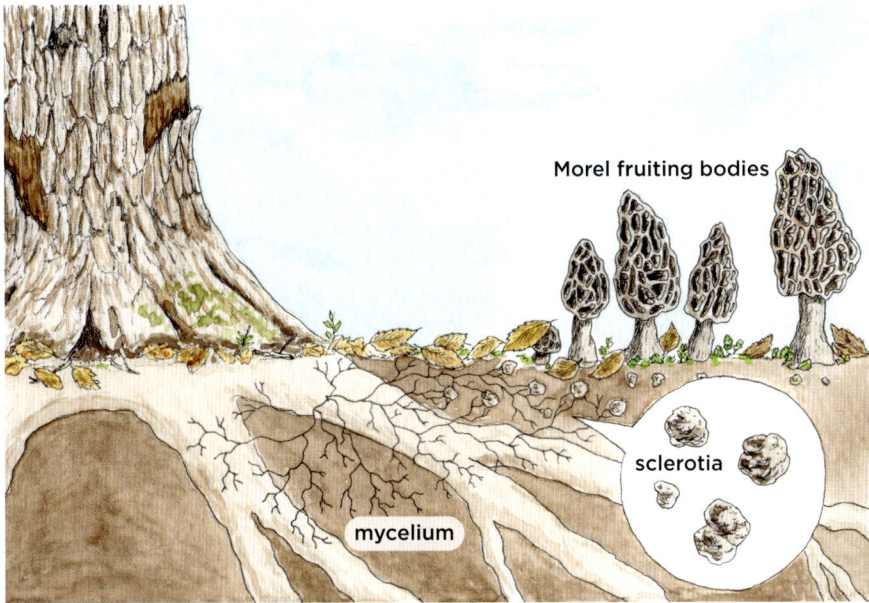

Figure 1.6. The growth stages of morels, a terrestrial saprotroph.

from places with high-density bacteria. Additionally, the fungus kept some bacteria as "seeds" that could be used to initiate the next farming cycle, just like human farmers do.

This study shows how similar fungi are to us in cultivating, harvesting, and dividing tasks to farm bacteria. The bacteria benefited by increased dispersal through the environment and by feeding to produce more growth. The fungus benefited by an additional carbon source. This study happened in the lab. We can only imagine how much more complex the cycle is in soil with links to many other microorganisms and plants. The researchers suggest this type of fungal-bacterial interaction plays an important role in soil health.

Humans mine minerals for use in everyday objects, technology, and things of beauty. This ornamental aspect is something that fungi do not participate in, as far as we are aware. As discussed earlier in this chapter, though, mycorrhizal fungi do participate in the mining of minerals they need for their own cellular functions or for the partnerships they have developed with plants. The minerals that plants need would otherwise be available only through weathering and exfoliation of the Earth's rocks.

Fungi are known as master chemists in part because they are able to respond to environmental conditions quickly and efficiently to create enzymes, acids, and organic compounds that allow them to attract or fight off organisms or to mine metals and minerals. Through the production of organic acids such as citric acid and oxalic acid, they can solubilize metals, including minerals such as phosphorus that are otherwise difficult for plant roots to take up. Solubilization of minerals allows the fungi to utilize nutrients that are otherwise unavailable to their plant hosts. In exchange for these minerals the plants feed sugars to the fungi.

We know fungi have been present on Earth longer than plants and animals, and that their tendency toward transformation and collaboration shaped early soils and plants. We don't know to what degree the farming, mining, and chemistry activities of fungi have shaped the evolution of all life on this planet, but we suspect that they have had, and continue to have, a significant impact.

Humans in Ecosystem Collaboration

Collaboration, resource sharing, diverse and distributed networks of relationships, and resilient communities characterize the way fungi have evolved on our planet. This way of being is reflected in the values and social organization of all Indigenous human cultures we have come across. By *Indigenous* we mean, "peoples who remain on their ancestral lands and practice the ways handed down to them by previous generations."

We as Indigenous people carry the land with us, we acknowledge the systems that support us, and we are constantly showing gratitude for these connections. This sense of being in sacred relationship is the basis of most Indigenous perspectives. All life is connected yet different; each being holds its own unique node in the vast and diverse network of life. Each one of us is needed and respected, and each one of us has a responsibility to do whatever we can to support the great web of life, to feed back into it at least as much as we receive. Indigenous communities are much less human-centric than others, understanding that this responsibility also applies to the beyond-human—the soil, sky, water, forests, grasslands, mountains, deserts, insects, animals, fungi—all of it.

One early fall I was bow hunting and stalking a group of half a dozen deer. As they came out into a clearing, three of the deer were all close enough for me to take a shot. I asked, "Who will come home with me tonight?" As soon as this inaudible question was finished the largest deer looked directly at me, leapt over a small hill and disappeared. The second deer followed. The third deer stepped out and turned broadside toward me. This would be the deer that I later tracked and found under a small pine tree. In this case I asked someone to come home with me for food. Asking permission for what we need is of the utmost importance. It closes a loop of which we are a deeply connected part, even though some of us are unaware of the connection. I did not force my will upon any of these deer. Respect, skill, gratitude, and permission are what allowed me to bring a deer home that evening.

Later, a person tried to criticize me for not taking the largest deer. He was a hunter whose goal was simply to bag the biggest set of antlers he could hang on his wall. He had killed several related bucks in one area. A four-point, six-point, and eight-pointer. There was a ten pointer that he was trying to kill. I replied that I was not trying to kill a whole lineage of deer. I was not taking the most fit and productive bucks from the herd. I was not in it for sport, but to feed myself. I pointed out that he was making the herd weaker by not selecting the weaker and less agile deer. This is what the other predators of the world do. When big cats chase game, they isolate the weakest from the herd. This shows an awareness for the health of the entire system, not solely for individual gain.

The mindset of this other hunter is the same one that led to the deforestation of Europe and to five hundred years of developing deforestation in the Americas. This is the same mindset that places profit and the hoarding of power and resources over the health of the entire community. Is this the mindset we want to encourage in those who manage our forests?

The forests of North America were giants that native peoples supported, encouraged, and shaped for generations. What does clearcutting do in the forest? It strips out all of the healthy and genetically strongest trees, leaving only the weakest to reproduce. This makes for a weak forest. Our forests are now severely suffering and becoming fragmented because of this mismanagement. After razor-sharp clearcutting happens, the native trees are often replaced with hybrid tree plantations. This destroys the soil relationships for many canopy, understory, vine, and herb layer plants. A forest is a complex system and its diversity should be protected. Within a pine-tree monoculture desert, the diversity that supports a forest ecosystem aboveground and belowground collapses. It is time to change this unsustainable model and return to a model that supports strong resilient forests, with all of the parts operating in concert.

Here in the Southern Appalachians, in the early 1900s, before the chestnut blight wiped out our giants, it was estimated that over half of the forest canopy was American Chestnut. This mighty tree was a dominant force from the Ohio River valley, with the spine of the range running the Appalachian Mountains up to Maine. This magnificent, nut-bearing tree was the dominant biomass in the region. This was not by accident; this was by design. Our ancestors intentionally created disturbances to allow for the flourishing of species that supported game, and species that were significant for human use. The American Chestnut gave us a protein- and fat-rich source of food, a habitat for small mammals and birds, and strong, beautiful lumber. Over countless generations, our ancestors in North America and around the world had slowly changed the landscape to suit our needs, all the while working in collaboration with the nonhumans instead of against them, just as the fungi do. This is a relationship we think of as wild co-tending.

Food and forest systems were set up and fed people for thousands of years. Humans were an essential part of the systems that fed them and other wildlife. It is only in modern times that we have separated ourselves from the land and think that food production is inherently destructive to the natural world. Those of us raised in a lineage that has maintained this connection to the more-than-human world do not see ourselves as "other" or "apart" from our environment. It is this mindset of separation that will devastate our Earth, making it uninhabitable for us and countless other species. This may be the case even if we do play our cards right. Would it not be a much better existence if we worked with our environments to make things greener?

The romantic story of pre-European invasion North America being a vast wilderness untouched by humans—known as the pristine wilderness myth—is false yet still held by the majority of non-natives in the United States. In the Amazon it is widely known, although not quite yet accepted by Eurocentric academia, that the rainforests were not huge swaths of wilderness "untouched" by humans. The opposite is true: these forests were encouraged with species that benefited humans in forms of medicine, food, and wildlife. The Amazon was a huge food forest that supported millions of people before European interference.

Tropical jungle forests are not known for their rich fertile soils. Most of the fertility lies in the biomass and the cycling of nutrients throughout the life situated in these regions. Yet, throughout the Amazon region, we keep finding patches of soil that hold an amazing fertility. *Terra preta* is an Amazonian black earth that was created by ancient Indigenous peoples and that we still cannot recreate today. This is a natural technology superior to modern-day farming practices. Terra preta is sought far and wide in the Amazon, with people travelling great distances to take some of this black earth to increase the fertility of their own soils. It is rich in microbial life, fungi, nitrogen, and phosphorus and it has the ability to retain high levels of moisture.

When Europeans first arrived in the late 1400s and early 1500s, there were estimated to be more than 110 million people in North and South America, and maybe up to 200 million. Europe had a population of only about 50 million at that time. The land was covered with trade routes, creating vast exchange networks for food and seeds; these routes mirrored the mycelium underground. Indigenous peoples managed the forests and grasslands as well as the herds of deer, elk, and bison that provided food, bone, and hides. The abundance of fish, wildlife, and food was incomprehensible for some of the new arrivals from Europe. Hernando de Soto's expedition into eastern North America was said to have traveled not through a thick tangle of virgin forests but through savannahs, open old growth forests where fire was used as a constant tool to shape the lands. De Soto traveled through what is now the state of Florida with what started out as a group of 620 people. No difficulty in travel was mentioned, except in crossing rivers. There was no centralized government agency involved in fish and wildlife enforcement, and yet there were flocks of birds so plentiful that their migrations would block the sun for several days. Huge herds of megafauna roamed the savannahs, plains, and forests of the continent.[15]

When sustainability is woven into the culture, it becomes consensus, approved and celebrated. The culture asks: How do we feed everyone? How do we house everyone? It does not ask: How do we charge everyone for everything? How do we make money off the basic decency of human existence? This notion of profiting from nature is a mind virus that has taken a foothold only during the last five hundred years in North America. We exist in its wake. It is up to us to change that.

Beginning in the early 1600s, forests in the United States were being destroyed. The destruction reached its pinnacle in the late 1800s, and by 1920 the US Forest Service estimated that more than 700 million wooded acres had been clear cut. The topsoil that had been built by people, plants, fungi, and other fauna over millennia washed away. The streams, rivers, and land became a human-created disaster.

We could mourn this history and believe that human destiny is to create destruction and drive species extinct. Scientists would say that it must have been the actions of native people that led to the extinction of ancient megafauna in the Americas. But this conclusion reflects the viewpoint of a few select groups of people and does not consider the Indigenous perspective, nor the Indigenous management of the land. It is a Eurocentric view that ignores native stories and ways of interacting with the land. Yes, many bonds in our ecosystems—including the bonds that have held our humanity together—have been broken, polluted, and fragmented. We can argue about who is responsible for the damage, but is that the way forward?

All too often, it is only when we are on the cusp of losing something that we realize how important it is. When our children develop cancers, become asthmatic, or contract polio from lead and mercury poisons in insecticide sprays, then we realize how important health and the mitigation of pollution is.

In 1871, the human population of North America was only 39 million. By 1940, people came to recognize a rapid decline in the abundance of fish and wildlife and their habitats. We have come to understand that a significant reason for this decline was that the native population had been murdered, removed, fractured, and displaced, which prevented many nations from tending the forests and adhering to traditional farming techniques. One example of this is the Dawes Act of 1887, which forced Indians into small plots of land, which was a huge break from their tradition of communal-style agriculture. The best hunting grounds and farming lands were sold to European settlers.

Many people starved to death as native traditions and ways of gathering foods were stamped out. Meanwhile, the forests declined in productivity, and the US Fish and Wildlife Service was created to reverse that decline. Has that been a real solution?

We still are not allowed to gather wild foods on our native land, some of which is now called the Great Smoky Mountains National Park, or we must pay for a permit from the United States government. Personally, I have been told not to pick wild foods such as Sochan (cone-flower leaves), nuts, and various mushrooms from government-controlled lands. But these wild foods depend on human interaction and relationships to continue to flourish.

We all have a responsibility to participate in the regeneration of our natural ecosystems. As you explore forests looking for wild mushrooms, or sites for mushroom cultivation, know that you are an integral part of this magnificent, life-giving, habitat. In chapter 7, we offer suggestions for how to wild-harvest specific mushrooms ethically and regeneratively. The attitude you bring, the intention you hold, the choices you make, and actions you take, can be part of bringing this abundance back to our now-shared lands—or you can perpetuate the legacy of extraction and damage. It is up to you.

CHAPTER TWO

Outdoor Mushroom Cultivation

Outdoor cultivation is typically how people first grow mushrooms. It is relatively easy because you are working in tandem with the forest. By introducing prepared spawn (plug or sawdust) to a log, or adding a spore slurry to wood chips, you are simply encouraging what could happen naturally in that ecosystem. The downside of most outdoor cultivation methods is that it takes anywhere from a few months to several years before the mushrooms appear. That will help you work on your patience! And just about the time you have forgotten and moved on to other projects, the mushrooms will fruit. We hope you will be as delighted as we are each time we harvest.

Being a mycologist and a native person, I have spent a lifetime watching and listening intently, especially to elders, and make careful observations. These skills have served me and have helped me connect the dots along my journey into the of mystery of mushroom cultivation. So, take your time—there is much to learn about outdoor cultivation. There's no need to rush into lab work and indoor mushroom production if you don't feel ready. The more you grow outdoors, the more you will learn about each type of mushroom, their preferred habitats and conditions, and when they like to fruit. These observations will help you become a better grower and a more successful wild mushroom hunter.

Most mushroom growers start their journey into the world of mycology with outdoor mushroom cultivation. It is a simple and effective way to begin cultivating your favorite culinary and medicinal mushrooms. Outdoor cultivation can take many forms: growing on logs, wood chip beds, and sterilized substrate blocks, with spore slurries, cardboard spawn, stem spawn, and many more. In this book, we focus on the methods most applicable to growing medicinal mushroom species. This is by no means an exhaustive guide; we simply cover some of the easiest methods to get you started.

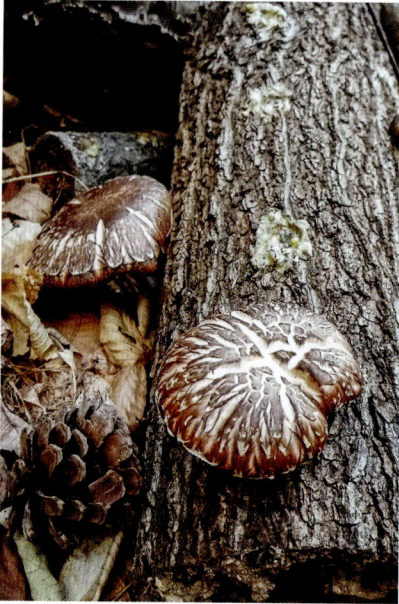

Figure 2.1. Donko Shiitakes on oak logs.

When I first learned about mushroom cultivation at the age of fourteen in that fortuitous high school forestry class, it was, to me, amazing that I could inoculate oak logs once and reap harvests of mushrooms from them for up to eight years. It was addictive! I've always felt the urge to grow plants, and I have good memories of participating in my father's and grandparents' gardens. Growing things came easy to me, and growing mushrooms seemed like a "lazy" way of farming. Of course, leave it to the fourteen-year-old mind with an underdeveloped prefrontal cortex to find lazy ways of doing things.

Spending time in the natural habitats where mushrooms occur and observing the ways they take advantage of opportunities in various forest niches gives you not only the medicine of being in the forest but also clues into how to become a better cultivator. I learned this more than twenty years ago when I had my first encounter with Lion's Mane mushrooms on a dead log on the forest floor. After that, I could never find more. I told another member of the Eastern Band of Cherokee Indians (EBCI) that Lion's Mane kept escaping me in the forests. I had never had such a rough time trying to find a mushroom. He told me, "You are looking in the wrong place. They are *Uguku*; they are up in the trees."

Uguku is also the Cherokee word for Barred Owl (*Strix varia*). I was looking in the wrong place. As I began looking up in the trees while mushroom hunting, it became very clear that Lion's Mane likes to fruit on dead snags. And not only do they like dead snags, they seem to prefer the ones that angle up at about 45 degrees. This observation would come in handy when I wanted to start growing Lion's Mane mushrooms. I continue to learn from the forest; it makes my cultivation more successful and enjoyable.

Growing Mushrooms on Logs

Log cultivation is a way to cultivate many kinds of saprotrophic (wood-eating) mushrooms in areas where suitable species of trees are located and where the climate is satisfactory. What we know of the history of log cultivation begins with the story of Wu San Kwung, a woodcutter in the time of the Sung Dynasty (960–1127 CE) in China, whose careful observations led to the successful cultivation of Shiitake (*Lentinula edodes*) on logs. (We tell this story in the Shiitake profile on page 206.) The technique of growing Shiitake on logs has evolved since that time, which was more than a millennium ago, but Wu's discovery was a big gift to the world.

WHEN TO CUT LOGS

Understanding the annual cycle of trees and knowing the optimal time to cut wood for the purpose of growing mushrooms is important to your success. Late winter and early spring are the best times for cutting. The sap is up in the trees at this time and that small amount of sugar content gives the mycelium a bit of a "jump." Many growers will not accept logs cut any other time of the year, but keep in mind that this is not the *only* time of the year when you can cut wood for mushroom production.

On our farm in western North Carolina, we have an opportunistic perspective, and so we also use logs cut in late winter through early fall, taking a break in early summer. We stop harvesting logs around the last week in May and wait until the second or third week in June to resume. We pause because this is when the soil is coming out of its winter slumber and is bursting with energy. Nutrients are rushing up through the xylem in the tree trunks. Leaves are fully out, photosynthesizing and pumping sugars down through the phloem to feed the mycorrhizal fungi in the mycorrhizosphere. As a result, the tree is beginning to

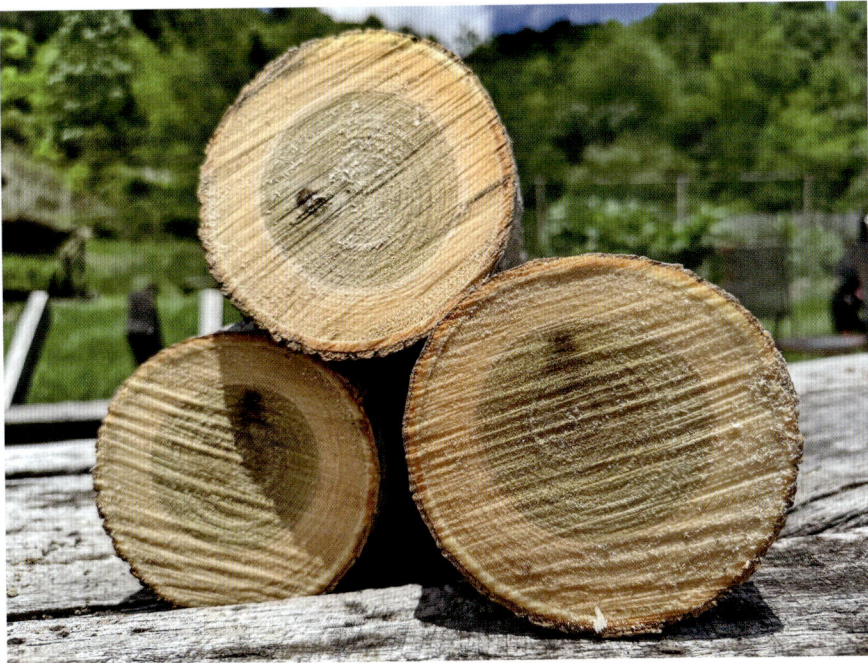

Figure 2.2. Freshly cut and disease-free Tulip Poplar logs.

grow quickly to take advantage of the season. The rapid growth makes the bark loosen. If you cut trees at this time, the bark will start to fall off the logs within six months or so. This six-month timeframe is just the point at which the mycelium becomes well established within the wood and becomes strong enough to keep out competitor fungi. Since the timing depends on your location, you will need to talk to locals or do your own research to learn when this time of rapid tree growth occurs for your region. If you make bark baskets, early summer is the perfect time to cut wood and to peel bark. Everything has a season.

Because we are in Zone 6, we stop cutting logs for mushroom production in late fall. We do not inoculate logs after mid- to end of November, and we begin to inoculate again around March 1 according to weather conditions. In some parts of the United States, in Zone 7 and warmer, it is possible to inoculate logs year-round.

SELECTING TREES TO CUT

When selecting trees to harvest for mushroom production, look for trees that are not diseased or dying. This cannot be stressed enough. It is your first line of defense for keeping competitor fungi at a minimum.

Once you have decided on suitable trees to take, keep in mind that you are causing a disturbance in the forest. During tree judging in my high school forestry class, the goal was to determine how suitable the trees would be for lumber and to estimate how many board feet said trees would produce. So, what would we look for? Nice straight trees, for one thing. Straight trunks would rest more easily on logging trucks, would yield nice straight-grained lumber, and would handle better at the sawmill. But once the straight trees are cut down, what gets left behind? That's right—all the trees that are not straight. When we cut all but the weakest trees, we are selecting for the weaker genes. So, the gene pool that is left is less suitable for lumber. They are gnarled with undesirable growth patterns. With this approach, there is no true regard for the health of the forest, which in turn means little regard for the health of the animals, for water quality, for air quality, or for us humans.

Matching Tree to Mushroom

Knowing which mushrooms you can grow on which types of logs is crucial to successful cultivation. Learn the preferences of the mushroom species you want to cultivate before you cut down any trees!

Appendix 1 on page 258 is a table of tree and mushroom species combinations that we find to work well here in the mountains of Western North Carolina (USDA Hardiness Zone 6). It may be different in your region.

When consulting with new mushroom enthusiasts, whether they have two acres or one thousand acres, we encourage them to pause and study the forest as a whole, to take into consideration the health of the forest, as they decide which trees to cut. We need to reconsider our tendency to seek instant gratification. Seeing the whole system as a living entity, not a resource, makes a difference in how we interact with the forest. Mushrooms do not care if the trees they grow on are bent or crooked or gnarled, so select those trees for your mushroom production.

MUSHROOM-LOG INOCULATION TECHNIQUES

There are many ways to inoculate mushroom logs, and I describe three methods: the standard inoculation method, the totem method, and the envelope method. Whatever method you try, you can be confident that mycelium wants to grow. Given the proper opportunities, they will often outperform our expectations.

Standard Inoculation Method

Once trees are selected and cut, take as much care as possible to keep them off the ground. Imagine cutting a tree and dropping it on top of the leaf litter on the forest floor. If you leave the tree there for several weeks while you gather your materials for inoculation, you may discover that some unknown type of mycelium has grown between the leaf litter and the tree's bark. And even if you cannot see any rhizomorphic mycelium (thick mycelial threads) growing there, it's certain that various types of fungal spores are distributed across or in the leaf litter layers, just lying in wait for the opportunity to germinate and get to work. These forest fungi will compete with whatever mushroom species you plan to grow. This is why keeping your logs elevated off the ground until inoculation is very important. We find that wooden pallets work great for this. Wooden pallets are typically free and abundant. We always use pallets that are not chemically treated.

Pre-Inoculation Log Care: The Resting Period

When I first started plugging mushroom logs in the early 1990s, the common practice was to let the logs rest for six weeks, then inoculate, making sure they were inoculated by the eighth week. It was only a two-week window; we had to work fast. We now know that you can inoculate as early as two weeks into the resting period. That is our rule on the farm: we wait at least two weeks but no more than eight weeks. Even when we have hundreds of logs to plug, this is enough time; we are not burdened by having to hurriedly plug them all at once. Waiting for the first two weeks to pass is important because there are compounds in tree sap that are allelopathic, or repellant, to saprotrophic fungi, which can make it hard for the mycelium to get established. These compounds will have

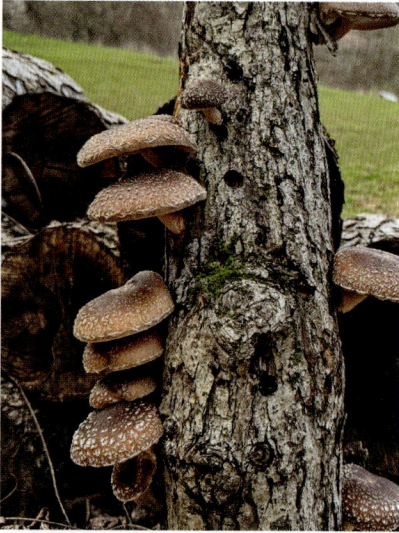

Figure 2.3. Fall flush of Shiitakes from a strain we cloned from the wild in Western North Carolina.

started to break down after a couple of weeks. By the eight- to ten-week mark, they are mostly dispersed. At this point the logs are open to competitor fungi. In our region of the eastern woodlands, common competitors are Split Gill (*Schizophyllum commune*), Parchment Fungus (*Stereum complicatum*), Turkey Tail (*Trametes versicolor*), and Mazegill (*Daedalea quercina*). You may deal with a host of other contaminants.

Log Inoculation Procedure

The basic steps in log inoculation are drilling holes in the logs, inserting mycelium in the holes, and applying wax over the holes to seal in the mycelium. These steps should happen in quick sequence to ensure that the mycelium is exposed to as few possible contaminants. The holes drilled in the sapwood are vulnerable openings that spores from the surrounding environment can infiltrate.

Use a corded drill (cordless ones tend to run out too quickly) with an appropriately sized drill bit. If you are using plug spawn, you will need a drill bit that matches the diameter of the plugs—most likely that will be $5/16$ inch. If you are using sawdust spawn and an inoculation plunger, then use a drill bit that matches the plunger, most likely $7/16$ or $1/2$ inch.

EQUIPMENT NEEDED

Logs

Corded drill

Drill bits

Spawn—either sawdust or plug (wooden dowels)

Inoculation plunger (optional)

Small slow cooker

Wax

Wool daubers or foam paint brushes

1. Set up the logs on a table or other device that will make it easy on your back while you are drilling holes.
2. Drill holes about $1/2$ inch deep if using sawdust spawn, and 1 inch deep for plug spawn. There is no benefit to drilling deeper; you just end up using more spawn but will not receive any more mushrooms. The simplest and most common drilling pattern is the diamond pattern. This pattern results in even distribution of inoculation into the sapwood of the logs, which should help ensure uniform establishment of mycelium.

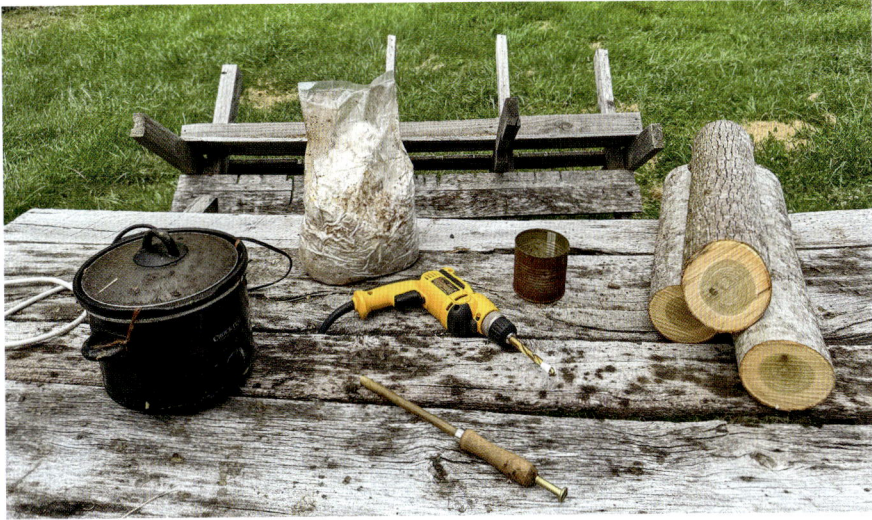

Figure 2.4. Equipment for standard inoculation using plug spawn.

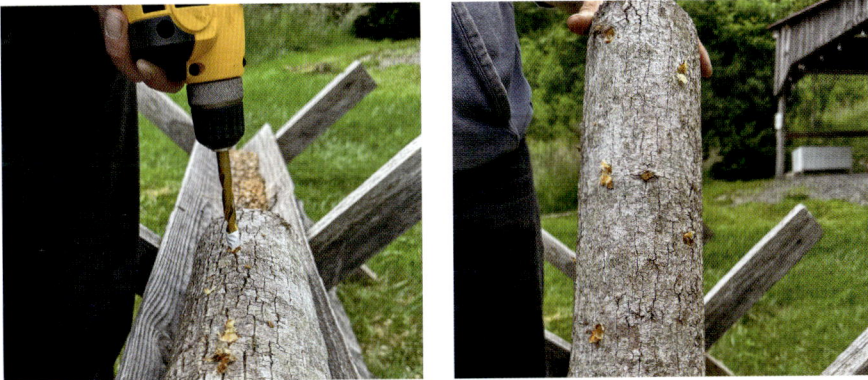

Figure 2.5. Drilling holes in a log in a diamond pattern.

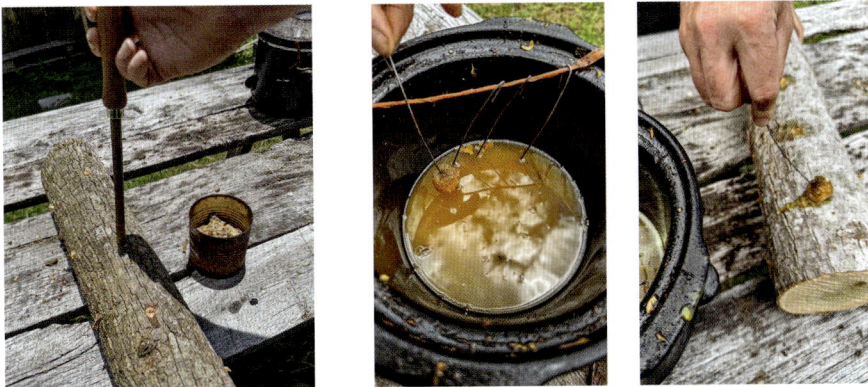

Figure 2.6. Inoculation with sawdust and plunger.

Figure 2.7. Covering inoculation holes with wax using wool daubers.

3. Once holes are drilled, fill them quickly with spawn inoculated with the type of mushroom you want to grow. You can pinch some sawdust spawn into each hole with your fingers. If you are inoculating more than a few logs, use an inoculation plunger (see figure 2.6). If you are using plugs, place the plug in the hole and hammer gently until the plug is flush with the bark.

4. Seal each hole with melted wax to prevent any insects from getting in and eating the mycelium (figure 2.7). You can use a variety of chemical-free waxes (such as soy) or paraffin-based waxes. Beeswax works, but for us, it's too precious for this purpose—we save it for making salves. A small, inexpensive slow cooker is a great way to melt the wax. Turn it on high for thirty minutes or so before you begin inoculating logs. We keep wax in the pot at all times—we don't clean it out between uses. To apply the wax, we use small wool daubers, which we hang from a piece of string over the melted wax. Make sure not to drop them in the wax!

It is easy to set up an assembly-line system to inoculate logs. Ask people from the community to help, or invite a couple friends to visit. One person drills holes, the next person plugs holes with spawn, and a third covers holes with wax. You can switch jobs as each person grows weary of their post.

Post-Inoculation Log Care: The Incubation Period
With your logs inoculated now comes the first part of playing the waiting game. Try to remember that this is a long game. Those handy pallets where your

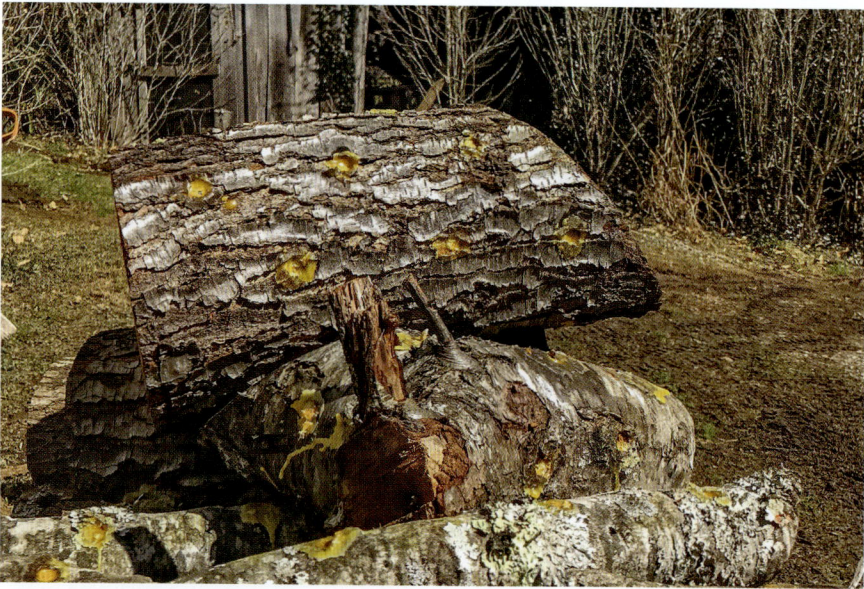

Figure 2.8. Logs incubating on pallets in the forest.

logs rested will now become the place where your logs will incubate for the next two to three months. The incubation area needs to be as shady as possible and exposed to rainfall. Make sure you either soak your logs before, or quickly after, they have been inoculated. In the spirit of simplicity, our preferred method is to inoculate logs on a day before rain is predicted, so the rain does the job for us. This also has the advantage of using less water from your home well or municipal water system. Plus, when you water down logs before inoculating, you make those logs much heavier. Personally, after lifting logs for thirty years, I am not interested in making logs heavier.

If possible, set up this incubation staging area close to the logs' permanent home where they will live out their productive lives. Also consider where the nearest source of water is. During the two- to three-month incubation period, you'll need to make sure that your pile of logs receives water at least once every two weeks. If you live in a rainy climate, this is taken care of by nature. Otherwise, you'll need to give them a good soaking every two weeks.

Permanent Location and Fruiting Phase

When the logs have completed the incubation period, the fungi should have enough of a hold to keep contaminants at bay. Where and how these logs should be placed in their permanent location varies according to the species and variety of mushrooms you are cultivating. Pay attention to where these mushrooms appear in the wild: this will help you know where to best place your logs. This will give you clues to what the fungi needs to proliferate in the permanent spot

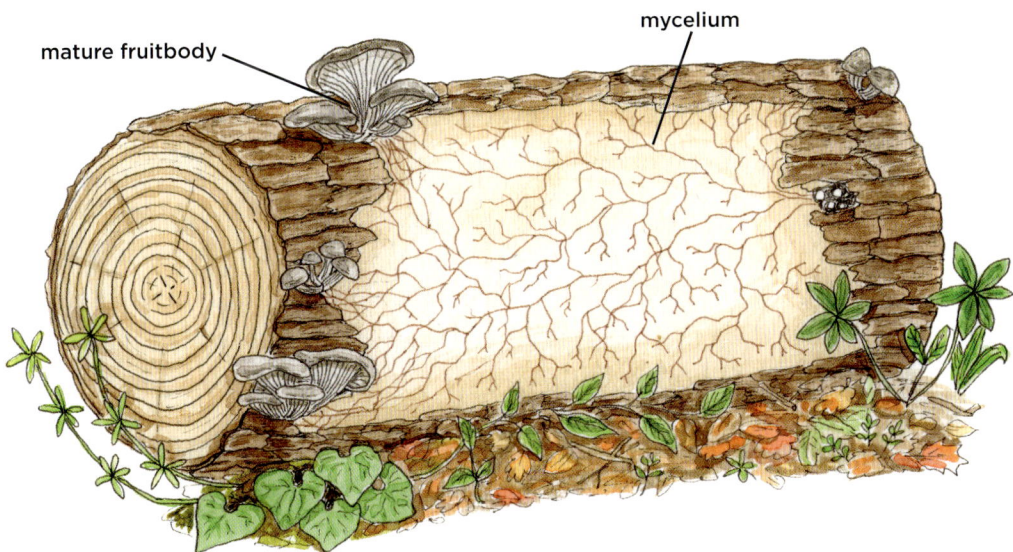

Figure 2.9. Mycelium running through a log.

you have set up for them. For example, if you find Maitake mushrooms growing wild in dry open areas in local forests, then aim to place your Maitake-inoculated (*Grifola frondosa*) logs in a similar environment. If you are finding wild Golden Reishi (*Ganoderma curtisii*) on ridges or south-facing slopes, then try to place your Reishi logs in that type of microclimate.

Totem Method

One of the most satisfying ways to inoculate a massive number of logs at once is the totem method. With this method, you build an upright totem by stacking cut segments of a tree trunk one atop another, with a layer of spawn between each section. We use sections of freshly cut trees for making totems. This method has one disadvantage. The logs you start with will be larger in diameter than those typically used in the standard log inoculation technique, and it's just more difficult and tiring to move these large pieces of wood. We cut each log into 10-inch segments for constructing a totem. We find that size reasonably easy to work with.

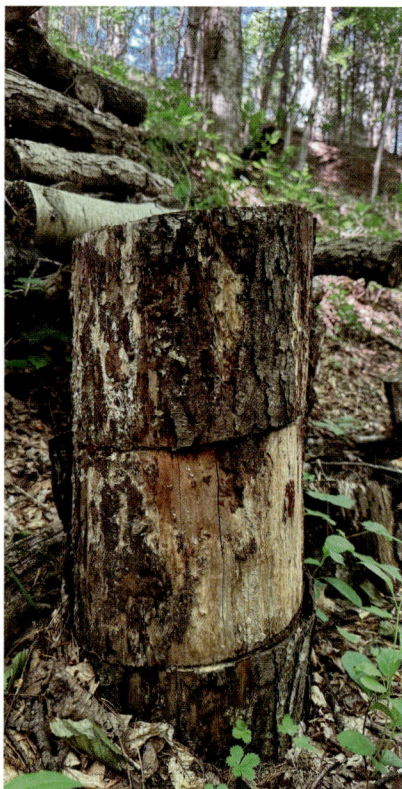

Figure 2.10. Wild Cherry log totem.

EQUIPMENT NEEDED

Logs, 12 to 20 inches in diameter
Chainsaw

Cardboard
Sawdust spawn

1. With your freshly cut tree still lying on the ground where you cut it, use a chainsaw to slice a three inch "cookie" off each end of the tree trunk. This three-inch section on each end will serve to protect the assembled totem against competitor fungi.
2. Cut the rest of the log into 10-inch segments.
3. Place a piece of cardboard larger than the diameter of the log on a prepared and leveled spot on the ground near the log. With the cardboard in place, top it with a layer of sawdust mushroom spawn, approximately 1 inch deep. The spawn should cover just the footprint of the bottommost cookie.
4. Set the bottommost 3-inch cookie in place, then spread spawn over its upper surface, approximately ½ to ¾ inches deep.

5. Repeat this process of adding a segment of log and topping it with spawn approximately ½ to ¾ inches thick until you have used up all the 10-inch segments.
6. Put the second 3-inch cookie on the top of the totem.
7. Occasionally, we add one last layer of spawn on the surface of the topmost cookie and then staple cardboard to the log to act as a cap. This method of placing spawn on top of the last cookie is not strictly necessary.

The reason for the difference in the thickness of the tiers that are sandwiched between the layers of mushroom mycelium is that the top and bottom pieces are the ones most likely to be exposed to outside contaminants and be the vectors of competitor fungi becoming established. Imagine you set up a totem that has sections that are all 16 inches long. From those layers of myceliated spawn, the hyphae need to burn through 8 inches of wood before reaching their sister mycelium. The very top of the totem is exposed to the elements. Wild spores have the potential to land on the exposed surface and start the journey down into those logs you have worked so hard to install. However, if you put the 3-inch cookie at the top of the totem, any spores that land there can only grow down 3 inches before reaching a wall of mycelium that is already established, and the wild mycelium will not be able to penetrate its defenses.

How tall can you make your totems? We suggest making them as tall as it becomes comfortable to reach. Stability also depends on the diameter of the log. It would not be wise to build a totem 8 feet tall and only 15 inches in diameter. These totems would have the possibility of falling over and would pose a health risk! We are growing medicinal mushrooms, not trying to cause health risks. So build them as tall as feels stable. The totem method lends itself to the set-it-and-forget-it approach.

Certain wild mushrooms that fruit *en masse* are great for making totems. Once, in the summer of 2005, I was floating in an inner tube down the Oconaluftee on the Qualla Boundary where many of the Eastern Band of Cherokee live. We were tubing from the Big Cove community toward my Uncle Don's campground. Adawehi was about ten months old and sleeping on my

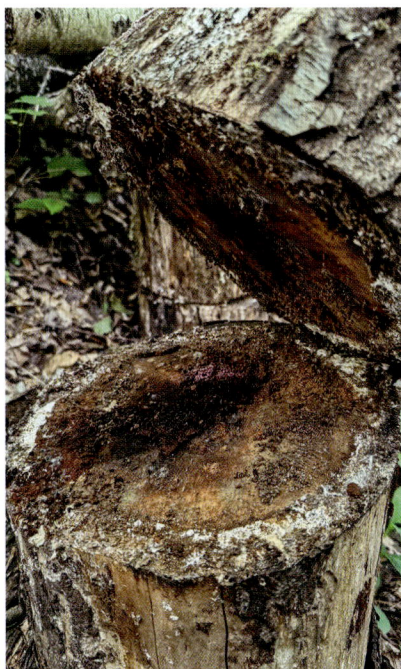

Figure 2.11. View of mycelium between totem layers.

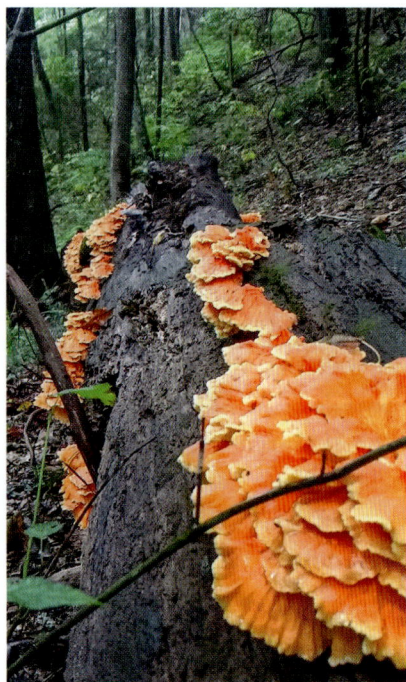

Figure 2.12. Large flush of wild Chicken-of-the-Woods.

chest. Rounding a bend in the river, we came upon an enormous oak nearly 4 feet in diameter. The massive trunk was about 40 feet tall and from there its splintered top was reaching for the sky. Covering the trunk, from soil level up to around 25 feet high, were layers upon layers of Chicken of the Woods mushrooms (*Laetiporus sulphureus*). I nearly popped off my tube at this sight. After finishing my float, Adawehi and I went back to my grandma's house in Birdtown, grabbed an old bedsheet, and drove to the oak tree. We picked mushrooms from head height down to the ground, gathering about one hundred pounds of mushrooms and leaving the vast majority on the tree. We cooked, froze, and ate those mushrooms and shared them with friends and anyone we came upon who liked them.

Chicken of the Woods is the perfect example of a species suited to be cultivated on totems. In a totem stack, the fungi have more cellulose and lignin to consume than on a small log, and so have the potential to produce larger flushes of mushrooms. The other species that are befitting of totems are Lion's Mane, Oysters, Brickcaps (*Hypholoma lateritium*) and, to a lesser extent, Shiitakes. Which ones will you experiment with?

The Envelope Method

Stumps of recently cut trees are another great place to put into mushroom production. Stump cultivation is simple and effective. A stump from 1 to 8 feet tall is plenty to work with. One of the first and most important things to do is girdle the stump with a chainsaw. Girdling is basically making a surface cut in an unbroken circle all the way around the tree. To be safe, be sure to cut through the sapwood layer because doing so cuts off all supply of chemical compounds from the root system. (Remember, many of those compounds are allelopathic.) This reduces the probability that the mycelium with which you inoculate the stump is neutralized by the allelopathic compounds and has a better chance of perpetuating itself through the stump.

One way to inoculate a stump is the wedge technique, but we have always found it cumbersome. The basic wedge method is to cut a wedge out of the tree trunk, remove the wedge, stuff sawdust spawn into the opening, and then replace the wedge and nail or screw it in place. However, we find that most of the sawdust gets lost. Plugging the stump with sawdust spawn or plug spawn is a great alternative. We also like using what we call the envelope method, shown in figure 2.13. We use this method on stumps or large logs lying in the forest that are difficult to get to.

EQUIPMENT NEEDED

Chainsaw   Paper envelope
Log   Sawdust spawn

1. Use your chainsaw to cut a shallow-angled slice into the stump, cutting only as deep as the depth of the chainsaw bar.
2. Continue making angled cuts around the full circumference of the stump, spacing the cuts evenly 1½ to 2 feet apart (see figure 2.13).
3. Fill the envelopes with enough sawdust spawn so that the envelopes will fill the cuts in the log.
4. Slide one spawn-filled envelope into each cut. The edges of the envelopes that stick out of the wood can be tacked down using nails or staples to help secure them in place.

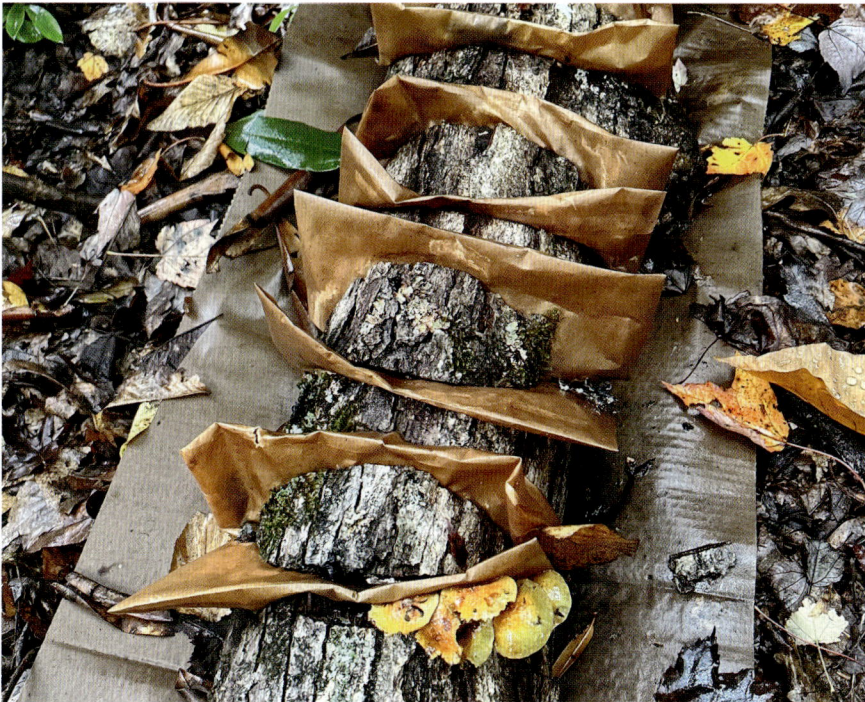

Figure 2.13. Chestnut mushrooms growing from the envelope method. Photo courtesy of Rose Russo

Of course, it is best to set up this inoculation technique right before it rains. This method is mostly used to grow fungi in hard-to-reach areas where bringing in equipment might be challenging.

Straw Cultivation Techniques

Oysters are one of the easiest mushrooms to grow, and most people have access to materials that will serve as substrate. In our region straw is easily accessible. It is an agricultural waste product.

Straw cultivation involves heating straw in hot water to pasteurize it and neutralize potentially competing fungi. Spawn is mixed with the pasteurized straw and put into bags or buckets. In a few weeks' time, mycelium colonizes the straw, and then moisture is added to stimulate fruiting.

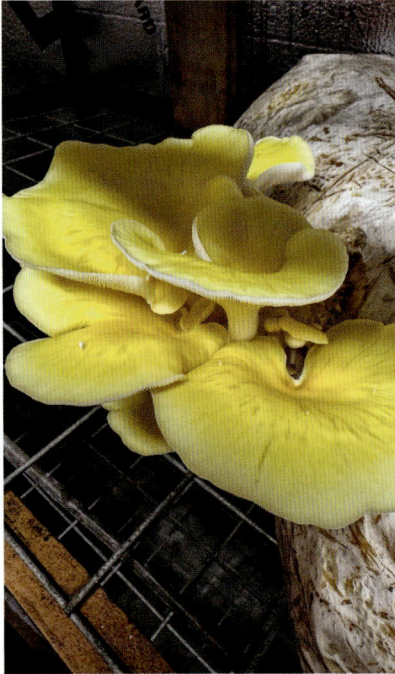

Figure 2.14. Oyster mushrooms growing from straw.

Don't worry about whether or not the straw was produced organically. Oyster mushrooms will break down any pesticide remnants into useable carbon and hydrogen. The mushrooms will be safe to eat, and the spent straw will be great mulch for an organic garden.

Although it's okay to use straw with pesticide residues on it, make sure that the pot or barrel you use for cooking the straw was not previously used to store toxic material.

EQUIPMENT NEEDED

Large metal pot or barrel

Water

Propane burner or concrete blocks

Propane fuel or firewood

Meat thermometer with extended range probe

Straw or dried, high-cellulose grasses (such as *Miscanthus* or pampas grass)

Cement blocks or other heavy weights

Pitchfork

Clean table or tarp

Spawn of the appropriate species of mushroom

Poly tubing bags or clean food-grade buckets with lids

Zip ties (if using bags)

Straight pins (if using bags)

Fiberfill (if using buckets)

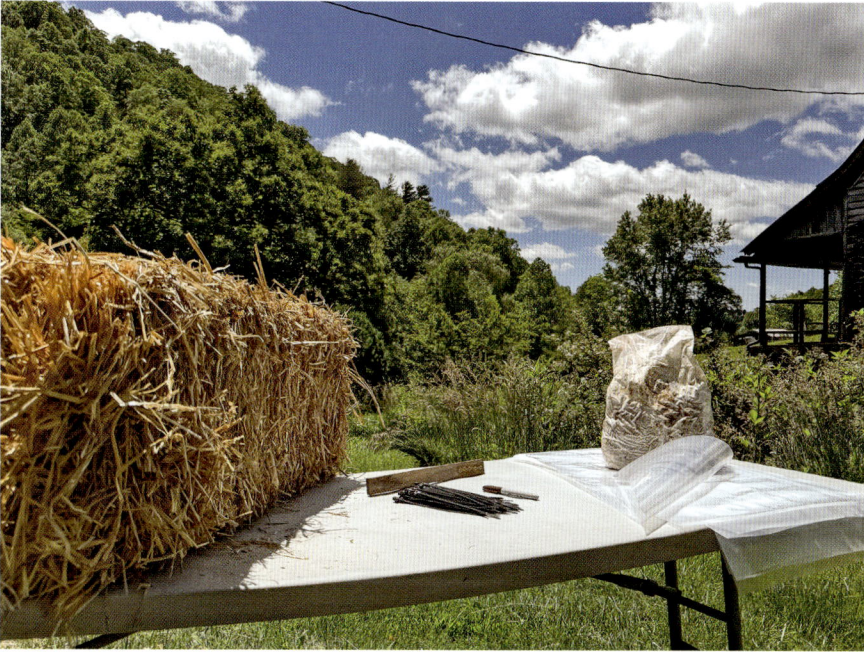

Figure 2.15. Straw production setup.

1. If you plan to use buckets for growing, prepare them by using a drill to make holes in the bucket sides.
2. Fill the pot or barrel with water to about two-thirds full.
3. Set up the propane heater. Or, to use wood heat, position the concrete blocks as a base for the pot or barrel and build a wood fire in the area between the blocks. Set the barrel or pot on the concrete blocks.
4. Using the thermometer to check the temperature, heat the water to 170°F (77°C), which is pasteurization temperature.
5. Sink the straw into the heated water, being careful not to add so much that the water overflows from the container.
6. Cut off the heat source and place the cement blocks or other heavy weight on top of the straw to keep it submerged.
7. Monitor the water temperature and make sure it does not fall below 155°F (68°C) for the next ninety minutes. As long as the volume of water is large enough, it should have enough thermal mass to maintain temperature. Otherwise, restart the heat and bring the temperature back up, keeping it under 170°F.
8. When the ninety minutes is up, remove the weights and then use the pitchfork to remove the straw from the water and place it on a clean table or tarp to drain and cool. When pasteurizing a small quantity, you can pour off the water through a strainer instead.

9. Once the straw is cool to the touch, it is time to inoculate it with sawdust spawn. Clean your hands, and then sprinkle spawn evenly across the cooled straw. We find that a 6-pound bag of sawdust substrate will inoculate one full bale of straw weighing 40 to 60 pounds (18 to 27 kg).

10. Gather the inoculated straw and stuff it into poly tubing bags or the prepared food-grade buckets. Seal the bags with zip ties after packing or place the lids on the buckets.

11. Use pins to poke pinholes into the bags to allow for fresh air exchange. We poke two lines of holes on opposite sides of the bag. If using buckets, cover the holes with micropore tape or stuff the holes with fiberfill to keep out insects and allow for fresh air exchange.

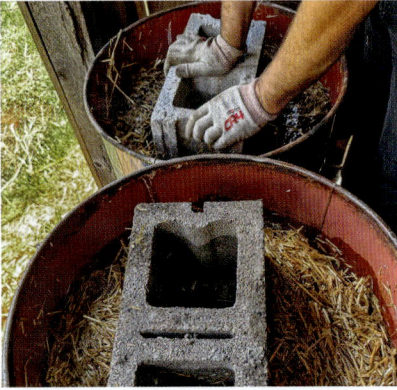

Figure 2.16. Straw submerged in water with block as weight.

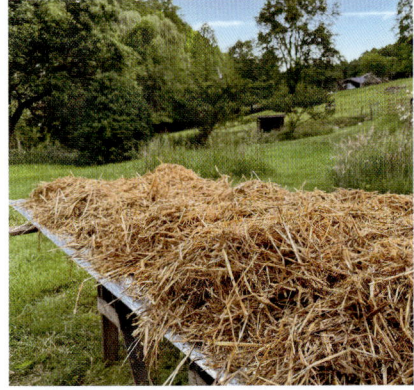

Figure 2.17. The moment before inoculating the pasteurized straw.

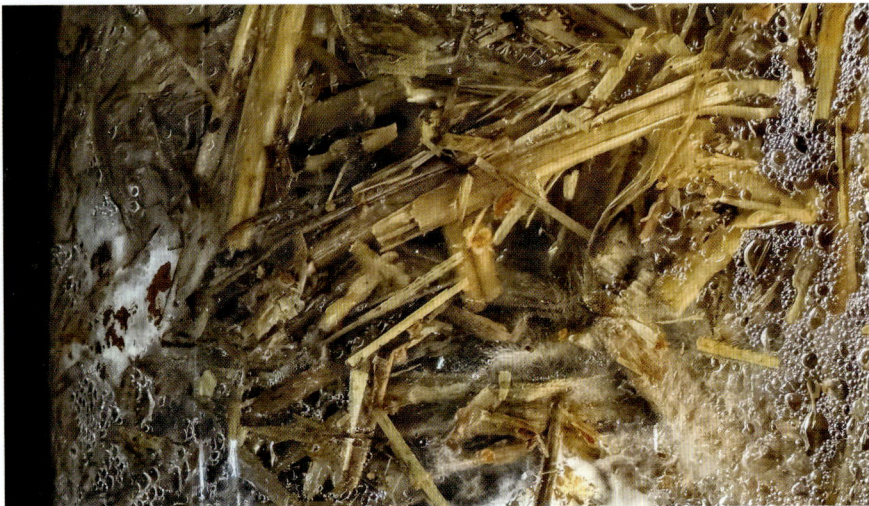

Figure 2.18. Inoculated straw incubating.

Let the bags or buckets sit in a spot where temperature will not drop below freezing. The cooler the temperature, the longer it will take the straw to be colonized. When the straw is fully colonized, which will take about twenty days, cut bigger holes into the bags or remove the fiberfill or tape from the bucket holes. Add moisture to encourage fruiting.

Species-Specific Techniques

Inoculation of wood for mushroom cultivation is basic and mostly the same across species. Here we discuss a few key medicinal mushroom species that require some special attention to the types of wood, the size of logs, and the orientation and treatment of the logs. All of these details have an impact on success.

SHIITAKES

Shiitake logs are typically stacked in log cabin stacks or set upright and leaned up against another in long rows. The Japanese have developed a technique of stacking logs called the hillside stack, shown in figure 2.19. This clever method makes it possible to produce mushrooms even in very steep areas.

REISHI

Most Reishi like to be in contact with the ground. Incubated logs should be partially buried: set large-diameter logs vertically, logs of smaller girth horizontally. We have found that 2-foot-long logs are about the maximum effective length for Reishi production. With longer logs, you reach a point of diminishing

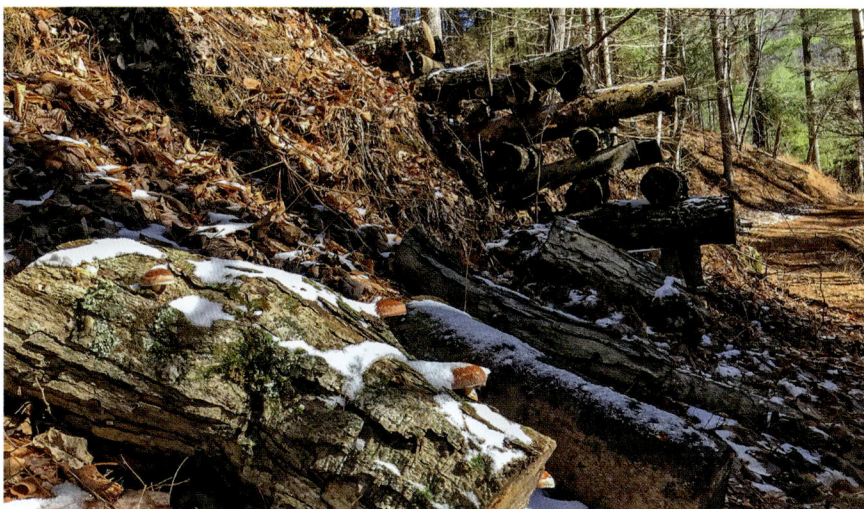

Figure 2.19. Hillside stack for optimum land use.

return. From my study of Golden Reishi in the wild, I've concluded that they prefer large leader roots, the kind that serve to anchor trees into the ground. Sometimes around large dead oak trees, I have found a winding trail of Golden Reishi extending many meters in several directions away from the base of the tree, following large leader roots, where the soil and wood interface.

The great thing about producing Reishi on buried logs is that they can be incorporated into your current landscape without drawing attention from your homeowner's association. Partially buried logs can also be used as a border for plant beds.

LION'S MANE

Observations over time have led me to cut logs for Lion's Mane shorter than I once did. I had observed that logs 4 to 6 feet long would produce the same number of mushrooms as logs only 2 feet long. Thus, we now cut larger-diameter logs, up to 20 inches, no longer than 2 or 2.5 feet. After Lion's Mane logs have safely incubated, place them with one end in the ground at an angle of about 45 degrees. For large logs, place pieces of rot-resistant wood, such as cedar or locust, under the Lion's Mane logs as a support. This is the perfect way to line pathways on your farm or forest. Set the incubated logs up so that the

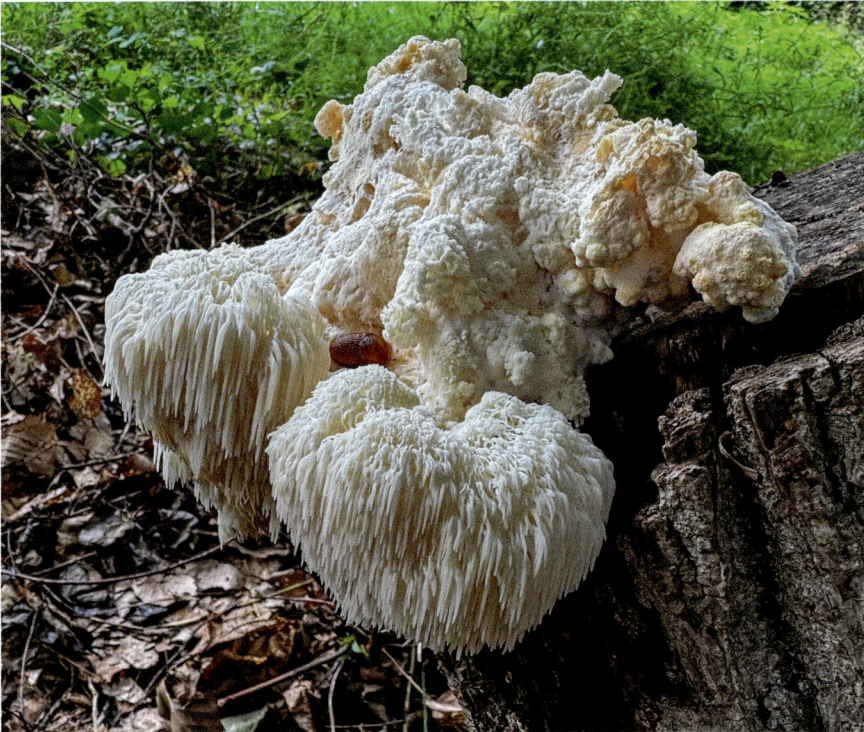

Figure 2.20. Logs for Lion's Mane production.

exposed cut ends face toward the path. The first flushes of fungi will happen right on those 45-degree upward angles, and you can saunter along the path with a basket in hand, picking Lion's Mane.

OYSTERS

If we had to pick one method to cultivate Oyster mushrooms, it would be totems. Softwood species are best for quick flushes and large yields. Totems typically produce larger flushes of mushrooms compared to Shiitake-sized logs. If you use small logs (3 to 6 inches in diameter), the mycelium will eat through the wood very quickly, producing only a few scanty flushes over a year and a half maximum. We tend to find this not worth the effort. Totems (using logs 12 to 20 inches in diameter) are an easy way for your farm to create passive income and have large amounts of fungi to sell to wholesale accounts, markets, or farm stands.

Oysters have a wide range of fruiting temperatures, from tropical to cold climate. If properly set up, Oysters can be produced with consistency for three seasons of the year. In our region we can grow cold-weather varieties such as Blue Oysters and Pearl Oysters in late winter through spring, and again in fall into early winter. In summer we can grow Golden Oysters (which are tropical, but the mycelium will survive the winter here). Pink Oysters are also a tropical species, but they won't survive our mountain winter, so they are limited to hot weather climates.

TURKEY TAIL

Turkey Tail mushroom is the perfect candidate for production on smaller logs that are not suitable for other species. We have used oak logs 1.5 to 2 inches in diameter for Turkey Tail. The big advantage we see is a flush in the first year; after that the logs are finished. This can be an annual practice to make sure your needs for this powerful medicine are met. When larger logs are used for Turkey Tail, they also typically give just one large flush. Rarely to occasionally, there will be another flush the following year. Thus, we recommend saving your large logs for mushroom species that will produce for several years before petering out.

MAITAKE

The Dancing Mushroom is more challenging to cultivate than some other species. Tree-stump Maitake culture can be successful, and you can double-up production by cutting off the stump top, leaving approximately 2 feet of the stump intact. Use the cut tops for producing other species; inoculate the stump with Maitake. Girdle the tree near ground level and then inoculate with plug or sawdust spawn above the girdle. As the lower portion of the stump dies, the mycelium will move into the larger leader roots. Depending on the diameter of the stump, it may produce Maitake mushrooms for up to twenty years. The larger the diameter of the stump, the longer it will produce.

The other method that works well for Maitake is standard log production. Use logs that are at least 12 inches in diameter. Once inoculated, and the incubation period is over, bury these logs vertically or horizontally in the ground with approximately 50 percent of the wood above soil level. It can often take a couple of years until mushroom production starts. Once the Maitake is established, it will produce for many years.

Working with Spores

Capturing spores and using them to make a spore slurry is an easy way to get started with the process of cultivating mushrooms from those you find in the wild. It is also an essential technique to learn for correctly identifying wild mushrooms, which is crucial if you plan to grow more of them.

There are three main reasons to capture spores from wild mushrooms. First, you can use spores to develop cultures and improve species that you find in the wild. You can take a spore print (see below) and then transfer those spores to petri dishes to select for the traits you want in a culture. Different mycologists choose traits for different reasons. They may be looking for mushrooms that perform well in a commercial farm, or in specific environmental conditions, or on a novel substrate.

Second, for King Stropharia (Wine Cap) mushrooms (*Stropharia rugosoannulata*) and a few other species, we use spores as part of a low-tech cultivation method such as a spore slurry without the need to breed them on a petri plate.

Third, spores can be used as a means to transplant ectomycorrhizal species back into areas that have been deforested and need a jumpstart to reestablish the partnership connections between trees and mycorrhizal fungi.

TAKING SPORE PRINTS

There are three relatively simple methods of taking spore prints. You can use spores collected by spore printing to then make a spore slurry that can be sprayed on wood chips as an easy cultivation method.

Spore Prints on Aluminum Foil

The first and most simple method of taking spore prints is to use aluminum foil. Aluminum foil is easy to procure and does not serve as a food source for contaminants. After taking the spore print, you can fold up the piece of foil and label it with the species name, the date, the area where the mushroom was gathered, and any other notes needed. Then file it away for later use. Depending on the species of mushroom you are taking prints from, the mushroom may

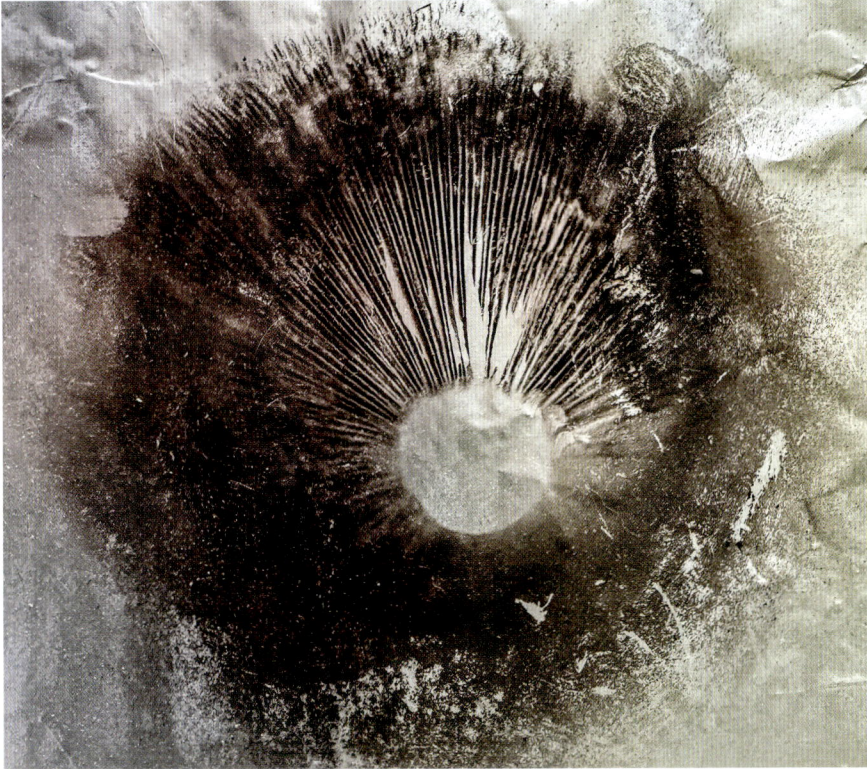

Figure 2.21. King Stropharia spore print on aluminum foil.

release the majority of spores onto the foil in only a couple of hours, or it could take from twelve to twenty-four hours.

EQUIPMENT NEEDED

Paper towel

Isopropyl alcohol

Metal or (unused) bamboo
  chopsticks

Mushroom of desired species

Knife

Aluminum foil

Bowl, slightly larger than the
  mushroom cap

Marker pen

1. Wet a piece of paper towel with alcohol and use it to wipe the top of the mushroom cap to remove any contaminants. If using metal chopsticks, clean them by dipping them in alcohol.
2. Lay the chopsticks parallel to each other on the foil; they will serve as a platform for the mushroom cap.
3. Trim off the mushroom's stem as close to the cap as you can. Place the cap hymenium (spore-producing) side down, straddling the two chopsticks and raised up off the foil.

4. Turn the bowl upside down and place it over the cap. The bowl should be large enough to not touch the cap and small enough to rest on the chopsticks. The bowl creates a stable environment without too much air movement underneath, but does allow enough air exchange so that moisture does not accumulate on the spore print.

5. After the expected period of time for spore release has passed, carefully lift off the bowl and then the mushroom cap. You may see spores on the foil. If not, then replace the cap and bowl and leave overnight. When the spores have released, you will see a patch of spores laying thickly on the foil. Fold up the foil, capturing the spores inside, and use a marker to label the foil with the species, date, and other information. Spores of some species will remain viable for much longer than others.

Spore Prints in a Canning Jar

The glass jar method of collecting spores is also simple. We teach this method because it is accessible for people who do not have access to a lab or are not ready to build out equipment to deepen the journey yet. With this method, you suspend a mushroom cap in an open jar so that the spores release and fall to the bottom of the jar. Any clean glass jar with a canning lid will do. Half-pint jars work well, and pint jars with wide mouths are good for larger caps. We modify the lids as described below.

EQUIPMENT NEEDED

Paper towel

Isopropyl alcohol

Mushroom of desired species

Knife

Thread

Needle

Half-pint or pint canning jar with ring and modified lid

Tape

1. Wet the paper towel with alcohol and wipe the mushroom cap to remove contaminants.

2. Trim the stem.

3. Thread the needle and then carefully pull the threaded needle horizontally through the cap. Be sure there is sufficient thread protruding from each side of the cap to drape over the edge of the jar.

4. Position the mushroom cap to hang in balance with the spore-producing surface facing down into the jar. Pull the ends of the thread down on either side of the jar and tape them in place. Place a heavyweight paper towel over the top and screw the ring (but not the lid) onto the canning jar to hold the paper towel in place. (Screwing on the lid would result in too much condensation inside the jar, potentially ruining your spore print.)

5. Once spores have dropped onto the bottom of the jar, carefully remove the ring, paper towel, and the mushroom cap. At this point, screw on a modified lid. Write the date and species on a label and stick it on the jar.

Once you have successfully collected the spores, you can then inject sterilized water into this jar through a port and create spore syringes.

We alter plastic canning-jar lids to suit our needs; the finished lids are easy and cost effective to make. We like to use plastic lids on jars that contain spores because they do not rust and can be reused many times. We drill two ⁵⁄₁₆-inch diameter holes in the lids 1 to 1½ inches apart. Then we roll a bit of fiberfill between our fingers (washing our hands beforehand) and stuff it into one hole as tightly as possible to provide a little airflow. In the other hole, we use a caulk gun to apply a generous dab of 100 percent silicone and let it set. This creates a self-sealing injection port. The silicone should cure within twenty-four hours.

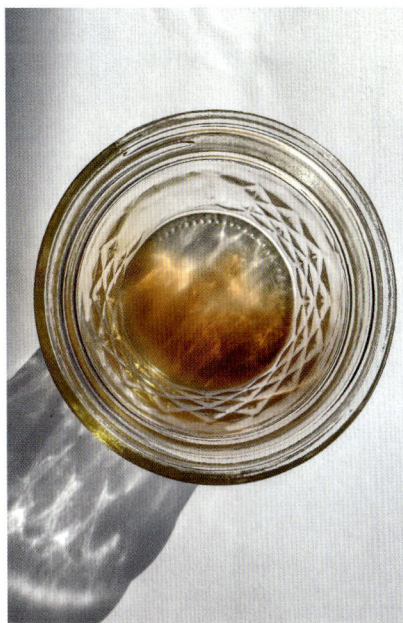

Figure 2.22. Taking a spore print in a jar.

You can insert a syringe needle through this type of silicone port to remove liquid culture from the jar or to inoculate the jar. When you withdraw the needle, the hole seals right back up.

Spore Prints on a Petri Plate

This method is one that should be done in a lab or still air box. We typically use it to collect Cordyceps, but it can be used for other fungi that are small enough that their respiration does not cause enough moisture formation to interfere with spore release. Cordyceps spores are not known for remaining viable over a long period of time. Thus, this method is a good choice because it is simple, quick, and streamlined.

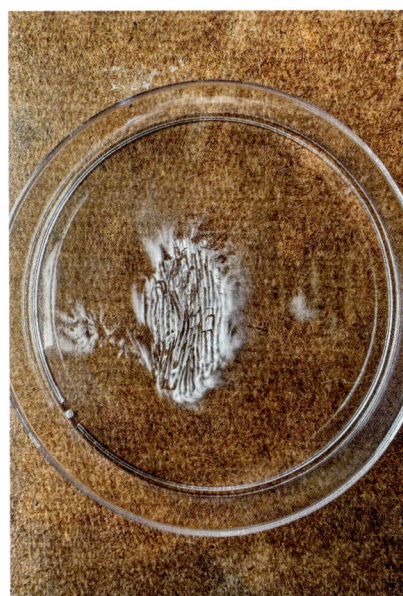

Figure 2.23. Lion's Mane spores.

EQUIPMENT NEEDED

Knife

Cordyceps club

Paper towel

Isopropyl alcohol in spray bottle

Petri plate

Parafilm

1. Trim the fruiting body of a Cordyceps club away from the host species. Wet a paper towel with alcohol and lightly clean the fruiting body, then place the fruiting body inside a petri plate. Do this deliberately and swiftly.
2. Place the petri plate on a table in front of a flow hood with the hood off for several hours or overnight.
3. Remove the fruiting body to reveal the spore print on the plate. Cover the plate, wrap with Parafilm, and label accordingly.

Another entomopathogenic fungus that we have used in a more immediate spore-capturing process is *Isaria tenuipes*, a type of Cordyceps that has a more arbuscular appearance than other Cordyceps species. It produces spores in copious amounts. The powdery dusting of white spores will be apparent on everything it touches. For these we simply touch the fruiting body to the empty petri plate and then lift the fruiting body off. It is an immediate spore print. Replace the petri plate lid. Wrap with Parafilm, add a label, and file away for later use.

Making a Spore Slurry

Using spores that you have collected to make a spore slurry is another easy way for beginners to jump into cultivation. A spore slurry is simply mushroom spores suspended in water. You can use a slurry to spread spores into new areas. If you have enough outdoor space to lay down a few square feet of wood chips on soil or a grassy surface, that's a great place to start. If you don't have that type of space available, you can grow Oyster mushrooms and some other kinds of mushrooms in wood chips in a plastic tub or bucket. You just apply the slurry to the wood chips and leave the tub outside in a shady area.

A student of mine once successfully grew Blewits mushrooms (*Collybia nuda*) under his bed in a storage tote. He was pretty secretive about the methods he used, but he did show me pictures of the Blewits growing in the tub. I was surprised because we have never grown Blewits indoors.

Understanding what conditions the mushrooms need and want to grow in is important. This is one of the advantages to growing fungi indoors—they can be grown in a variety of ways, and even a small space can produce a lot of mushrooms for the home grower. Growing mushrooms from spores in a less-controlled environment than a petri plate is easier in certain aspects because you are less involved. You will allow the microclimate to select which

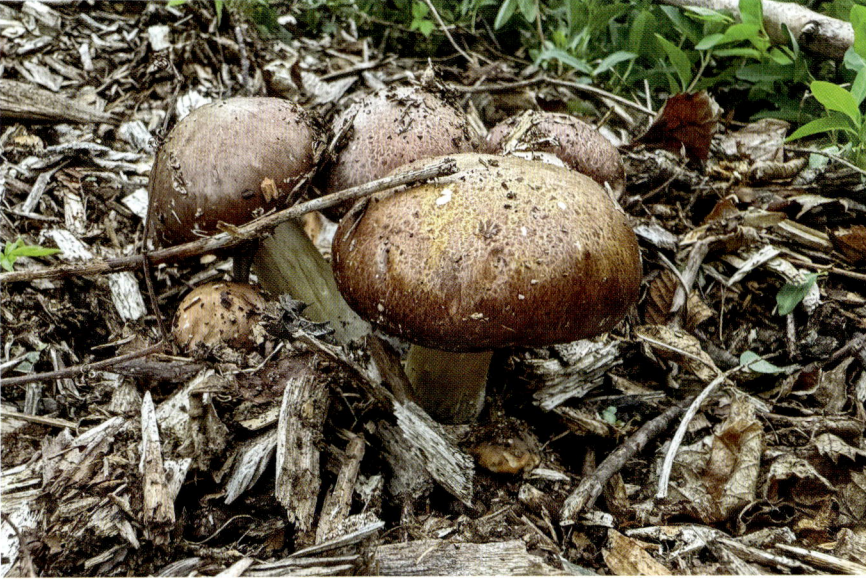

Figure 2.24. King Stropharia growing on wood chips.

spores germinate and become successful. This most certainly requires less equipment as well.

To get started making a spore slurry, wash a spore print off the aluminum foil into a clean bucket (1 to 3 gallon). The more water you use, the less concentrated your spore slurry will be and the larger an area you can inoculate. Use the volume of water needed for the area you want to cover. Keep in mind, though, that the more concentrated the slurry, the higher chance you have of establishing the target species. We have used this method to establish Wine Cap mushrooms in piles of wood chips on the farm. Some of these patches are in the forest, and others are close to creeks, around fruit trees, and even in the garden beds. Once we have created a spore slurry, we just walk down the pathways slowly pouring out the spore-laden water as we walk. We have found that spreading the spore slurry thinly and watching to see what happens informs us on how to do it next time. Even though I am pushing thirty-five years of experience in mycology, I am still surprised to find that mushrooms often produce better than expected in areas that I thought would be too harsh.

Because the wood chip piles break down relatively quickly, we need to keep making new piles and inoculating them with *Stropharia* spores. Thus, we regularly collect spore prints from the mushrooms growing in the piles so we'll have a continuous supply of spores for making slurries. We don't collect the spores randomly though; we select from various piles for differing reasons. For the piles in the forest, we select mushrooms that produce in the early spring and are productive. In the garden beds we are more interested in collecting spores from

Fungi Feed the Garden

In our vegetable production areas, we use manure from our farm animals—goats, a horse, a donkey, and sheep—to make a range of compost. The nitrogen from the manure speeds up the decomposition of the wood chips, and the *Stropharia* spores use that nitrogen to produce mushrooms. The part of this equation that is important for the health of the soil, waterways, and humans is that metabolites produced by the *Stropharia* fungi destroy fecal coliform bacteria (such as *Escherichia coli*) that may be present in the manure. The intertwined web that fungal mycelium creates in the soil also helps keep garden soil from washing away. In this way, the nutrients that you put into your garden are retained, and so this reduces the need for outside inputs. The use of fungi in the garden has a ripple effect. Fewer inputs equal less driving to the garden center, and less money spent on organic fertilizers, and even less work overall. This is a win–win–win on all levels.

mushrooms that are growing well in the full sun. For some situations, we want spores from mushrooms that will decay the wood chips quickly, to build topsoil as quickly as possible.

For those who don't have enough outdoor space for such adventures, gather a plastic bin with drainage holes and fill it with a mix of about 80 percent fresh wood chips to 20 percent decayed wood chips. Containers designed for collecting recyclables typically have drainage holes in the bottom. If you are using a container that does not have holes, drill a few holes in the bottom. Mix the fresh and decayed wood chips together well, and then pour a concentrated version of spore slurry on the wood chips. Place the container in an area out of direct sunlight, and cover it with a trimmed-to-size piece of cardboard or something similar to keep moisture in but allow for fresh air circulation. The spores will germinate and begin to colonize the wood chips. Once the chips have colonized, you can take them to your community garden or spread them around to friends and neighbors.

Oyster spore slurries can also be used to inoculate pasteurized straw by simply soaking the straw with spores without the need to continuously purchase spawn. This of course will require finding Oyster mushrooms in the wild or purchasing the spawn to start with and later capturing the spores from the cultivated fruiting bodies. Using Oyster spores from the wild can be beneficial for selecting the genetics that perform well in your region.

Collecting and distributing the spores of ectomycorrhizal fungi is a strategy to reestablish the native fungi in the forest, especially into areas that have seen disturbance from human activity or natural disasters. Collecting the spores of species that work in unison and tandem with the forests deepens your

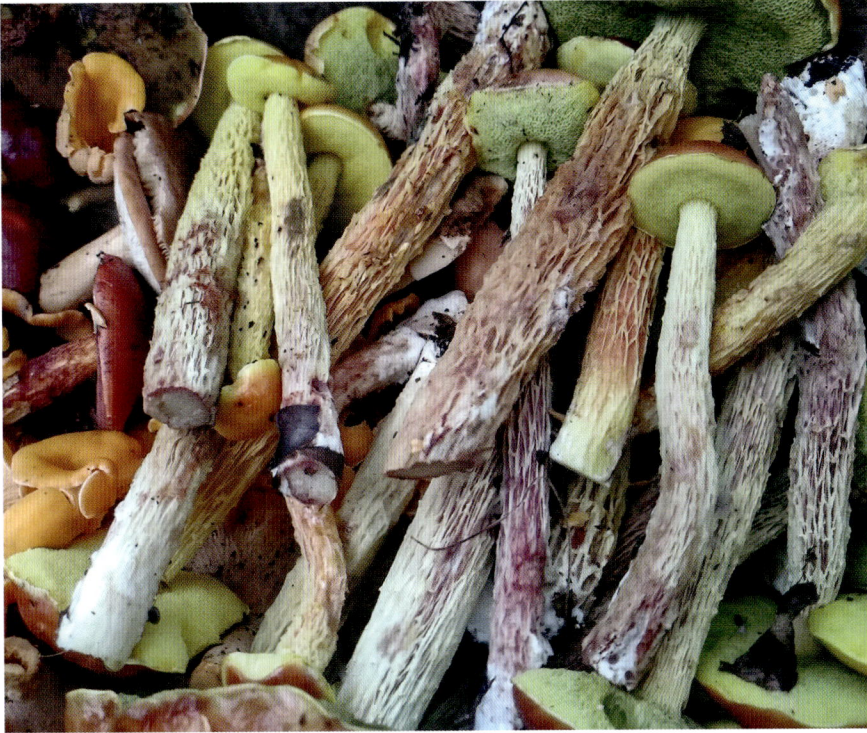

Figure 2.25. Scaly Stalk Bolete, an ectomycorrhizal species.

understanding of the forests. In our experience this work will lead to happier, more fulfilling lives. The ectomycorrhizal communities that we humans observe and pay attention to are typically the edible fungi, such as Chanterelles, Milky Caps, Russulas (*Russula* spp.), morels (*Morchella* spp.), and boletes (*Boletales* spp.). Some of these are highly sought after and demand high prices.

The Southern Appalachian forests where we live are subtropical rainforests. In the modern era, since rainforests are no longer managed by Indigenous communities, the forests have low fertility in the soil because the fertility is in the living organisms that make up the forests. Most of these trees depend on mycorrhizal partnerships for survival. When a section of forest is cleared to build a house, occasionally a large oak or a few large mature trees are left in place, but those trees usually die within a couple of years. The scraping away of the topsoil removes the nutrients the trees need and kills the vast network of mycelium that is crucial for the health of the forest. The partnerships these trees depended on have been stripped away; the trees are expected to live in isolation like we humans do, but they cannot. Collecting and redistributing spores is a way to jumpstart the underground mycelial network essential to healthy forest ecosystems. I encourage you to slow down and study the area where you live to understand the living systems that are associated with the soil and the plants of the understory and canopy. By understanding the patterns in the natural world, you can help to heal them, and you can also incorporate those interdependent ways of being into your personal life.

One tip we can offer is to remember that mushrooms have been repeating the cycle of growth, spore production, and decomposition for longer than humans have been on planet Earth. Mushrooms produce and release spores at the perfect time of the year to ensure that those spores will germinate, find a suitable connection, and become established. For this reason, try your best to harvest spores and then promptly apply them to their desired host plants so the fungi can become established during the time of year that is the most advantageous. Using a spore slurry is the quickest way to inoculate an area with ectomycorrhizal fungi.

CHAPTER THREE

Setting Up a Mushroom Lab

Setting up a lab may be something that brings you a lot of happiness, or causes you some problems. The advantages of having a lab are that it gives you control of the full process of mushroom cultivation, and it gives you the ability to make long-term observations that inform your cultivation and improve your mushroom strains. If you decide that having your own lab is not for you, then you'll need to rely on others for spawn and cultures. Fortunately, there are plenty of quality spawn and culture producers.

A lab space can be small. You can set up a lab in part of an existing room or in a well-lit closet. For a small-scale commercial operation, a 10 × 10-foot space can be sufficient. I've seen some setups with walls made of plastic sheeting hanging from ceiling to floor, with a split in the plastic for a door. As you plan your lab, think creatively and think clean. Hard surfaces such as hardwood, tile, or linoleum floors are best because they're easy to clean. Carpet or drapes or any kind of fabric can harbor contaminants, which will be disturbed if you touch or brush against them, resulting in particulates in the air that can contaminate your work.

Once you start on your journey as a cultivator, you will find that you need to dedicate a space or several spaces to your new venture. Be creative and set things up to suit your needs. You may need to work with multipurpose spaces until you become more serious about this adventure.

Basic Equipment for a Simple Mycology Lab

When you are a spore and not yet a full-fledged colony of mycelium, you can start your lab venture with some basic equipment that you can build yourself. As you become a more experienced cultivator or mycologist, the list of equipment you may want to acquire will expand. Here is the basic equipment you'll need as a beginner to set up your lab.

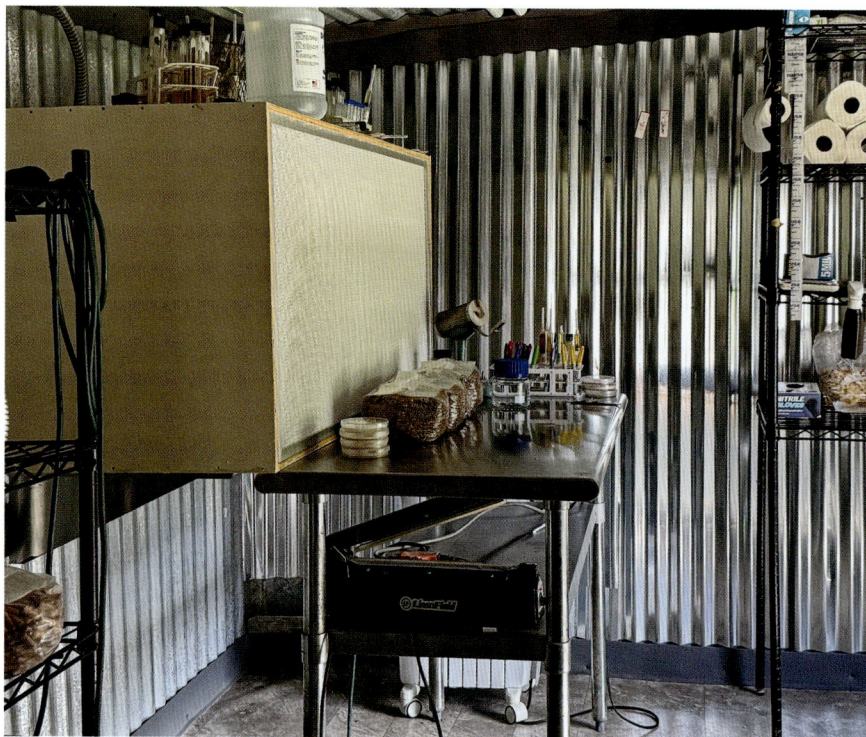

Figure 3.1. Basic mushroom lab.

A still-air box, also called a glove box, is essentially an enclosed box with rubber gloves inserted through one side into which you put your hands to manipulate items within the box. It is essential for maintaining a contaminant-free environment while working with spores and cultures. See "How to Build a Still-Air Box" on page 57–58.

Scalpels are available with different blade shapes, and a two-piece scalpel is best because the handle should last for your lifetime. We still use the one I have had for decades. Scalpel blades must be replaced periodically because repeated heating and cooling (to sterilize them) causes them to eventually lose their edge. Experiment with different blade shapes until you find the one that suits your needs best. Student scalpels, in my opinion, are essentially useless. The blades are thick and dull quickly, which is frustrating when you are dealing with small pieces of mushroom flesh or doing plate transfers.

Dental spatulas make your life easier when you are retrieving mycelia from media tubes. Unlike scalpels, they need not be sharp. Media tubes are narrow, and a scalpel just does not work well. The dental spatula is most effective if you adulterate it a bit by slightly bending the end of the spatula to a curved 45-degree angle. This shape makes it easy to snag a portion of mycelium and agar from a media tube without bumping the inside of the tube.

Lab Equipment Checklist

Still-air box or glove box
Scalpels
Media tubes
Dental spatulas
Alcohol lamp
Electric tool sterilizer
Isopropyl alcohol (70-91%)
Canning jars and lids
Autoclavable filter patch bags
Impulse sealer
Laminar flow hood
10cc syringes and needles

Polyester fiberfill (Polyfil)
Silicone caulk
Nitrile gloves
Paper towels
Permanent markers
Logbook
Glass serum bottle with rubber stopper
Erlenmeyer flasks, graduated
Aluminum foil
Parafilm
Pressure cooker

An electric tool sterilizer is a device that reaches temperatures of over 1400°F (760°C). It is used to sterilize scalpels or spatulas in under ten seconds.

An alcohol lamp, running on isopropyl alcohol, is useful for sterilizing scalpels and other tools. It is especially useful if you are doing sterile work in remote areas where there is no or limited electricity. If you are working off grid, running an electric sterilizer pulls a significant amount of electricity. It is good to have options. We do not like using an alcohol lamp in front of a flow hood because the lamp burns clean, and the flame can be hard to see. When used in front of a flow hood, the lamp's flame may be blown out without you noticing it.

Caution: Be careful if you use an alcohol lamp in a glove box. See page 57, "How to Build a Still-Air Box," to learn why this can be dangerous.

Glass canning jars (with lids) of various sizes, from pints up to a half gallon, are used for spore prints, grain spawn, and other materials. Mason or Ball canning jars work great because canning lids are easy to acquire and are replaceable, which helps to keep contamination levels down. White plastic lids are a better option than metal lids, which rust easily after a couple uses.

Autoclavable filter patch bags are for indoor production and withstand the temperatures required for sterilization. We highly recommend springing for the biodegradable option (Unicorn is a brand we've used and liked). Biodegradable are a bit more expensive but will break down even if they end up in a landfill. Be responsible.

An impulse sealer is a piece of equipment used to seal off autoclavable filter patch bags of grain or bulk substrate bags after inoculation in front of the laminar flow hood. This becomes important when the scale of your operation reaches a certain production capacity.

Laminar flow hoods can be purchased ready to plug and play. One of the highest quality hoods we have seen is produced by a company called Phenomenal Fungi. They are master carpenters. You can also purchase parts individually and construct a hood yourself, but this does require carpentry skills with an eye for detail.

10cc syringes and needles are an important part of the cultivator's toolbox because of their versatility. They are indispensable for liquid culture and for spore syringes. They can be used to transport pure cultures with little fear of contaminating them, which makes them particularly important and effective in environments that are less than ideal. In fact, when we teach classes outdoors using syringes and needles in open air, even our novice students are able to achieve sterile techniques with low contamination rates.

Polyester fiberfill is used for plugging holes in jar lids. Polyfil is a brand name of this material, but it has become the generic term most cultivators use. Your intentions for a lid will determine the number of holes it should have. An injection lid will need two holes, one of which will be stuffed with Polyfil as tightly as possible. This allows for gas exchange but does not allow microbes or spores to enter. We used to purchase filter patch lids, but they are expensive and can't be reused. Making our own lids using Polyfil is a more effective and cheaper alternative. We also use Polyfil to fill puncture holes in poly tubing for growing mushrooms on pasteurized straw. The Polyfil allows gas exchange through the holes but keeps pesky fungus gnats or fruit flies out of the substrate.

Silicone caulk or 100 percent silicone is the perfect substitute for self-sealing ports, as described in "Spore Prints in a Canning Jar" on page 46. The ports cost between one and two dollars each, depending on the supplier. A tube of silicone will cost up to ten dollars but will provide you with about one hundred self-sealing ports. This is at least ten times cheaper than purchasing self-sealing ports.

Nitrile gloves are a must-have for lab work, especially once you start working in front of a laminar flow hood. If you are working from a glove box, it may be possible to use nitrile gloves, but if the glove box is constructed using chemical gloves, then nitrile gloves are not needed. For a glove box made with Tyvek sleeves, the nitrile gloves are required. They are an essential barrier against all of the microorganisms on the surface of your hands and wrists.

Paper towels are a simple and effective way of cleaning work surfaces. We do not use them in our everyday lives because of the inputs required to produce them; however, in the lab, cleanliness and avoiding cross-contamination are essential. Working with reusable cloths increases the probability of bringing in or harboring contaminants. Cloth has so much surface area where spores can become caught—it is not worth the risk.

Permanent markers are an indispensable tool in the lab. We always have a variety of them on hand for different applications.

A storage bottle with a wide mouth is used to speed up the process of quenching tools that have been heat sterilized. The quench speeds up the work in the lab because one doesn't have to simply stand and wait for a hot tool to cool just in the airflow. It is important that the bottles have a wide-enough mouth. Not only so that a heat-sterilized tool can be inserted into the alcohol and be quenched, but we then place the tool across the top of the open bottle, with the working end of the tool as close as possible to the flow hood. This ensures that the tool will stay sterile while we make final preparations.

Erlenmeyer flasks, graduated, are important for pouring agar. This is the only task we use them for.

Aluminum foil is used to cover jars when sterilizing them so that excess moisture does not enter the jar when the water in the sterilizer is producing a boil or steam. Make sure to fold the sections of cut foil down over the lid, letting them extend slightly down the jar. We also cover media bottles or Erlenmeyer flasks with aluminum foil to keep water out during the sterilization process. Foil is also our preferred method of keeping spore prints.

Parafilm is a type of laboratory sealing film. This is a breathable, stretchy film that is used to cover the top, wrapping the edges of a petri plate after inoculation. Sealing the plates allows you transport the plates into non-sterile environments without risk of contamination.

Pressure cookers are essential for sterilizing substrates. This piece of equipment will serve you well for a very long time. We recommend buying an All American–brand pressure canner. All American makes equipment so sturdy you will be able to pass it along to your grandchildren. (We do not have an affiliation with this company.) We have an All American 921 ½. They are machined to be metal-to-metal and have no rubber gaskets, which would eventually fail. (Be sure to use a cheap vegetable oil to lubricate the metal-to-metal surface between the lid and the main body of the pressure cooker.) A 5- to 15-pound (2.3 to 6.8 kg) "jiggler" weight on top of the cooker is sufficient. Some models have a valve that remains sealed even after it returns to atmospheric pressure. The All American 921 is a good starter model. It will cost you upfront, but you can likely find a used one in good shape at a much cheaper price than brand new.

HOW TO BUILD A STILL-AIR BOX

The still-air box, also known as a glove box, is the most economical way to work in an aseptic environment unless you have access to a complete lab.

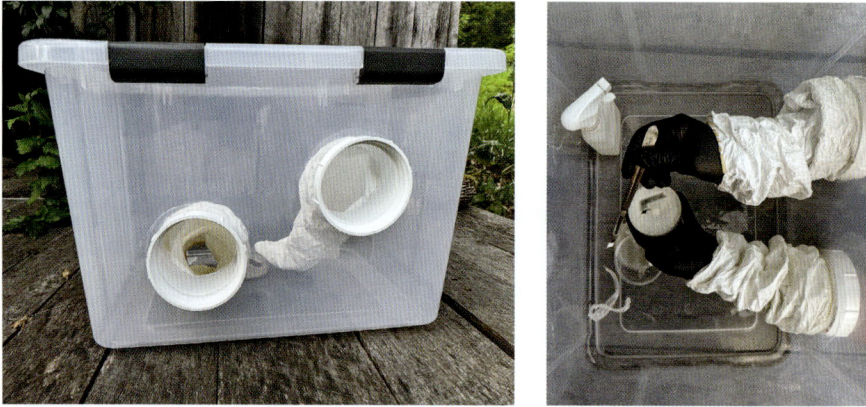

Figure 3.2. Simple glove box.

The first glove box I built from scratch was a disaster! It is much easier to start with some type of ready-made box, such as a plastic tub or storage tote. The construction of a glove box is relatively straightforward. The lid must be transparent so that you will be able to see your hands as you work with items inside the box.

Construct your glove box so that the hole on your dominant side where your arm is inserted is higher than the hole for the nondominant-side glove. I discovered that doing this gave me an ergonomic advantage while working in the box, for example, when I was pouring grain from a jar or transferring agar wedges into jars. It allows you to use your dominant hand when you need to lift one item higher than another.

EQUIPMENT NEEDED

Plastic tub or storage tote with lid
Box cutter
1 small sheet plexiglass
Two 4-inch-diameter PVC couplings

1 pair elbow-length, chemical-
    resistant gloves
Silicone caulk

1. If the lid for your box is solid, use a box cutter to cut a rectangular piece out of the top slightly smaller than the sheet of plexiglass. You will need to make many passes when cutting so as not to split the top of the box. Take your time and be careful.
2. Use silicone caulk to secure the plexiglass in the rectangular hole in the lid. Set the lid aside.
3. Hold a PVC coupling against one long side of the box and use the permanent marker to trace the outside for the placement of the coupling. (Recall the tip about positioning the dominant-hand hole higher than the other.)

4. Use the marker to trace the placement for the second hole.

5. Cut through the box along the traced circles. Insert the couplings into place through the holes.

6. Use caulk to secure the couplings in place and let them cure.

7. Place the open end of one glove (be sure they are oriented properly—that is, left to left and thumb to center, etc.) over each coupling inside the box. Peel back the wrist edge of each glove to expose more of the coupling.

8. Caulk the glove edges, making sure they have full contact with the coupling, and unfold the edges back over the caulk on the coupling surface. Give the glove edges a little squeeze to make sure they have made full contact with the coupling and are seated with no gaps. This complete seal is crucial. Allow to cure for twenty-four hours.

Please be careful when you are sterilizing instruments in a glove box. Typically, sterilizing instruments in a glove box can be as simple as spraying the inside of the box and all instruments with isopropyl alcohol. But if you are using a scalpel, you will need to flame-sterilize it, so be sure to not spray isopropyl before this. Using isopropyl alcohol after the flame sterilization of any tool is perfectly safe.

Once, a guy came to talk with me about mushroom cultivation, and I noticed he had scanty eyebrows and a couple of burns on his face. He told me he had sprayed his scalpel and other tools with 90-percent isopropyl alcohol inside a glove box and then proceeded to strike a lighter, intending to sterilize the scalpel with an alcohol lamp. The box immediately blew up in his face. Luckily, he had no lasting ill effects. It had slipped his mind that the alcohol fumes built up inside the box and had nowhere to dissipate. You may think that this could not happen to you. And indeed, if he had been working in front of a flow hood instead of inside a glove box, then this protocol would have worked fine. Please be careful, y'all! Working out of a glove box can be cumbersome, but once you get used to it, it is surprising how much you can accomplish with so little space.

CHAPTER FOUR

Sterile Lab Techniques

In chapter 2, Outdoor Mushroom Cultivation, we introduced low-tech methods for capturing the genetics of wild mushrooms and bringing them into cultivation. In this chapter, we provide a basic foundation in sterile techniques for capturing genetics, and for beginning to experiment with strains of wild mushrooms through culturing spores, cloning fungi, and creating your own grain spawn.

When fungi release spores into the environment, the spores of any given species are either asexual or sexual. (Most of the species we cultivate are sexually reproduced. For that reason, we focus in this chapter on the sexual reproduction of fungi.) When sexual spores are released into the environment, they will need to land or be deposited in a suitable place. After they germinate, they then become exploratory in finding food and looking for partners from the same species. When these partners are found, they go through a process called the "marriage of cytoplasm." This union creates the next generation of fungi, which carry slightly different genetics from the parents, just as it is with us humans.

When you *clone* a fungus, though, you replicate genetic material precisely, so the mycelium (that is, the tissue culture) you have captured has exactly the same genetic makeup as the initial mushroom you started with.

Culturing spores and cloning fungal tissue are multistep processes that require a sterile environment (a lab) and some specialized skills, which are described in detail in this chapter. If you are not ready to try culturing spores or cloning, feel free to skip ahead to the "Grain Spawn" section on page 84 or to chapter 5 for instructions for making bulk substrates. Keep in mind, though, that even if you plan to wait until a later time to try sterile techniques, it can be helpful to understand the process. With that in mind, let's dig into a discussion of the techniques involved.

Working with Agar

Agar is a jelly-like substance made up of polysaccharides. It is sterilized and poured into a petri plate, and then it becomes the substrate on which the mycelium feeds and grows. You can make agar from readily available ingredients.

AGAR RECIPES

We use several recipes for agar, and we rotate through them in our lab. Different recipes are used for different reasons. Switching them up is important to prevent stagnation and senescence of mycelium. We cover more about this in "Maintaining Your Slants" on page 84. These recipes can be mixed in bulk and kept on hand in the lab in dry form in airtight containers.

Agar powder can be found from many lab supply sources online. Soy peptone is a nutrient supplement used to provide partial proteins to feed the mycelium.

We recommend keeping all ingredients for agar recipes in sealed containers. Do not open them to the air for longer than necessary; this is important to reduce the likelihood of spores being introduced into agar ingredients.

Agar Recipe 1: Dog Food and Agar Powder (DFA)

20 g agar powder
20 g dry dog food

DFA is the easiest recipe that we use. Use the highest quality all-natural dry dog food you can find. Do not use dog food that contains any type of fish or fish products. In our experience, using dog foods containing fish increased the likelihood of salmonella contamination on agar plates.

Agar Recipe 2: Potato Dextrose Yeast Agar (PDYA)

20 g potato flakes
20 g dextrose
40 g agar powder

4 g nutritional yeast
2 g soy peptone or pea protein
    powder

This recipe is comparable in nutrient content to the malt yeast peptone agar (MYPA). Thus, we do not follow these two recipes back-to-back when we are preparing petri plates. After we pour plates with PDYA, we pour plates with DFA, and then we follow that with MYPA and then DFA again. This gives the mycelium varying nutrient profiles to consume.

Agar Recipe 3: Malt Yeast Peptone Agar (MYPA)

20 g agar powder	2 g nutritional yeast
20 g light malt extract	1 g soy peptone or pea protein powder

We include this recipe because of the importance of rotating recipes to avoid stagnation of the mycelium, but malt extract is our least favorite ingredient to work with. We buy light malt extract from a local brewer's supply, and it comes in bags of various sizes. Once a bag is opened, it tends to start to become gummy and sticky because it absorbs moisture from the air. If left open for an extended period of time, it will become one solid mass. It can still be used; the mass must just be cut into smaller chunks.

Some mycologists add food coloring to an agar recipe when adding water to the flask before sterilizing. This helps identify which agar recipes they used on those plates. This is a good idea if you are going to pour two different types of agar plates in one visit to the lab. For us, this approach seems like an unnecessary complication. Instead, just after we pour agar into a stack of petri plates, we run a permanent marker down the edge of the plates to mark them and make a note of which color marker we used for which agar recipe. This is an easy way to determine which kind of agar recipe is in a plate later on.

Any of these recipes can be scaled up to the amount necessary to satisfy your needs. For our small commercial operation, we tend to use quart jars to store the dry mixes. This is convenient because we have dry ingredients ready to go when we want to pour plates, and that reduces the tasks we have to do on any given day.

MIXING AGAR AND POURING PETRI PLATES

Pouring petri plates is a task that I always find enjoyable. It is a practice of hurry up and wait. On our farm we create between forty and fifty plates at a time. This should be sufficient for an operation of considerable commercial capacity. Poured plates don't need to be used immediately. It's common practice to refrigerate plates after pouring. In the formative years of my lab work, I was told it was industry standard, but that notion never sat well for me. We don't refrigerate plates. Instead, we sustain our plates at room temperature in the lab on a shelf, stored in a sealed container or in bags with a zip seal. We prefer to see how well we have done with our sterilization of agar and to test how reliable our technique is. If you use one large container and it becomes contaminated, it could possibly spread to the rest of your plates. It is easy to keep them on a shelf inside of a container. If plates are put in cold storage, any contaminants on the plates will not show up until they are brought out of storage and placed into service with the addition of mycelium or spores. This creates confusion: it is

Petri Plate Choices

Plastic sterilized plates are a cheap and easy way to start producing and expanding fungal cultures. The biggest disadvantage is the waste of plastic, because they cannot be reused. Another less wasteful but more expensive option is borosilicate petri plates. Borosilicate glass is used for all good quality lab glassware. The advantage of borosilicate is that it will withstand the extreme temperature swings from an autoclave or pressure cooker directly to room temperature and not suffer the thermal shock. We use 100 × 15-mm plates. You may want to purchase smaller diameter plates, depending on what your operation will require. The advantage with these plates is that, unless you break them, they can be used for decades. The biggest hurdle is the price and the time to clean and resterilize them. We have used both plastic and glass, and if you get into the business of trading cultures or selling them you may want to consider using both, too.

The alternative to petri plates is 4-ounce regular-mouth canning jars, which are easily found at local hardware or grocery stores. They do pose a few disadvantages, including the need to adulterate lids to allow for gas exchange with the growing mycelium in the jar (this is described in "Spore Prints in a Canning Jar" on page 46). Beware that canning jars do not withstand thermal shock as well as borosilicate petri plates.

difficult to figure out where the origin of the contamination is. And regardless of how good you are, the issue of contamination will arise!

Regardless of the agar recipe you use, you will start by combining the dry agar mix with water in a clean Erlenmeyer flask or media bottle. Use graduated flasks or bottles that have a 1000-ml capacity and fill them halfway. Do not ever fill a flask or bottle to full capacity. If you do, it will undoubtedly boil over during the sterilization process and ruin the batch.

A sleeve of petri plates usually contains twenty plates. You'll add about 25 ml of liquified agar to each plate, so two flasks containing 500 ml of sterilized agar is enough to fill forty plates. We use a thermal, insulated, polyester glove with waterproof latex coating when pouring agar. This glove should be bought brand new and have never been used for any other purpose. We also strongly recommend wearing nitrile gloves underneath this glove. If you don't, over time, you will inadvertently introduce sweat, dead skin, and other contaminants into the glove. This will cause contamination problems down the road.

Procedure

With this procedure, it is possible to pour twenty to thirty plates. The final number will be determined by the size of the plates and how deep you pour the agar into the dishes. Some prefer pouring agar from media bottles. We find media bottles are hard to use with hot liquified agar because the bottles are thick and retain heat in the neck, which is where they are held.

Steps 1 through 10 below can be done in a kitchen or work area. Then the pressure cooker should be carried or wheeled on a cart to the lab. Carry the cooker into the lab while still hot. Before starting to work in the lab, we shower and change clothes. This timing works out, because it gives the pressure cooker some time to cool down.

Keep it Clean!

Once you move into the lab to pour the plates, keep in mind this tip to provide security against contamination: Assume *everything* is contaminated. Clean *everything* well. This cannot be overstated.

Set up your lab workspace in the arrangement that suits your needs, according to your dominant hand. All of our tools in the lab are on the right side of the hood and our open workspace is on the left.

Note that the instructions below describe the procedure for plastic petri plates in sleeves. If you use borosilicate plates, you will sterilize them before use. They will not be packaged in plastic sleeves.

EQUIPMENT NEEDED FOR MIXING AGAR

Prepared agar mix of your choice
Water
Two 1,000-ml Erlenmeyer flasks or
    media bottles
Aluminum foil
Pressure cookers

EQUIPMENT NEEDED FOR POURING THE PLATES

Flow hood
Isopropyl alcohol, 70 to 90 percent,
    in a spray bottle
Nitrile gloves
Paper towels
Petri plates
Thermal glove
Permanent marker

1. Gather the equipment you'll need for mixing the agar.
2. Weigh out 20 g of agar recipe mix into each flask.
3. Boil slightly more than 1000 ml of water (a little extra is needed to compensate for evaporation).
4. Pour the boiling water into each of the two flasks, filling them only to the 500 ml mark.
5. Swirl the water around until the agar mixture dissolves. Do not worry if there are lumps ¼ inch (1 cm) in size or smaller that do not dissolve immediately. Those will dissolve during the sterilization process.
6. Place aluminum foil over the flask opening; the foil piece should be large enough to cover the opening and extend down the sides so it won't fall off.

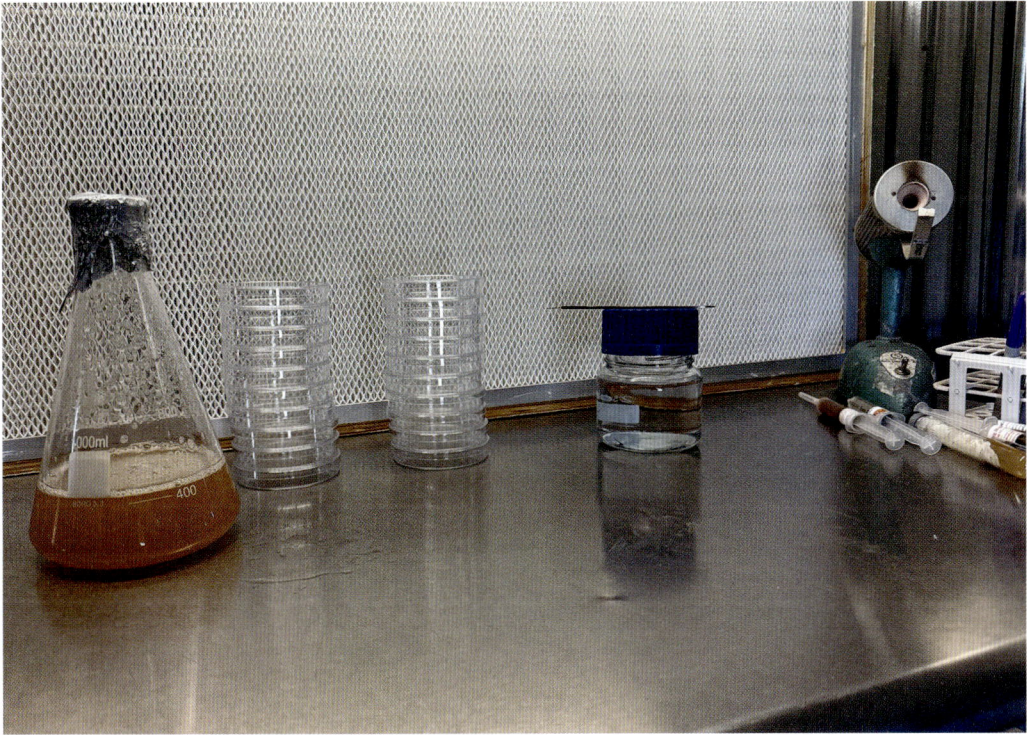

Figure 4.1. Items needed to pour petri plates.

7. Place both flasks in the pressure cooker, making sure the baffle is in place in the bottom of the cooker. Then add water to approximately the level of the liquified agar in the flasks.

8. Lock the lid on the pressure cooker, place it on the heat source, and heat sufficiently to bring the pressure up to 15 PSI.

9. Maintain this pressure for 45 minutes. Passing the 45-minute mark risks caramelizing the sugars in the agar mixture, which will make it more difficult for the mycelium to run across the agar.

10. Turn off the heat and let the pressure cooker cool for 30 minutes to 1 hour. Do not allow the cool down period to last too long. Many problems can develop if you do. Worst case scenario is that the agar completely sets up in the flasks. Or it may remain liquid but begin to set up as you are pouring the plates, making the plate surfaces chunky. Sometimes the agar will cool to the point that it is impossible to effectively pour the last portion out of the flask, increasing waste by reducing the number of usable petri plates you'll end up with.

11. Bring your pressure cooker into the lab. Turn on the flow hood to scour the air in the lab for at least a few minutes, and up to 30 minutes, before beginning to work.

12. Open the pressure cooker and crack the lid, but do not take the lid off.
13. Alcohol your hands and rub them together until the alcohol dissipates.
14. Put on nitrile gloves and wipe the work surface in front of the hood clean with alcohol.
15. Place the sleeves of plates in front of the hood. Spray alcohol on the outside surfaces of the sleeves and wipe with a paper towel.
16. Flip each sleeve so that the plates inside it are upside down.
17. Cut the upside-down sleeve from one edge to the other. Then invert the sleeve again. The plates are now upright and you can simply slip the bag off.
18. Divide each stack of plates in half, so you have four stacks of about ten plates each. Slide the empty plates up to the hood and pull one stack as close to your dominant side as is comfortable.
19. Remove one flask of hot agar from the pressure cooker. The flask will be very hot. If you are using a thermal insulated glove, simply put it on over the nitrile glove.
20. Set your flask on your dominant side, ready to be poured. Note the foil should still be over the top.
21. Alcohol off your gloves and work surface once more.
22. Wrap a folded paper towel around the neck of the flask to catch any agar that accidentally drips down from the opening when you pour.
23. Gently peel off the foil from the top of the flask.
24. Grab the lid of the petri plate at the bottom of one stack and lift up that lid and the other nine plates balanced on top of it. Lift with dedication and intention. Gently and methodically. This is a game of concentration.

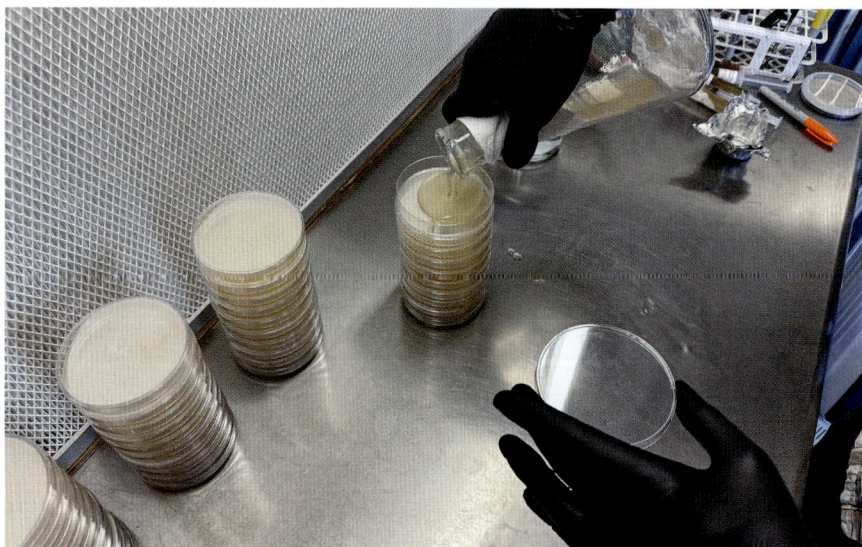

Figure 4.2. Top plate being filled with agar.

25. Pour some hot agar into the open plate, just enough to fill the plate to 90 percent full. The liquified agar will slowly drift and fill the last 10 percent without you needing to add more. It's wasteful to fill plates 100 percent full—so this method increases the mileage of our agar.

26. Replace the lid on the full plate. Grasp the lid of the next plate up the stack and repeat the filling step.

27. Continue working your way up the stack until you have finished filling the top plate.

28. Set down the flask and slide the stack of still-warm poured plates over to the far side of your work area, making sure to keep it as close to the flow of the hood as possible.

29. Continue filling plates one by one until you have successfully poured all of the agar. Once your plates are stacked and cooling, use a permanent marker to run a strip up the outside edge of the plate to identify the type of agar recipe inside. Leave the plates in front of the hood for a couple hours to help dissipate excess condensation in the plates.

Filling plates is like the board game Operation, which requires some hand-eye coordination to remove the tiny parts from the patient on the operating table without touching the sides of the opening. I remember playing this as a child, and if you did hit the edge, the board would buzz and the nose of the patient would light up. This kind of hand–eye coordination is exactly what we practice with sterile technique, because regardless of how much you sterilize, the ideal is to work smoothly and with efficiency to avoid bumping anything unexpected. This is a practice in mindfulness, in staying aware of your movements and where your body is at all times. The more moves you make and the more you overthink, then the higher the likelihood of contamination and failure.

Some people make stacks of only three or four plates. We find this time consuming; and it takes up too much workspace. Also, condensation ends up on your plate lids. Ambient air in contact with the lid of a plate will be much cooler than the freshly poured agar inside the plate. The temperature difference will lead to condensation forming on the inside of the lids of the plates at the top of each stack. The rest of the lids cool more slowly, which reduces the likelihood of developing condensation on the lid. For us, the solution to this problem was to pour stacks of ten plates, thereby exposing only one of every ten plates to the direct cooling laminar flow. Another little trick is to place the empty flask from pouring agar on top of a stack of plates, which will slow the cooling as well. In this way, you will end up with only two plate lids with condensation. (When pouring plates in a still air box, condensation and space will obviously not be a problem, and it will result in pouring a much smaller number of plates.)

Once the plates have cooled sufficiently, place them in your preferred containers. They are now ready to use. Locking-lid small plastic boxes that seal are a good place to store these plates. We keep these boxes on a shelf in the lab ready for use.

A Low-Tech Pouring Method

An alternative method of pouring plates that we have used in the past is simpler but much riskier. We call this the range oven method, and it follows similar protocols to the standard method, with the exception that you will use your kitchen range as an improvised flow hood. To do this, set your oven at its highest setting (approximately 475°F or 250°C) and let it continue heating as you make a batch of liquified agar on the stove top. When you are ready to pop the lid on your pressure cooker, cut the heat from your oven and open the oven door fully flat. Place some type of nonporous flat material on the open oven door. A 14 × 14-inch clay tile works great. Alcohol it off. From there, set up your plates on the tile and follow the procedure for pouring agar as described starting at step 15 of the standard procedure (see page 66). You will pour agar into plates just like you would in front of a flow hood.

The notion with this method is that the thermal updraft coming out of the oven and then flowing up is a sufficiently microbe-free stream of air to simulate a laminar flow hood for a short period of time. We have used this method many times in the past because it is less cumbersome than trying to pour plates in a still air box. However, the probability of contamination runs extraordinarily high. One must work much more quickly and with care and deliberate movements. There is very little room for error.

Culturing from Spores

Cultivating fungal strains from spores you have collected is an essential technique that allows you to grow mushrooms already adapted to your local region. Now that you know how to pour petri plates, we will guide you through the entire culture process. Inoculation loops are often suggested as a good tool for introducing spores to a petri plate, but we find that the thin wire of inoculation loops is just too weak and pliable and does not offer the rigidity needed. Instead, we use a dental spatula adapted to serve the purpose, as described in "Dental Spatulas" on page 54.

Procedure

EQUIPMENT NEEDED

Dental spatula
Electric tool sterilizer
Isopropyl alcohol in a quenching
    bottle

Prepared petri plates
Parafilm
Permanent marker

1. Prepare your aseptic environment.
2. Sterilize the dental spatula in the tool sterilizer for 7 to 10 seconds.
3. Quench the end of the spatula in isopropyl alcohol making sure to not cool the spatula off completely. You want to remove the spatula as soon as the isopropyl alcohol stops boiling.
4. Quickly withdraw the spatula, remove the lid from the plate, and then push the spatula into the agar on the petri plate. You will notice that it slightly melts the agar. This is exactly what you want because some of the cooled agar will remain on the spatula.
5. Run this agar-tipped spatula across a very small section of a spore print.
6. Streak the spore-charged tip of the spatula in a zigzag across the agar on the plate in the largest Z shape you can make. This gives the maximum amount of space on the plate to watch the mycelium start to grow out.
7. Put the lid back on the plate. Sterilize the spatula again and then quench in isopropyl alcohol.
8. Wrap the petri plate in Parafilm.
9. Write the date, species name, and other relevant info on the bottom of the plate.

You will then play the waiting game to see what transpires, as described in "Monitoring Petri Plates" on page 76. I think this is the best part. You are giving spores that you have harvested a chance to show how they can perform. Once the mycelium starts to grow, you will notice that some spores have germinated quickly, while some areas on the plate are still bare. Some of the mycelium may

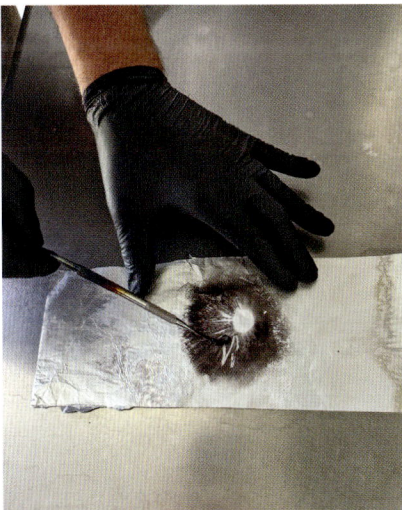

Figure 4.3. Agar-tipped spatula gathering spores.

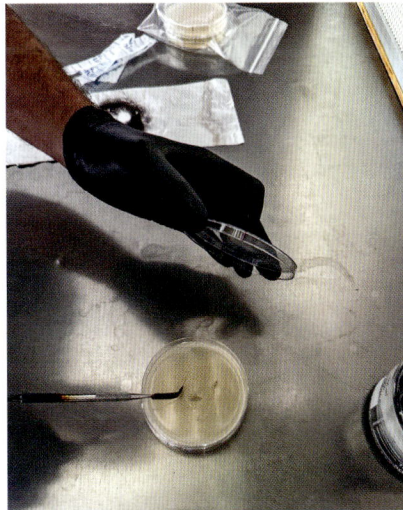

Figure 4.4. Spore streak across agar on plate.

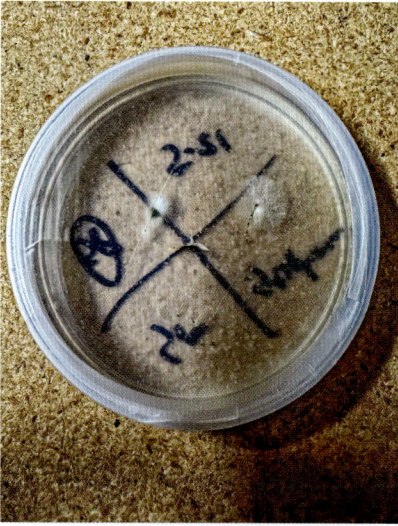

Figure 4.5. Mycelium growing from streak pattern.

become aerial, cottony, or rhizomorphic, or show other traits.

You will be selecting for certain traits depending on the species and your needs. *Hericium* species, for example, tend to have wispy mycelium that is more prone to contamination than other species. Therefore, we always look for stronger, heavier *Hericium* mycelium that does not fruit prematurely (premature fruiting results in spores dumped on the plate, which then changes the culture by introducing new genetics). With Wine Cap (*Stropharia rugosoannulata*), Reishi (*Ganoderma* spp.), and *Lentinula* species we look for a strong, full mix of cottony and rhizomorphic mycelium. In our experience these traits are an indicator of strains that are best able to fight and overcome contamination. Sometimes they are good mushroom producers, sometimes not. This is where growing out the mycelium to fruition is important. Keeping records and naming isolates is of the utmost importance.

Cloning (Tissue Culture)

Cloning mushrooms, also known as tissue culturing, is one of the most powerful tools you have when becoming established as a mushroom grower. Lab work is where I find the most pleasure and excitement. There are many ways of growing mycelium out for cultures. My favorite approach has always been working with agar in petri plates. Some folks prefer to work with liquid culture, which is a legitimate and effective way of growing mycelium. But we find that petri plates provide a much more detailed view of the mycelium. Some mycologists use a combination of both. There are advantages and disadvantages to both, and your choices will be up to you.

The surefire way to extract a pure culture from a mushroom is by cloning. This is a simple process but not always easy. We recommend that beginners start with mushrooms that have a relatively large fruitbody, like Shiitake (*Lentinula edodes*).

CHOOSING MUSHROOMS TO CLONE

When choosing a wild mushroom to sample for cloning, it is important to find one that is not decaying or riddled with larvae tunnels. With some species, such as Oysters (*Pleurotus* spp.), this can be difficult because the insect damage can be extensive. Gathering fungi when they are young is best; gather several mushrooms if they grow in clusters or troops. This helps you beat the insects to the mushrooms you are interested in cloning and increases the likelihood that you will end up with something productive. Select only fruiting bodies that are young and firm. Examine the margins. Is the cap upturned, and has the mushroom already dumped the majority of its spores? This could mean that it is past its prime and may fail when cloned. Is there enough mushroom flesh to provide a clean piece of tissue for culturing? If not, then you may need to collect the fungus with the host material still attached. Once you have determined that you have found a suitable mushroom for cloning, pick the mushroom.

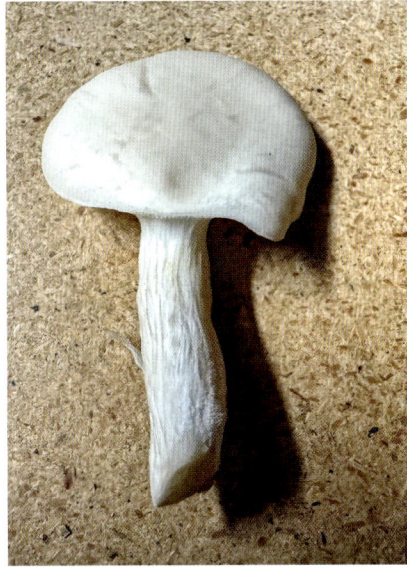

Figure 4.6. Suitable young Oyster mushroom for cloning.

Procedure

Once you locate a fungus you want to work with, if it has a cap and stem, trim off the base of the stem and trim off the cap so you can work with the middle section of the stem. Place this portion of stem into a plastic bag to keep it as clean as possible. Some species, such as Turkey Tail (*Trametes versicolor*), have stems that are too thin to get a clean piece of tissue. In this case we bring a small part of the branch or the host substrate with us in the plastic bag.

We recommend setting up three tissue culture plates for each mushroom you plan to clone. This gives you a higher chance of getting a good sample. You can make more

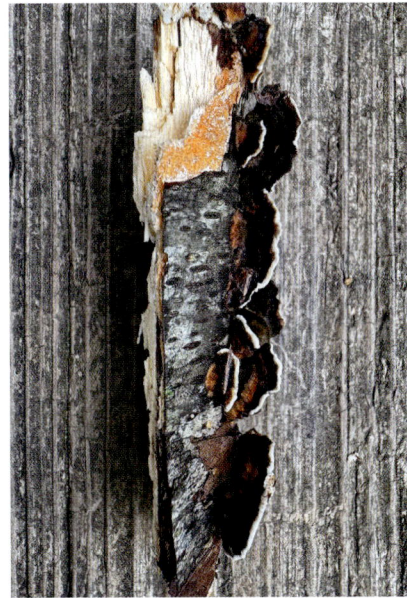

Figure 4.7. Turkey Tail on host substrate.

plates if you would like, but we do not advise using less than three plates per mushroom. We also recommend using a fresh scalpel blade when cutting wedges of mushroom tissue for cloning.

EQUIPMENT NEEDED

Scalpel

Zipper-locking plastic bags

Flow hood

Nitrile gloves

Tyvek sleeves

Isopropyl alcohol in a quenching bottle

Paper towels

Storage bottle

Prepared petri plates

Parafilm

1. With the scalpel, cut the spore-producing surface away from the specimen and trim off the base of the stem. Trimming these parts away before bagging helps keep dirt and other objects away from the sample you have gathered. Cutting the hymenium away removes the opportunity for the mushroom to produce spores, increasing the chances you will get a pure culture.

2. Place your sample in a small zipper-locking plastic bag, but make sure not to completely zip the bag closed. This sample is alive and still needs to breathe.

3. Take your samples into your sterile environment and flip on the flow hood. Turn on your tool sterilizer. Suit up with nitrile gloves and Tyvek sleeves and wipe down the work surface with alcohol.

4. Set up at least three petri plates in front of the hood for each individual mushroom you are going to clone.

5. Tear off a paper towel, spray the paper with alcohol and, without touching it, drop the mushroom sample onto the paper towel.

6. To clean the mushroom, slide one hand under the paper towel so you can cradle the mushroom sample without contaminating your gloves.

7. With your other hand, use the paper towel to wipe off the mushroom tissue.

8. With both hands, pinch the mushroom using your first fingers and thumbs and gently pull to split the stem open (figure 4.8), as if you were peeling it right down the middle.*

9. Examine the opened stem and decide which part of the flesh is most pronounced and looks the best to you. Ideally the flesh will look vibrant. You will develop an eye for this.

10. Use a sterilized, cooled scalpel (preferably a fresh blade) to make a series of cuts in the vibrant flesh. You can use the scalpel tip to pick up one wedge of tissue (figure 4.9). While lifting the petri plate lid slightly to provide the least opening for contamination, move the tip of the scalpel and the small wedge of tissue into the opening and gently drag the scalpel tip across the agar to place the small wedge in the center of the plate.

---

* Most people instruct students to sterilize a scalpel and use it to slice into the mushroom flesh, but we prefer our method of using fingers because there is less risk of introducing contaminants.

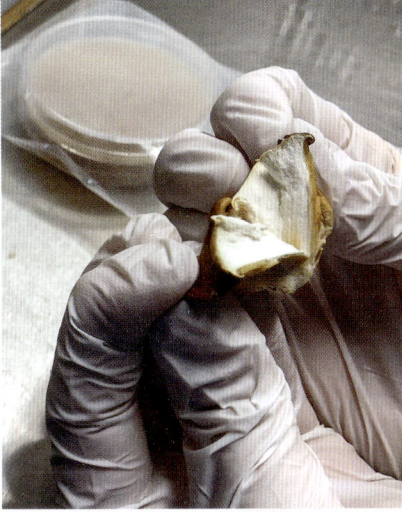

Figure 4.8. Opening mushroom to expose inner flesh.

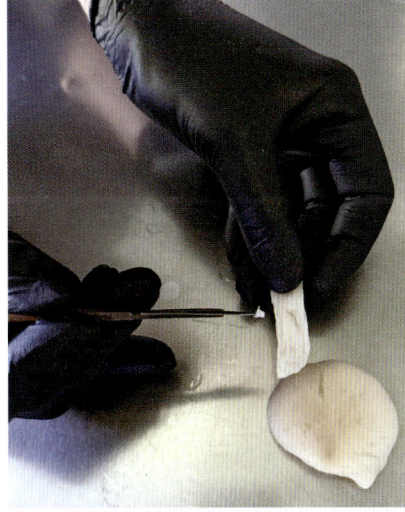

Figure 4.9. Removal of tissue wedge from wild mushroom.

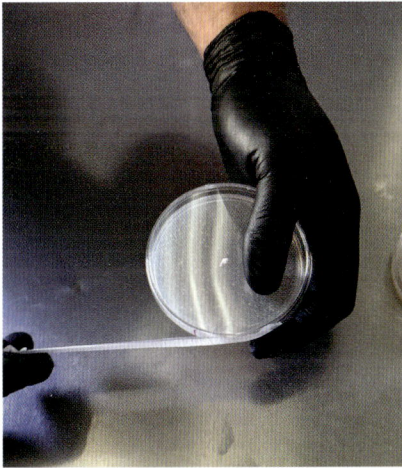

Figure 4.10. Correct technique for wrapping the petri plate with Parafilm.

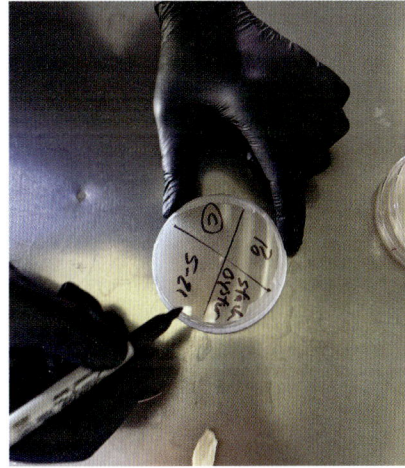

Figure 4.11. Labeled petri plates.

11. Remove the scalpel from the plate and replace the lid.
12. Repeat steps 11 and 12 until you have placed all the wedges into petri plates.
13. Place your scalpel back into the sterilizer. Once it is sterilized, quench it in the alcohol in the storage bottle and set the scalpel on the top of the bottle with the blade pointing toward the flow of the hood.
14. Cut a piece of Parafilm to wrap around the edge of the plate and cover the opening when the lip of the lid overhangs the plate. Leave the paper

intact on the Parafilm and pinch the Parafilm between the plate and your forefinger.

15. Stretch the Parafilm and wrap it around part of the plate as you spin the plate (figure 4.10). The Parafilm will stretch, and if you pull too hard, it will snap. There is a sweet spot that you will get to know quickly, but it is not uncommon for the Parafilm to develop occasional holes while being stretched. Because of this, we wrap each plate two times around. The double coating is insurance against accidental contaminants.

16. Wrap all plates, place them in a group, and set them to the left of the table.

17. Continue cloning more samples or doing your other tasks involving plates until you are finished.

18. Label the petri plates (figure 4.11). I label our plates in quadrants. It is a simple and effective method I learned from Paul Stamets's books decades ago. From top left, and moving clockwise, I record the species name, strain, date, and generation (or "P value," as Stamets called it). See "Inoculating Grain in Jars" on page 93 for an explanation of the importance of keeping track of generations.

Occasionally you will encounter a fruiting body that you cannot collect mycelium from in either of the ways described above. In these cases, you can gather mycelium from the stem butt. I use this method often for morels (*Morchella* spp.), Blewits (*Collybia nuda*), and Shaggy Mane (*Coprinus comatus*). This method can work with other species too; with a little experimenting you will get a feel for when to use this method. It works well for any mushroom that decays quickly, has thin flesh, or is for one reason or another hard to get a clean piece of tissue from. Harvest the mushroom, stem and all. Cut the cap and most of the stem away from the base. This is especially important for a mushroom like Shaggy Mane and morels because the Shaggy Manes will deliquesce overnight and morels also can begin to decay quickly, which will contaminate your sample.

Use the base of the stem where it was emerging from the soil. Place the stem butt in a small plastic bag, leaving the bag barely open to allow air exchange. Place this bag in the fridge. Once the stem butt is in the fridge, the mycelium will become exploratory, looking for new substrate to colonize. Because the mycelium is in a protected environment that is continually moist, it will become aerial and grow away from the substrate it was previously growing in, as shown in figure 4.12.

At this point you can gently place this bag in front of a flow hood and cut tissue pieces for cloning. Follow the instructions above, but rather than dumping the stem butt out onto a paper towel, you will leave it in the bag. Use a sterilized scalpel or spatula to reach into the bag and grab some of the aerial mycelium, which you'll then place on a petri plate.

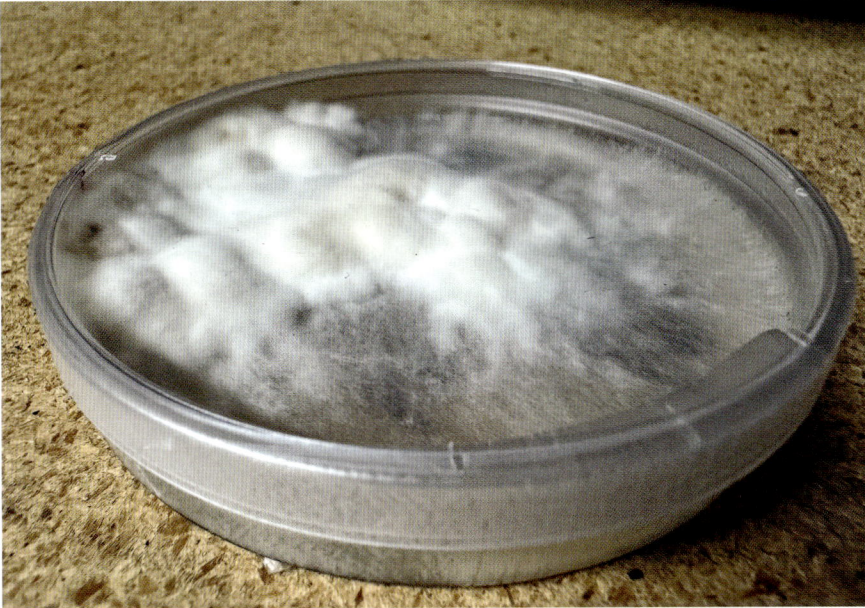

Figure 4.12. Thick, cottony Shiitake mycelium.

We developed this little trick when using morel stem butts to transplant back into non-morel producing areas of the forest. These stem butts also harbor other microbes that are important for soil health as well as the communities that are important for the species we are cultivating, that is, *Morchella*.

This is also a selective process, something you will learn to observe. Let's theorize that you have picked twenty morels of the exact same species from approximately the same area. They are the same, but they also have genetic variation. You take the stem butts of all twenty of the carefully selected mushrooms from the wild. You place them in a plastic bag to let the mycelium begin to run away from the stem and become aerial. Not all of them will do this. There will be some that do nothing. There will be specimens that the mycelium runs from, but they will not be impressive. There will be some that run and will run faster than the others and the mycelium will be stronger and thicker. These will be the ones you choose to cultivate. These will be the ones that have already provided telltale signs that they can exist in a natural environment as well as an environment that is artificial. The signs aren't foolproof, but this is what we keep a lookout for. Do not be discouraged if you choose to cultivate mushrooms on this level. Hold the line, stay with it. The fungi will reveal themselves and their secrets the more you study them. This kind of patience and persistence is the same as was needed when our ancestors first domesticated grain and vegetable crops many millennia ago. This difference now is that we can make use of much more technologically advanced equipment than our ancestors had access to.

MONITORING PETRI PLATES

After everything is labeled, place the plates on a shelf in the lab to keep an eye on them. Within two to seven days you will be able to see if any contamination shows up. If bacterial contamination occurs, it appears as little greasy-looking colonies. They will continue to enlarge until the edge of the fungal mycelium reaches the colony. The mycelium can recover from some contamination. Occasionally, mycelium will simply grow right over the bacteria, never showing signs of slowing down. This usually is an indicator that the mycelium has a memory of this bacteria and has overcome or used it as a food in the past.

Contamination by other species of fungi can pose problems. For example, *Trichoderma* species produce an enzyme called *chitinase* that has the ability to break the cell walls of other fungi. The mycelium of *Trichoderma* pops in through the broken cell wall, consumes the cytoplasm in that cell, and moves to the next cell. This is clearly a problematic contaminant. Some other fungi, such as *Penicillium* species, are not such a big problem. Some mycelia can overcome *Penicillium* contamination or at least surround it so that the culture can be cleaned up (isolated from the contaminate) and transferred over to different plates.

It is important to look at the petri plates once a day while they are colonizing. If a plate is contaminated but the mycelium grows over the contaminated area without you realizing it, the contaminant will be carried along with the

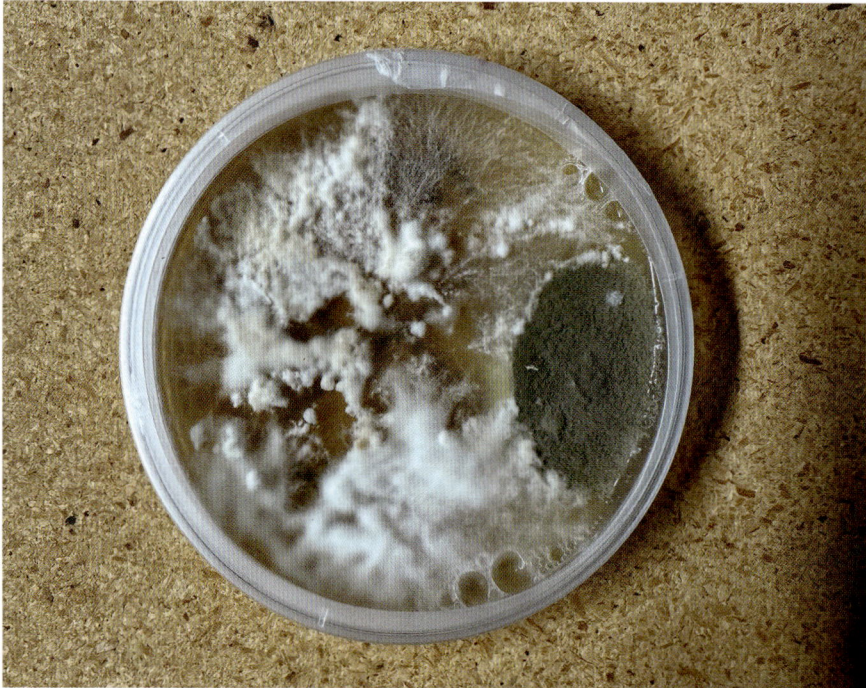

Figure 4.13. Contaminated petri plate.

mycelium to other plates when you do plate transfers. The contamination must be identified and isolated, so that the mycelium you take from the plate is clean. Marking the bottom of a plate with a permanent marker in the spots where you notice contamination occurring will help you avoid that area when you later take mycelium from the plate.

The other thing to watch for when tissue culturing is irregular mycelium. Each mycelium has its own unique patterns according to species; this is its hyphal phenotype. A seasoned mycologist is able to identify the species being cultivated by the appearance of the mycelium. If one area of the mycelium is growing out in a pattern obviously different from the other sections, this may be due to spores making their way into the mix when the tissue culture plates were first set up. This is not uncommon. The individual hyphal phenotype will be present on the plates. When this occurs with cloning, it is often only in one section. Isolate these phenotypes by transferring them onto individual plates and look for the consistent growing pattern in an outward radiating pattern. When consistency is achieved, this indicates the culture is pure. At this point you can back up the cultures in media tubes, as described in "The Culture Bank" on page 78.

Senescence

Senescence is an organism's loss of ability to continue the division of cells. Many factors play a role in fungal senescence. When you harvest a wild mushroom from a dead tree, consider this question: How long has this mycelium been consuming this tree and putting out fruiting bodies? For one year, ten years, twenty-five years, forty years? If the answer is forty years, you may discover that if you try to clone that mushroom, the mycelium will not run well in the plate or produce fruitbodies. It may be at the end of its biological ability to produce viable tissue for cloning. We all senesce at some point. It is the natural end of the process that starts with being born. We live and generate new cells to replace old ones for twenty, thirty, forty, or one-hundred twenty years, then we succumb to the transition of the death of our cells. Mycelium is no different. In fact, above all other beings on Earth, mycelium is all about death, as discussed in chapter 1.

Good labeling is important to keep track of the number of times you have expanded the fungal cells. A mushroom that is cloned is labeled in the 6-to-9-o'clock quadrant of the petri plate lid as "T" or "C." T stands for tissue, the original sample; C stands for clone. Once the mycelium grows away from the tissue sample, a small wedge of the colonized agar close to the leading edge is removed and transferred to a new plate. This next plate is labeled in the 6-to-9-o'clock quadrant as "#1". From plate one, it will be stepped up to another plate or plates and labeled as "#2". This will continue until the strain starts to senesce.

Different genera of fungi have different ceilings for senescence. Shiitake typically can be expanded by plate transfers from twelve to twenty times without cellular growth slowing down. On the lower end is Caterpillar Fungus (*Cordyceps militaris*), which will begin to senesce before hitting the fifth or sixth generational expansions.

The Culture Bank

A good, self-sufficient homesteader or farmer saves seed every year and keeps some of that seed for a couple of years so that they're not relying on just one year's seed—they not putting all their eggs in one basket. If a crop failure happens, or if a batch of seed turns out not true to type because of accidental cross-pollination, they know they will have backups. This is the purpose of setting up a fungal culture bank too. It's a reserve you can count on if some of your cultures don't turn out well.

Using petri plates is a way to encourage the fastest mycelial growth possible for the sake of expanding the amount of mycelium available for use to support your mushroom-growing work. Once we have developed a clean culture of a mushroom strain on petri plates, we back up the strain into media tubes.

Media tubes are another crucial part of a culture library. They are a way to continue to keep cultures in play for decades. Media tubes now come with screw-on caps, so it is easy to sterilize the agar inside the tube. Media tubes with agar added are called *slants* because, to cool them, we set up the hot tubes of liquid agar on an angle in front of the flow hood, and as the agar cools it solidifies on a deep slant down the length of each tube. Once you have mycelium running out across some plates and you have media tubes with clean cultures and in cold storage, you can then relax a bit and begin to play with the cultures.

Most of our slants are made with slightly different agar recipes than we use for petri cultures. When making slants, sometimes we simply mix agar powder and water, with nothing else added. If this is the case, we add a popsicle stick or bamboo skewer to the tube as an additional source of harder-to-access nutrients, as described in "Preparing Media Tubes for Slants" on page 80.

It is recommended to have at least three media tubes of backup for each strain in a culture library. In our library, however, if we do not have at least five, then my stress levels go up. You can set up your culture library however you like. Built-in redundancies are good insurance too. We recommend not keeping a culture library just in one fridge but dividing it up among at least two refrigerators.

We learned this lesson the hard way. At one point in our farm's history, we had over 250 cultures of medicinal and culinary mushrooms as well as

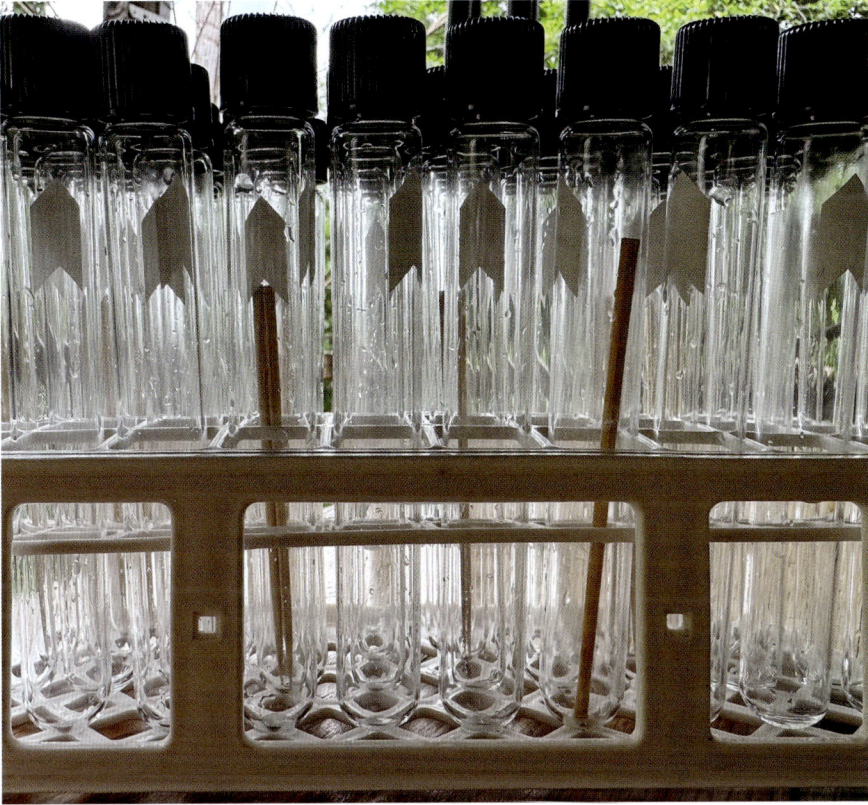

Figure 4.14. Media tubes ready for agar.

interesting species from our home region of the Southern Appalachians. We lost 99 percent of our cultures all at once from a flood event during a hurricane in 2018. A decade of work was taken away in mere hours. As we write this manuscript, a historical and geologically momentous event has just taken place here in my native home of western North Carolina. Record flooding has occurred in Asheville and the harder-hit surrounding counties. This is the type of event that happens only once in five hundred years. It is hard to plan for because no one alive remembers such an event. But something like this could happen where you live too. Be prepared: put some samples of your cultures into other people's hands, so they can continue to propagate those fungi if something happens to your culture library. When you share cultures with other mycologists, they will often share with you too, and the whole community benefits. We find this approach to sharing cultures exciting, not only as insurance against disaster but also because you can never tell what is going to happen with the fungi until they are grown out in an artificial environment or in outdoor cultivation. When you know you have good back up, you can relax and enjoy experimenting.

PREPARING MEDIA TUBES FOR SLANTS

Prepping slants is similar to filling petri plates with agar. But instead of sterilizing the agar before pouring it into the plates, you fill the media tubes with unsterilized agar, then sterilize everything together. You can fill twenty to thirty media tubes with 250 ml of agar.

The agar recipe we use for long-term storage contains less sugar. This less nutrified agar will keep the mycelium from having too many nutrients to grow, so it will remain in stasis. We never use DFA mix when making slants, ever. An agar recipe that is rich in nutrients such as DFA would stimulate too much growth, and the mycelium in the tube might extend all the way to the top of the tube and grow out. This is unwanted. The goal is for the mycelium to colonize the agar in the slant and immediately go into a state of the slowest growth possible without dying.

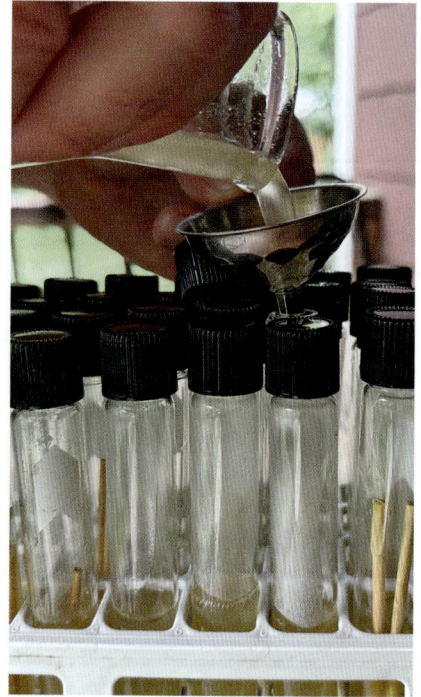

Figure 4.15. Adding agar to media tubes.

For all wood-decaying species, we add one or two clean new popsicle sticks or short bamboo skewers into the media tube before pouring in the agar. This provides an additional food source for the mycelium. Bamboo is harder than the wood of a popsicle stick, so it seems the mycelium will take longer to consume the bamboo than the stick. We propose that this is advantageous because the mycelium has to work harder for its food. It will be in cold storage, too, which slows metabolism further, possibly extending the life of the culture.

For species that are not wood loving, such as Cordyceps, medicinal molds, or some psychoactive mushrooms, omit the popsicle sticks or skewers.

Procedure

Steps 1 through 9 can be done in a kitchen or work area. Then transport the rack of sterilized tubes to your sterile lab to finish the procedure.

EQUIPMENT NEEDED

Agar

Bamboo skewers or popsicle sticks

Media tubes with caps

Small metal funnel

Aluminum foil

Metal test-tube basket

Pressure cooker

Plastic tube rack

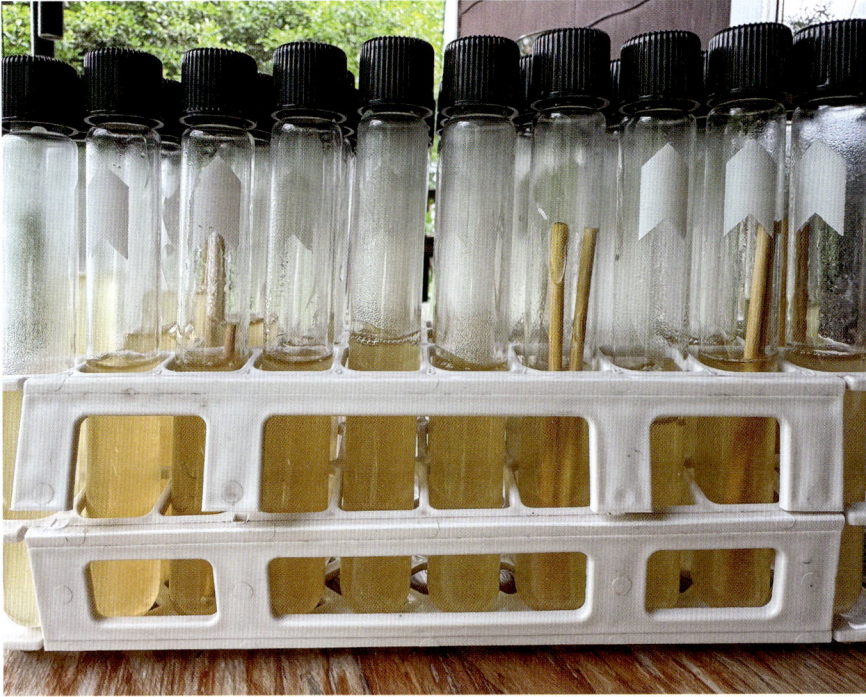

Figure 4.16. Tubes in rack.

1. Mix up an agar solution following steps 1 through 6 in "Mixing Agar and Pouring Petri Plates" on page 62.
2. Place a bamboo skewer or popsicle stick in each media tube, making sure the stick or skewer is at least 1 inch from the top of the tube.
3. Insert a small metal funnel into the top of a media tube and pour agar into the tube, filling the tube approximately one-third full.
4. Repeat step 3 for each tube.
5. Screw on the media tube caps loosely.
6. Place three tubes together, then cover the cluster of three with foil, as shown in figure 4.16.
7. Place the media tubes into a metal test-tube basket. We have one that is vintage, and we continue to use it today.
8. Place the basket in a pressure cooker with a few inches of water, and heat to achieve 15 PSI for 45 minutes.
9. Remove the tubes from the pressure cooker.
10. Prepare your aseptic environment and bring the media tubes in front of the flow hood.
11. Transfer the sterilized media tubes to a plastic test-tube rack, with the caps tightened. Prop up one side of the rack to create an incline, so that the agar in the tubes will solidify on a slant.

When the slants have cooled, we leave them in the lab at room temperature. We do not keep slants available at all times like we do plates. We discuss this in "Maintaining Your Slants" on page 84.

INOCULATING SLANTS

This procedure is done as soon as you can get a clean culture from a plate of tissue culture. Use a lab logbook to record your activities and anything that you notice about your cultures. For example, you might be making tubes for Chicken of the Woods, "Tall Pines" strain. Your logbook will serve as your memory of where you harvested the mushroom and when. It can also be a reference in case you are unsuccessful in culturing: you could possibly return to the location for another chance to capture the culture. You might even keep coordinates for future reference. It is essential to document and record activities. It is also just fun to look back on your entries and see where you have been and how far you have come. It inspires me to keep going and continue learning. Hopefully it will do the same for you. We keep clipboards with inventory in the lab: one in the spawn room, and one to record what goes out to the grow room (more about that in chapter 5).

Procedure

EQUIPMENT NEEDED

Nitrile gloves	Scalpel
Isopropyl alcohol in spray bottle and in a quenching bottle	Tool sterilizer
	Parafilm
Paper towel	Permanent marker
Culture plate of desired species	Logbook
Prepared media tubes filled with agar	

1. Put on nitrile gloves. Spray your gloved hands with isopropyl alcohol and wipe clean with a paper towel. Clean the worktable in front of the hood with alcohol and a fresh paper towel as well.
2. Place the petri plate on the clean table along with as many prepared media tubes as you will need (figure 4.17). Alcohol off these items. Assume everything is contaminated.
3. Sterilize the scalpel in the tool sterilizer, and quench in alcohol to cool off.
4. Use your dominant hand to cut a small wedge of colonized agar from the plate. The wedge should be small enough to comfortably fit in the mouth of a media tube.
5. Use your nondominant hand to remove the cap from a media tube. Tap the scalpel lightly with your finger so the agar wedge drops into the media tube. Move with precision so as not to touch the scalpel or agar to the inside of the tube. Replace and tighten the cap on the tube.

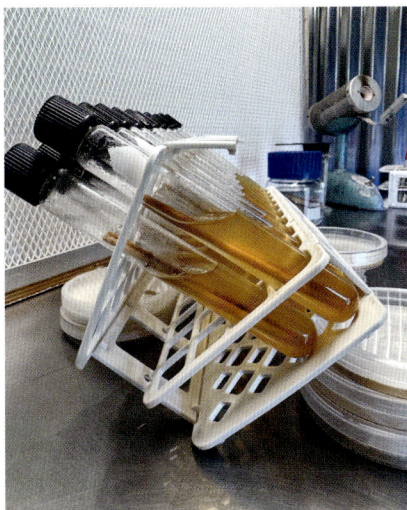

Figure 4.17. Slants cooling in preparation for inoculation.

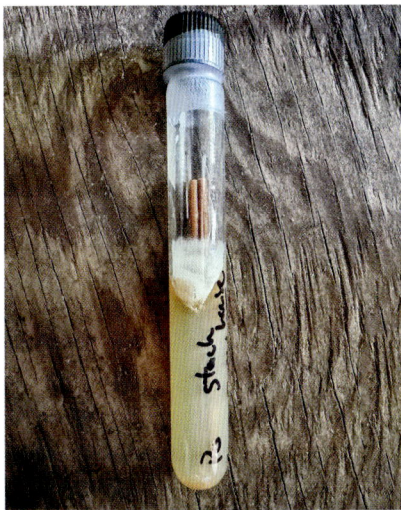

Figure 4.18. Inoculated, partially colonized, and labeled slant.

6. Repeat step 5 for each media tube you want to inoculate.
7. Once the inoculation of slants is complete, sterilize and quench the scalpel in alcohol again.
8. At the point where the tube meets the cap, wrap each tube with two layers of Parafilm.
9. Lay the tubes side by side on the worktable on your nondominant side (I put wrapped tubes on the left side of my worktable). Rewrap the used petri plate with a new piece of Parafilm.
10. Place the petri plate bottom-side up at one end of the row of recently inoculated slants. This allows efficiency in moving on to the next culture without the need to stop and label tubes in between inoculations.
11. When you are finished inoculating slants, use a permanent marker to label each tube with the date, species, strain, type of agar, and generation (figure 4.18).
12. In the lab logbook, a number and letter (such as A1, A2, A3) can be noted. Along with this code, record all the information about the slants you have just made. Any other notes or observations can be made to help with understanding more about the strain you have captured. This information will prove invaluable in the future.

As mentioned above, we recommend always making at least three slants for any one culture, and five slants is better. Redundancy is better than losing it all. Making more than five slants means you can share them with other mushroom enthusiasts for safekeeping.

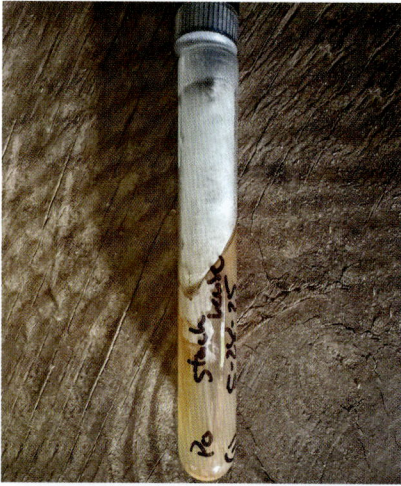

Figure 4.19. Colonized slants ready for cold storage.

The mycelium will colonize the agar in the slants and can then be placed in cold storage until needed. We often use a single quart-size container with a locking lid for each strain or genus. If you are storing multiple strains inside one container, group the slants together by strain inside zipper-locking plastic bags. This may seem like overkill; however, taking precautions to assure your strains stay without contamination is crucial to your culture bank. This will save headaches and protect the time you have invested.

MAINTAINING YOUR SLANTS

Approximately every eighteen months to two years, it's a good idea to pull your slants out of cold storage and wake up the culture. Do this by acclimatizing one slant for each of your cultures to room temperature for twenty-four hours. Then, using a sterilized dental spatula, reach inside the open slant, scoop up a small piece of colonized agar, and transfer it to a petri plate. Make two or three plates per slant because this will give you a better idea of the viability of the culture. If the mycelium picks up and runs within two to five days, you know the culture has vitality. If not, discard this slant and move on to the next slant for the species.

Use the new, viable mycelium in the petri plates to reslant the culture, as before. Again, to restate how to keep track of the generations, if your slant is the first generation, then the culture that grows in the petri plate becomes the second generation, labeled C2. Using mycelium from these plates to make new slants creates the third generation, labeled C3.

When you reslant a culture, change the agar recipe. For example, if your first slants were PDYA, then the next slants could be MYPA. Switching up agar recipes when reslanting helps the mycelium remain viable in storage.

Once you acquire many cultures, the task of maintaining them can be daunting. It is a good idea to set up a schedule that spreads out this necessary routine maintenance over time, instead of trying to do all your cultures at once. This will make maintenance more enjoyable.

Grain Spawn

Creating a large biomass of mycelium is the name of the game when your goal is to produce medicinal or culinary mushrooms. Grain spawn is the myceliated material used to inoculate substrate blocks for indoor growing, as well as plug spawn or logs directly for outdoor growing. Grain spawn production is often a demarcation for cultivators. Cultivating mycelium in petri plates is a necessary beginning, but making grain spawn is the first true step in expanding mycelium to production scale.

However, making grain spawn is one of the biggest hurdles to overcome. Many things can go wrong. If the grain is too dry, the mycelium will not colonize it. If it is too wet, bacterial contamination is almost guaranteed. There is a sweet spot that must be found, but it takes some time to master this process for consistent production. If you are not ready for producing your own grain spawn, you can simply buy some and jump ahead to chapter 5 to learn how to get started with indoor mushroom production.

CHOOSING GRAINS

Many kinds of grains can be used to create grain spawn. Rye, corn, and millet are the most popular. Choose one that makes sense in your region and to which you have easy access.

Millet is a tiny round grain with a relatively hard hull. For human consumption it is sold hulled; for spawn applications, you will need to purchase unhulled millet from a feed-and-seed store.

Corn is a good candidate for grain spawn, and sweet corn, field corn, dent corn, popcorn, and flour corn are all grown in western North Carolina. We have a tough time using corn that we have grown ourselves for making grain spawn because of my relationship with corn as a sacred food. On our farm we are continuing to raise a traditional Cherokee flour corn that has been grown in these mountains by my ancestors for thousands of years, though we don't use it for grain spawn.

If you decide to use corn, avoid large kernels and sweet corn seed. Smaller dent corn or popcorn are good choices. Popcorn is the best option because the kernels are small, and it is easy to find dark-colored varieties. Having a darker variety will allow you to see the mycelial growth on the kernels easier. Once you've seen the contrast of mycelium against the darker color of the corn, it becomes apparent why this is important.

We prefer to use rye, which is easy and quick to hydrate. Its small grains provide plenty of inoculation points. This grain crop also has a tougher outside hull than other cereal grains, so it is easier to hydrate without the grains bursting than it is when hydrating wheat or oats. Rye is also one of the grains most consistently available in our region.

COOKING THE GRAIN

Cooking grain to the proper moisture content can be tricky. If the consistency of the cooked grains isn't right—too wet or not wet enough—then the mycelium cannot thoroughly colonize the grain quickly enough, and contamination can set in. This often leads to many grains bursting during the sterilization process. Burst grains become a slimy mess, which leads to bacterial colonies proliferating, and the grain is ruined. Even if bacterial contamination does not become an immediate problem, the mycelium cannot colonize in an anaerobic environment, and eventually other contamination problems will develop. Finding the sweet spot takes time, but you'll find it as you get to know the grain you've chosen to use.

The method we describe here is not the only way to cook grain for spawn production, but for us, it has proven to be an easier way to get consistent hydration of grain. This method can be scaled up or down as much as you need.

For small- to medium-scale commercial production, you will need a container large enough to handle boiling 10 to 15 gallons of water at a time. Using a 55-gallon drum cut in half horizontally with a boiler drain installed is a cheap do-it-yourself way to heat a large quantity of water. At a smaller scale for home use, a large pot on the stovetop in the kitchen will serve the need. You'll also need 1-gallon, 3-gallon, or 5-gallon food grade buckets with lids to hold the grain and hot water. First off, wash the buckets and lids thoroughly with soap and water, then add the grain, filling the buckets approximately halfway. It is important not to overfill with grain, as explained below.

When the water boils, drain or pour the water into the buckets, filling them all the way to the top. Pop the lids on quickly to keep in as much of the heat as possible. The high ratio of hot water to dry grain provides enough thermal mass to keep the grain hot and absorbing water for hours. If you start out with too much grain in the bucket though, you will find that the grain at the bottom of the bucket will not be properly hydrated. Set aside the buckets and leave them to slowly hydrate the grain overnight.

The cooked grain should have a plump, full appearance and a slight opaqueness. The grain should be at the maximum limitation of hydration,

Equipment for Grain-Spawn Production

High-cost equipment is not necessary for producing grain spawn. Some of the items are things you'll have on hand anyway for other aspects of your operation. Here's what you'll need:

Sawhorses or folding table
Boards to span sawhorses

Corrugated metal panels
Container for boiling water
Plastic food-grade buckets (1-, 3-, or
    5-gallon capacity)
Grain
Jars with lids, or autoclavable bags
Impulse sealer (if using autoclavable bags)
Aluminum foil

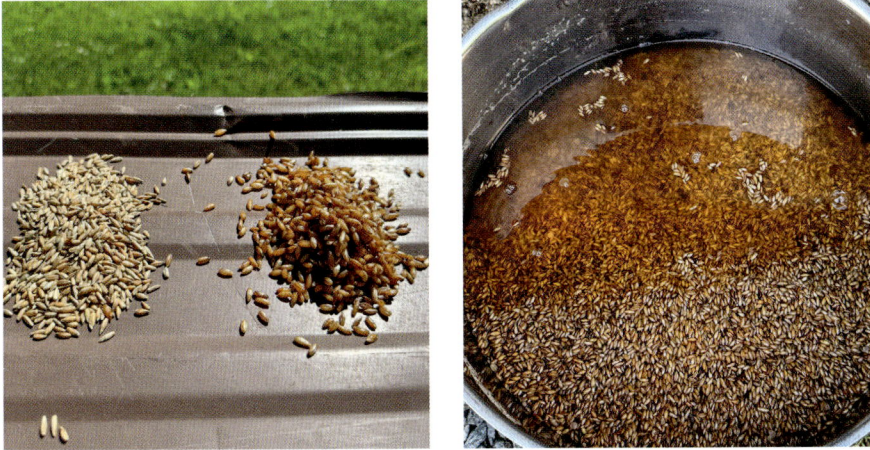

Figure 4.20. Dry grains (left); grains that have reached a state of ideal hydration (right).

which is referred to as *carrying capacity*. Ideally, the grain is intact but close to bursting. (Remember, you do not want the grain to burst.) It is impossible for the average cultivator to properly hydrate every last grain to carrying capacity and have zero grains burst. As long a batch of cooked grain has less than 5 percent burst kernels, it should still serve well for making grain spawn.

DRYING GRAIN

It's best to dry hydrated grain outdoors on a table or other flat surface. We set up sawhorses with boards spanning between them and topped with corrugated metal panels to create a temporary table. Wash the table surface or the metal with soap and water. Then unsnap one side of the lid of one of the grain buckets and place it on its side on the table to allow the excess water to drain out slowly. Once the water has slowed to a drip, open the rest of the lid and pour the grain out onto the table. Spread the grain evenly across the table and leave to dry. The amount of time needed will depend on the weather. During the winter in our region, we may have to leave grain on the table all day. On a windy summer day, the grain may be dry within two to three hours. Turn the wet grain a few times while it sits to maximize exposure to air.

When the surface moisture has dried from the grain and it still looks plump, remove the grain from the drying area and put it back in the buckets with the lids on to rest for anywhere from two to twelve hours, until moisture levels have evened out across the grains. Ambient temperature will determine how long this resting period needs to be. A bit of experience will quickly show you the sweet spot. Wait too long and yeast will start to grow. Not long enough and inconsistent moisture is still a problem. The resting period will allow the grain to equalize

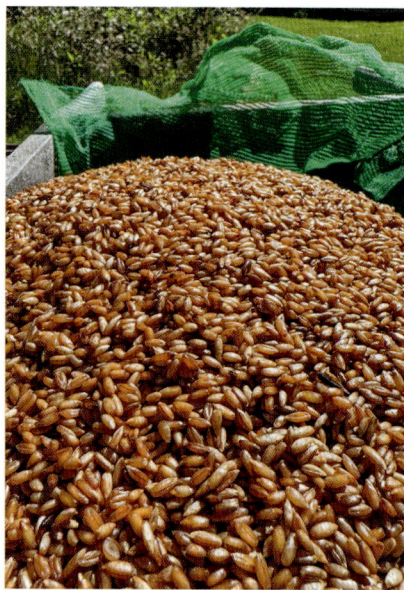

Figure 4.21. Hydrated rye grain.

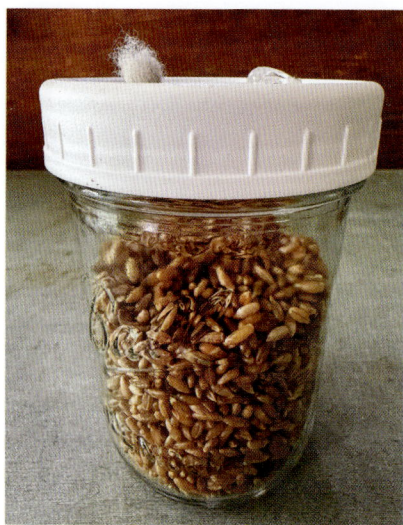

Figure 4.22. Grain in jar ready for sterilization.

the moisture content. If some of the grain became overly dry, moisture will transfer to it from the grain containing a slightly higher surface moisture content.

FILLING BAGS OR JARS

You can put hydrated grain into bags or jars. Then when you're ready to inoculate, you'll add mycelium to the grain in the bags or jars. The metabolic activity of the mycelium will generate heat as it colonizes the substrate. Packaging the grain in smaller amounts will remedy this.

Autoclavable bags have a limit of how much substrate they can safely carry (this limit is set by the manufacturer). We recommend to never approach this ceiling. We use bags that have a capacity of 4 pounds of substrate and we load 2.5 pounds of grain per bag. Grain bags that weigh more than 6 pounds tend to heat up and become contaminated more quickly. You can fill bags to your desired capacity according to your needs. Opting for smaller quantities in bags or jars also allows you more diversity in what you can grow.

If you decide to use jars rather than bags, be mindful that jars cannot be manipulated like bags. So, load jars only to approximately two-thirds capacity. That way, as the mycelium colonizes the grain in the jar, there will be plenty of headspace to shake and break up the colonized grain so that it may be poured out of the jar in a controlled manner. Once the jars are filled to the two-thirds mark, put the lids on, and cover the lid and down the sides of the jar with aluminum foil. This prevents excess moisture from entering the grain.

STERILIZING GRAIN

The next step is to put your bags or jars in a pressure cooker to sterilize the grain by heating it. This is an important step that reduces (though, not eliminates) the likelihood of contamination from other fungi and bacteria and gives your chosen fungi the best chance at getting established on the grain after inoculation.

When using grain bags, it is very important to *not* seal them before you put them in the pressure cooker—otherwise they can explode. After you load bags to the desired capacity, refold the pleats along the sides of the bag. The accordion-style pleats have three folds for the closure, and this is effective for keeping contaminants out. As the bags are being heated in the pressure cooker, the folds can expand a bit to release heat, but as the contents of the pressure cooker cool, the folds of the bags contract and tighten, creating a vacuum effect. This allows you to transfer the bags from the pressure cooker into a still-air box or to a table in front of a flow hood without risking contamination.

To prepare a pressure cooker for sterilizing bags of grain, place pieces of broken ceramic tiles between the bags and the inner wall of the pressure cooker. There will be just enough space between the cooker wall and the tile for boiling water to bubble up between and dissipate the heat from the wall, which will prevent the plastic bags from melting and sticking to the wall. If a bag melts, of course, it will ruin the bag and grain. Not to mention the energy it would take

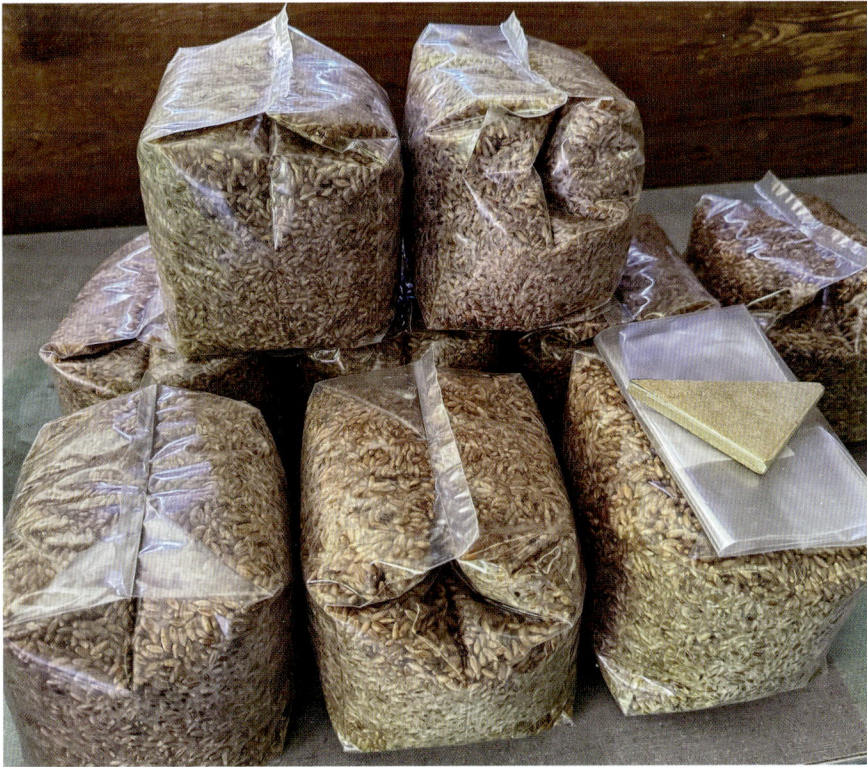

Figure 4.23. Folded grain bags ready for sterilization.

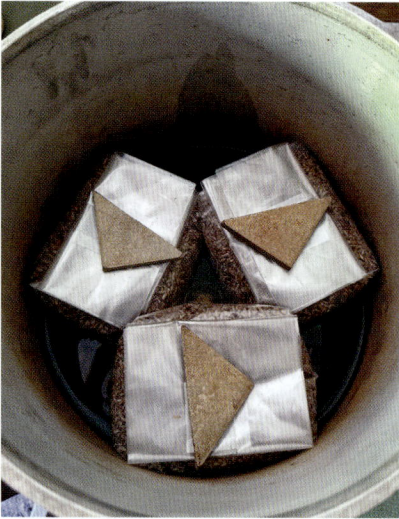

Figure 4.24. Correct orientation of first layer of bags in the pressure cooker, top up, opening facing center.

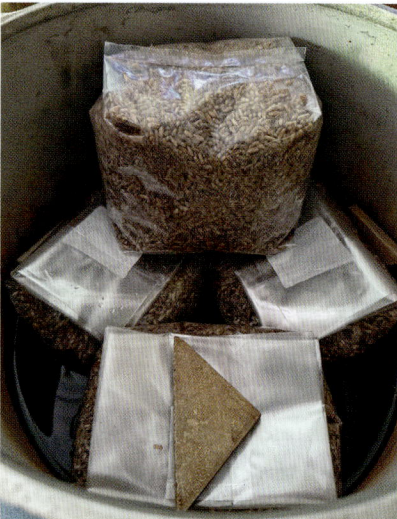

Figure 4.25. Second layer of bags added to the pressure cooker.

to scrape the bag off the wall and clean up the mess. Keeping the grain somewhat separated from the pressure cooker wall also helps prevent it from being overcooked.

After you have added grain to each bag and have carefully folded it closed, place it into the pressure cooker. Be careful not to snag the bags on the tile or they might tear.

Place the first layer of bags so that the top opening faces the center of the pressure cooker, with the folds of the plastic facing upward (figure 4.24). This prevents excess water dripping down the walls from getting in the bag and waterlogging the grain. Use a piece of broken tile to hold down the folds while loading the other bags. Once the first layer of bags is seated properly in the pressure cooker, pour water into the cooker to within 1 to 1.5 inches from the top of the bags.

Now you will add another layer of bags, and this layer is placed upside down (folds facing the bottom of the cooker) and the opening still toward the center, and it will hold the first layer of bags in place, so you can remove the broken pieces of tile as you put this layer of bags in place. Place this second layer of bags across the edges of two of the bags beneath, straddling those bags, as shown in figure 4.25. This allows for heat circulation through the cooker and thus the greatest chance of sterilization.

Loading jars of grain into a pressure cooker is less complicated. Simply arrange them for maximum capacity. If you use pint jars rather than quart jar, you can stack the jars in two layers. Place all of the jars upright. Fill the cooker with water up to the level of the grain in the first layer of jars. The water level should not surpass the grain level. If too much water is added, the jars may dance around in the pressure cooker during sterilization and break. Jars in the pressure cooker will clearly not melt, but the grain on the side closest to the wall can become overcooked. Even when the pressure cooker is no longer operating, the walls will retain heat and occasionally overcook the grain.

For both bags and jars, sterilize the grain at 15 PSI for 90 minutes. After 90 minutes, turn off the heat and allow the grain to cool inside the pressure cooker with the lid on. We typically let it cool overnight. The following day, we bring the pressure cooker into the lab before removing the lid, which is where we inoculate the sterilized grain with mycelium. There is no need to rush the process, which risks killing the mycelium if the grain is still too hot at the time you inoculate it.

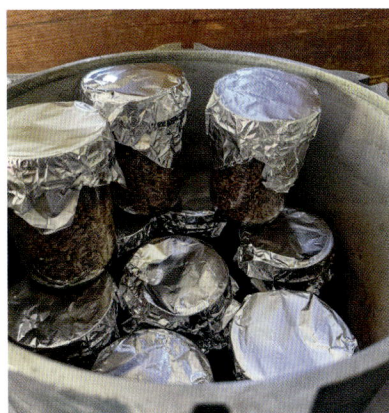

Figure 4.26. Jars in pressure cooker.

INOCULATING GRAIN IN BAGS

Inoculating sterilized grain with pieces of colonized agar is the next step in the process, and it must be done in a sterile environment to avoid contaminants like other kinds of fungal or bacterial spores getting inside the grain bag.

During this process, you will open a petri plate with a pure culture of mycelium inside. Once you remove the Parafilm seal, how you handle the plate will dictate whether you contaminate the culture or not. Being mindful of the flow of air and where your fingers are placed on the plate determines success or failure. Careful handling of the lid is also very important.

When making cuts in the colonized agar in the plate, you must stay clear of both the point where the original tissue sample sits as well as the edge of the plate. This reduces the risk of carrying potential contaminants into the grain. The original tissue sample could carry contaminants, and the edge of the plate where air flows under the lid or where gloved fingers have touched the edge of the lid are also potentially contaminated. Avoiding these two areas of the petri plates increases your chances of success. Take wedges from only approximately 80 percent of the surface area of a plate overall.

Procedure

EQUIPMENT NEEDED

Nitrile gloves

Isopropyl alcohol, both spray and
    quench bottles

Paper towel

Petri plate of cultured mycelium of
    your chosen species

Flow hood

Bags of sterilized grain

Scalpel

Tool sterilizer

Impulse sealer

Permanent marker

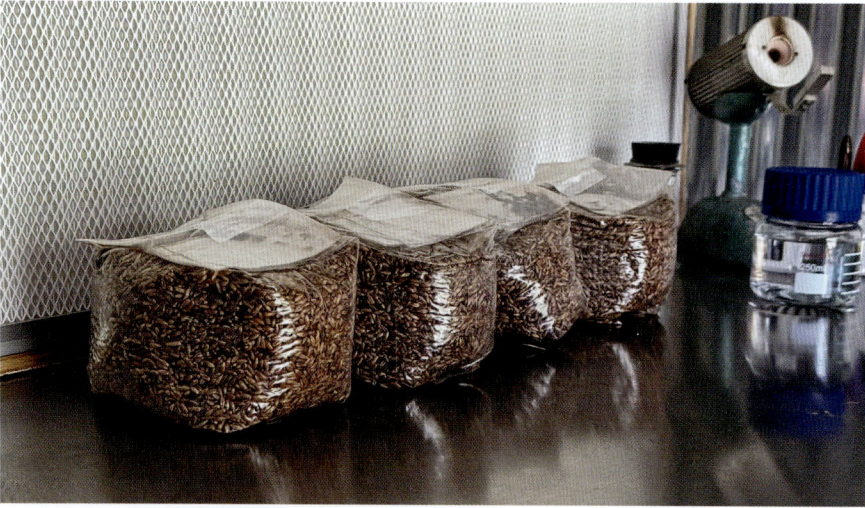

Figure 4.27. Sterilized bags ready for inoculation.

1. Prepare your aseptic environment. Clean the work surface with isopropyl alcohol.
2. Select the petri plate with the desired culture and place it at the center of the table. Push it as close to the flow of the hood as possible.
3. Remove grain bags from the pressure cooker and place them to the left of the petri plate(s). (If you are left-handed then the opposite work arrangement may be better for you.)
4. Spray the grain bags and petri plates with alcohol and wipe with a paper towel.
5. Sterilize the scalpel and quench in alcohol.
6. Rest the scalpel on the quench bottle with the blade pointing toward the flow of the hood.
7. Gently unfold the closures to open the grain bags.
8. Remove the Parafilm from the plate. Remove the lid and place it on top of another plate. Keep in mind that this lid must remain as close to the hood as possible and upwind from any movements you are making.
9. Use your non-dominant hand to hold the plate above the grain bags. I have found that tilting up the part of the plate closest to my body allows the flow of clean air to hit the lower edge. The clean air will pull up and across the plate, reducing the likelihood the air will drag across your gloved fingers, which could potentially introduce contaminants.
10. With the sterile scalpel in your dominant hand, slice through the colonized agar in a straight line. Then make another cut parallel to this first cut, about ½ inch (1 cm) apart. Make perpendicular cuts across these parallel lines according to the number of wedges you need to make overall.

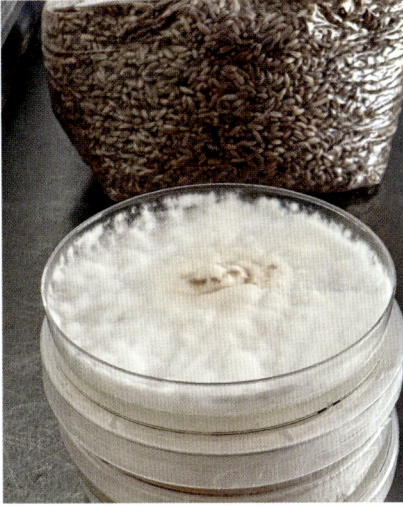

Figure 4.28. Myceliated plate ready for transfer.

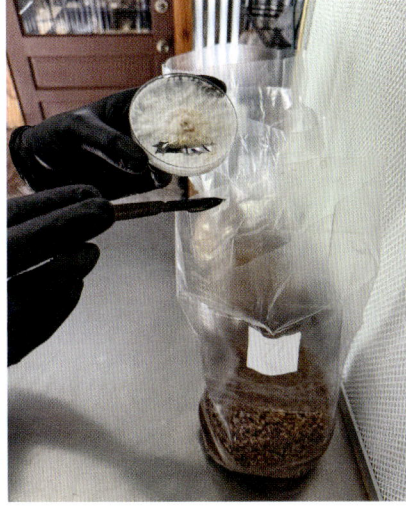

Figure 4.29. Transferring myceliated agar to sterilized grain.

11. Turn the plate 90 degrees and make cuts perpendicular to the previous cuts. Remember to avoid cutting close to the original inoculation point or close to the plate edges.

12. Use the scalpel to lightly skewer a wedge of the agar, lift it out of the plate, and hover it above the open bag of grain. It is important to make certain that the hand holding the scalpel never crosses the air flow in front of the petri plate. I start with the grain bag farthest to the left. I hold the plate (with my left hand) slightly to the left of that leftmost grain bag so that with my right hand I can cut agar wedges and drop them into the grain without ever crossing my right hand over the plate.

13. Lightly tap the scalpel with your finger so the wedge of agar drops into the grain. Repeat this as many times as necessary. A 2.5 pound bag of grain inoculated with five to seven wedges of agar is sufficient.

14. Move to the next grain bag to the right and repeat step 13 until all the grain bags are inoculated.

15. Seal the bags with impulse sealer.

16. With a permanent marker, label the filter patches on the autoclavable bags with a symbol or initial of the species of mushroom.

INOCULATING GRAIN IN JARS

The inoculation of grain in jars is done following the same process as described previously with bags. We would even say it is easier because you do not have to worry about the impulse sealer, and because the jars remain upright and they are reusable, costing the cultivator less money. You simply remove the lid of

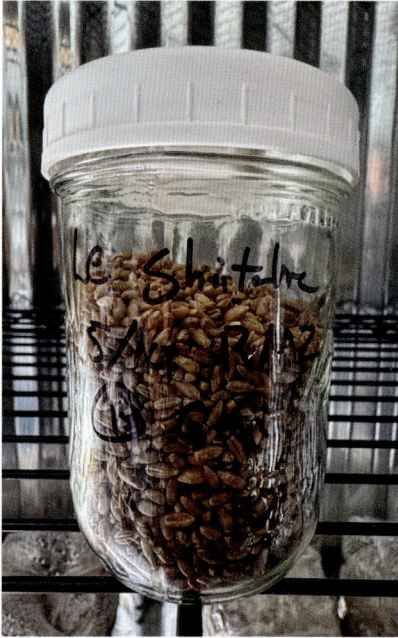

Figure 4.30. Jar labeled and ready for incubation.

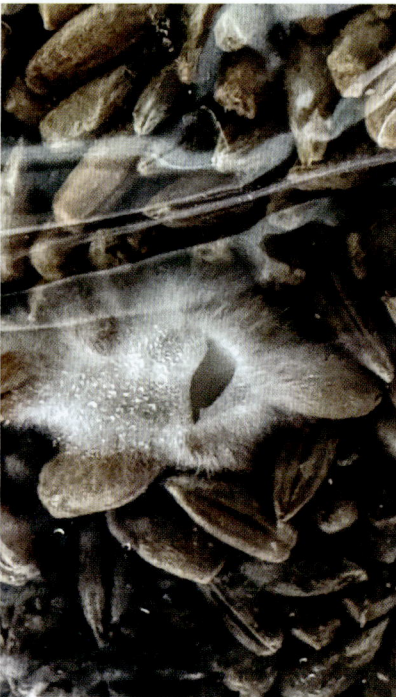

Figure 4.31. Mycelium leaping from agar to grain.

the jar and flip it upside down onto the neighboring jar. Inoculate as described above and replace the lid tightly. For a quart jar, use three to five wedges of agar. Use a permanent marker to label jars on the glass as you prefer with the date, species initials, strain, and generation. (Add the number 1 with a circle to denote the first generation.) We find this kind of code marking is easier for us to determine species and strain. Place the jar on the shelf in the incubation area and monitor for contamination until fully colonized.

GRAIN INCUBATION

Shelve the inoculated grain and pay careful attention to guarantee the mycelium grows out without contaminants. When the grain has colonized the bag, wipe the bag exterior with alcohol once more to clean it before you use it.

Occasionally, the grain will be slightly drier on the top than in the center or bottom. After inoculation, shaking the grain to evenly distribute the wedges of agar helps with even colonization. This also will distribute those dry grains into the matrix of perfectly hydrated grain. It is a good idea to try and manipulate at least one of the agar wedges to the edge of the grain so that you can observe the mycelium as it begins to become exploratory and colonize the grain.

The clean colonization of grain is the stopping point for grain incubation. Proceeding to the next steps becomes easier.

EXPANDING MYCELIUM ON GRAIN

When you expand mycelium on grain, you can safely make only two expansions. If we try to get greedy and expand the mycelium

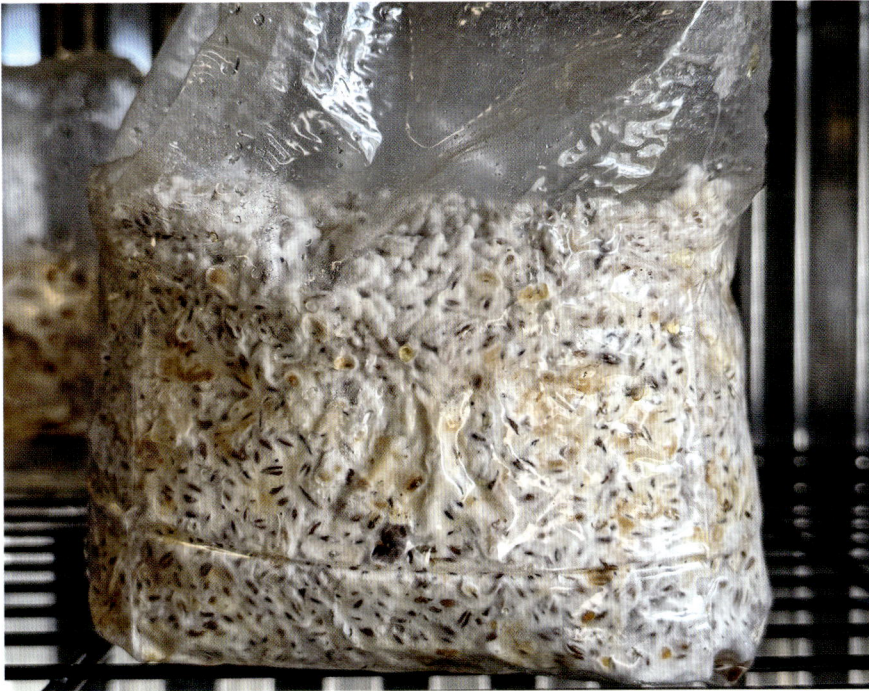

Figure 4.32. Fully colonized grain ready for use.

for a third time, it will often begin to run and then quickly fade—a sign of senescence. Mushroom mycelium loves a curveball. It prefers to have the substrate switched up from generation to generation; it does much better with diversity of nutrient sources. Remember, to get the most mushroom production success, you want to build as much biomass as possible before fruiting out.

When you inoculate colonized agar onto grain, the mycelium should "leap" or "jump" from the agar wedges to the grain quickly. A few days to a week are within acceptable range according to species. Once this first generation grain is colonized, we use it to inoculate more grain. A few tablespoons of first generation grain are sufficient to colonize second generation grain. The procedure is approximately the same as inoculating from plates to grain. The first-generation grain spawn should be massaged until well broken up but not crushed. For grain in jars, shake the jars until the grain loosens enough to be poured freely from the jar. You can also strike the side of your hand against the side of the jar to break grains apart. A potential hazard of this method is that a cracked jar may break when struck with the hand to loosen colonized grain. Inspection of jars after every use is important to reduce the hazard of broken glass. Please be careful.

To inoculate bags of sterilized grain with grain spawn, set up your materials as described before. But instead of petri plates, you will need a bag of first-generation grain spawn. Alcohol off the first-generation bag as well as the freshly sterilized grain bags. We advise opening only one side of the grain spawn bag. Slice under the seal on the bag past where the pleat is located. Bring the scalpel up at a sharp angle to make a clean cut.

Pull the pleat out, away from the grain, and it will open. It's like opening an old-style paperboard container of milk or juice—the kind that was common a few decades ago. (Who knew that this skill of opening a pleat would come in handy in your mycology career?) The grain is easy to pour, and the spout-like opening gives more control to manage the flow of grain out of the bag. Proceed to inoculate the sterilized grain with a small amount of the first-generation grain. Typically, a 2.5-pound bag of first-generation grain provides us enough to inoculate twenty to thirty 2.5-pound bags of sterilized grain, essentially turning 2.5 pounds of grain spawn into more than 60 pounds of grain spawn. When first starting out, beginners often use a higher rate of first-generation grain to inoculate the next generation. This is wise because if your technique has flaws, adding more spawn will lead the grain to colonize more quickly and run less risk of contamination. Label the bags of second-generation grain as you did the first generation, but with a 2.

CHAPTER FIVE

Indoor Cultivation

Indoor cultivation is where the rubber meets the road in intensive mushroom farming. It is the most predictable and plannable method of growing fungi, and the best way to ensure a consistent and predictable supply of mushrooms, either for your own consumption or to sell to others.

You have the option to either produce your own spawn or simply purchase spawn from a supplier for inoculating bulk substrate bags to grow indoors. The previous two chapters on setting up a lab and using sterile lab techniques explain how to produce your own spawn. If you are not ready for that, then you can just jump into this chapter by purchasing grain spawn.

At first, a simple pressure cooker is the only equipment you need to start growing mushrooms indoors. Once you have gotten your feet wet, you may want to dedicate a closet or a small room in your home to further your mushroom journey. Once you become more serious, you will want to move the operation out of your house into a space that is dedicated to cultivation. It is surprising how much you can do in a small space.

Every stage that is successful in producing mushrooms is exciting. The most exciting stage is arguably when we bring the culmination of all the work to fruition, literally. The choice of which medicinal or culinary mushrooms to grow is up to you. Just as with plants, each species of mushroom likes slightly different growing conditions and has habits that we have to adapt to. Substrate recipes are approximately the same across species, with a few minor changes in supplementation. All methods are tailored to get the most out of our indoor production.

Preparing Bulk Substrate

Bulk substrate simply refers to a bag of especially mixed, cellulose-rich material upon which the mycelium feeds before producing fruitbodies. Growing on bulk substrate can include sawdust spawn and what is referred to as a grow bag or kit. Sawdust spawn is simply sawdust that has been inoculated with mycelium, while a grow bag or kit contains sawdust with a nitrogen-rich supplement.

The kinds of materials used in a nitrogen supplement vary by region of the world and within local areas. This is also true for sawdust. It's a good idea to research the types of sawdust available in your area and whether they suit the needs of the types of medicinal mushrooms you want to cultivate.

Cultivating mushrooms from supplemented sawdust is a quick and consistent way of producing medicinal mushrooms indoors, an essential quality for a commercial operation. Bulk substrate can also be used to inoculate straw, wood chips, or logs for outdoor cultivation. (These growing methods were described in chapter 2.)

The equipment needed for growing mycelium in a bulk substrate is the same at that listed in the "Lab Equipment Checklist" on page 55. If you plan to scale up beyond producing a few pounds of mushrooms per week, though, you'll quickly discover that you need a more productive way to sterilize bulk substrate bags than using a pressure cooker. We have explored many different methods for this in the past, and we describe the method we now use in "Using a Low-Pressure Steam Sterilizer" on page 100.

BULK SUBSTRATE RECIPES

There are many recipes for bulk substrate. Hardwood sawdust or wood pellets work well. Pellets are easy to weigh and pour. The manufacturing process of sawdust into pellets heats them almost to pasteurization temperatures, and they are kiln dried, meaning the pellets will store almost indefinitely if kept dry. If loose sawdust is available, by all means, utilize this resource. Be mindful that a pile of moist sawdust is very inviting to fungi, which will begin to consume the cellulose and lignin. Use good judgment and a watchful eye to reduce contaminants.

The nitrogen supplement in a bulk substrate can also lead to contamination problems. It is usually easy to buy some form of nitrogen supplement from a feed-and-seed store. The most commonly used for grow bags are soybean meal, soybean husks, alfalfa pellets, beet shreds, rice bran, and wheat bran. Some of these are waste products from agricultural processes. Beet shreds are from processing sugar beets. Grain husks are leftovers from hulling grains. Alfalfa is grown as an animal feed. We have found that grain bran is the least likely to stimulate contamination. In our experience, alfalfa pellets led to high contamination rates, so we avoid them.

There are a couple of ways to test for contaminants. The main strategy we use to track down where contaminants come from is to place the sawdust pellets in the bag along with the supplement. We add water and sterilize *without* shaking the bags to homogenize. Once the bags have been sterilized and inoculated, we place them on the spawn room shelf. We watch the bags closely every day. Because they have only been slightly mixed but not homogenized, it should be

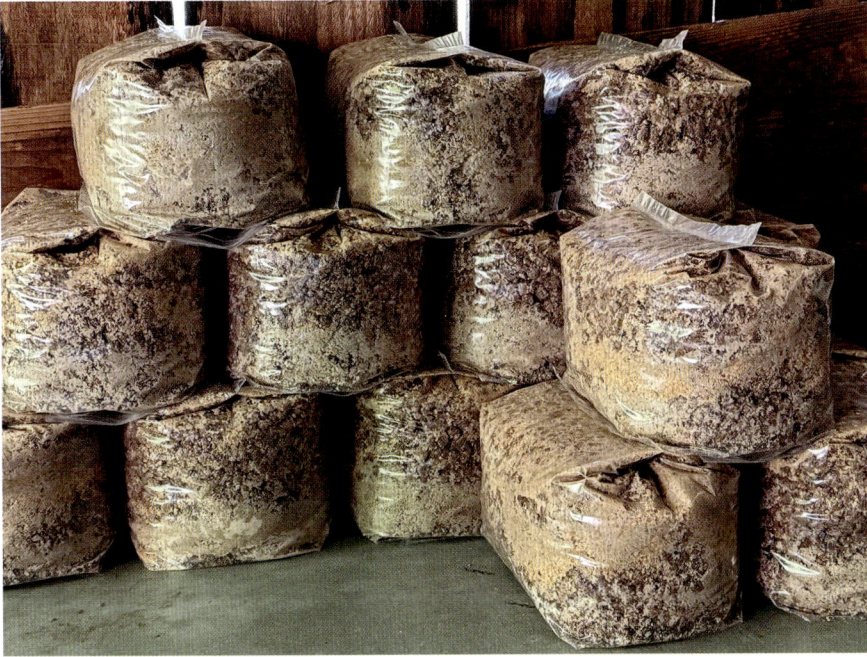

Figure 5.1. A stack of prepared substrate bags ready for sterilization.

clear where the grain, sawdust, and supplement are located, and it will be easier to determine which of these ingredients the contamination has grown from. This will help narrow down the problem.

Try this technique yourself. When you determine where the contamination is originating, check your supplier or your technique for preparation and sterilization. We once had organic alfalfa pellets that were the source of contamination. Since we were homogenizing the substrate after inoculation, we had no idea where the problem was originating until we used this detection method. We switched alfalfa pellet suppliers, and the problem cleared up.

Also be mindful of the storage containers you use for your substrates. Keep everything clean and dry. It will nip a lot of problems in the bud. Our main source of nitrogen supplements are organic cacao shells from a chocolate processing facility close by. Coffee grounds can be used if you have a local source, but you will need to provide clean containers for the grounds and pick up and use them all on the same day—otherwise the risk of contamination becomes unmanageable.

This basic bulk substrate recipe serves well for most wood-loving species of medicinal mushrooms. You can measure by weight or by volume.

70 to 80 percent sawdust pellets
20 to 30 percent nitrogen supplement

Some species, such as Shiitake (*Lentinula edodes*), will not tolerate a nitrogen supplement over 7 percent. For Shiitake production, the recipe should be at least 93 percent sawdust. Some fungi, such as King Trumpets (*Pleurotus erungii*) or Lion's Mane (*Hericium erinaceus*), can withstand a higher ratio of nitrogen supplement in the recipe, often 40 to 50 percent nitrogen. In those cases, reduce the portion of sawdust pellets to 50 to 60 percent.

These materials can be mixed by hand in a plastic tub or using a cement mixer. Add water to the full capacity of the materials to absorb it. You will need to experiment to figure out the right volume of water for the materials you are using. Some substrates, such as coffee grounds, are already full of water. Other substrates, such as cacao shells, will not absorb much water. Basically, when you squeeze a handful of homogenized substrate, it should yield only a few drops of water. (An alternate way to combine substrate ingredients is to add them dry to the bag first and then add water without mixing to homogenize.)

Mix and prepare as many bags as you need. For everyone from beginners to advanced cultivators, we recommend mixing your bulk substrate in one of the larger autoclavable substrate bags. If using a pressure cooker, the same folding rules apply as in "Sterilizing Grain" on page 88 in chapter 4. Sterilize at 15 PSI for 90 minutes in a pressure cooker.

USING A LOW-PRESSURE STEAM STERILIZER

Over the years we have experimented with many methods of sterilizing bulk substrate. Large autoclaves are pricey and out of reach for most beginners. We

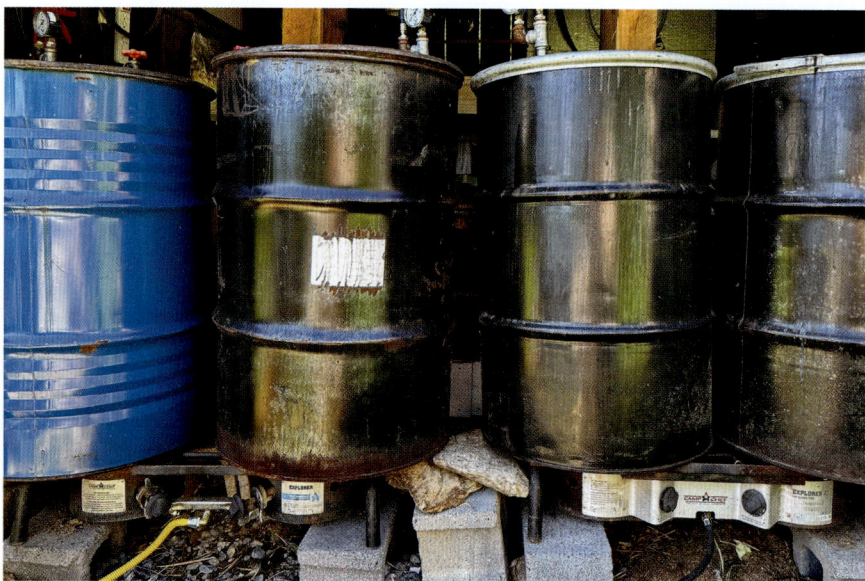

Figure 5.2. Low-pressure steam sterilizer with four barrels.

wanted a method that is more accessible, and we discovered that a low-pressure steam sterilizer made from 55-gallon drums works well. I have built a few of these backyard sterilizers myself. Once, I had one explode, distributing sawdust bags on top of the shed, spraying bags throughout the yard, and leaving the lid of the barrel driven vertically into the ground more than 6 inches deep. I'm not sure how high up it had to be blasted off to dive that deep into the soil. So, if you decide to make one of these sterilizers, heed my cautionary tale. Please follow the directions carefully. In our case, the problem was that we did not have a safety blowout valve on the barrel. Something had obviously clogged the boiler drain, which was the only pressure relief. This was clearly a bad idea. Safety blowout valves are important.

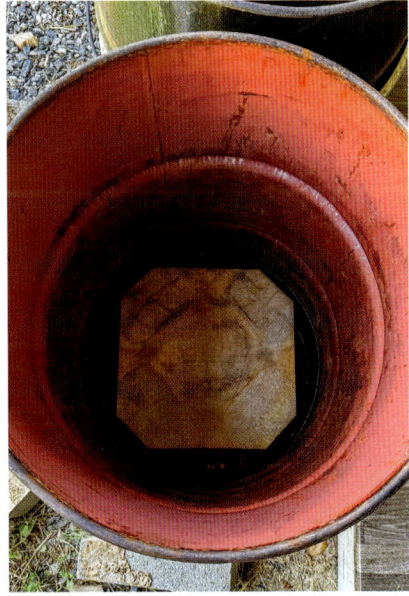

Figure 5.3. The inside of the barrel, ready to receive substrate bags.

Preparing the lid of the barrel is an important step in making it into a steam sterilizer vessel. The lid must have two bungholes. A boiler drain is installed in one of the bungholes to act as pressure relief. A splitter is installed in the other, with a pressure gauge attached on one side and a low-pressure relief valve on the other. These valves can be set from 1 to 10 PSI blowout. This will ensure a safer sterilization run. The lid needs a secure fastening system. A ring and bolt is more secure than a locking lid and can be tightened as needed.

We heat our low-pressure steam sterilizers over two propane burners—two barrels can sit on top of a two-burner camp stove with the legs removed. We use a 20-pound propane tank to fire the camp stove. One tankful of propane is enough to sterilize fifty bags.

Each barrel holds twenty-five 6-pound bags of bulk substrate. We stack two layers of bricks in the bottom of each barrel and add water up to the top of the bricks. We use large ceramic tiles with the corners cut off to form a raised platform, with one tile on the bricks in the bottom of each barrel. We load in the bags of bulk substrate, folded accordion-style as described in "Sterilizing Grain" on page 88 in chapter 4.

The first row of bags is placed on top of the tile upright and then the next row, which is inverted, straddles the first. This method of layering the bags is shown in figure 5.4. This arrangement allows the heat and steam to be evenly distributed throughout the barrel. We continue this alternating pattern with each level until we reach the top of the barrel. We then place the lid on top of

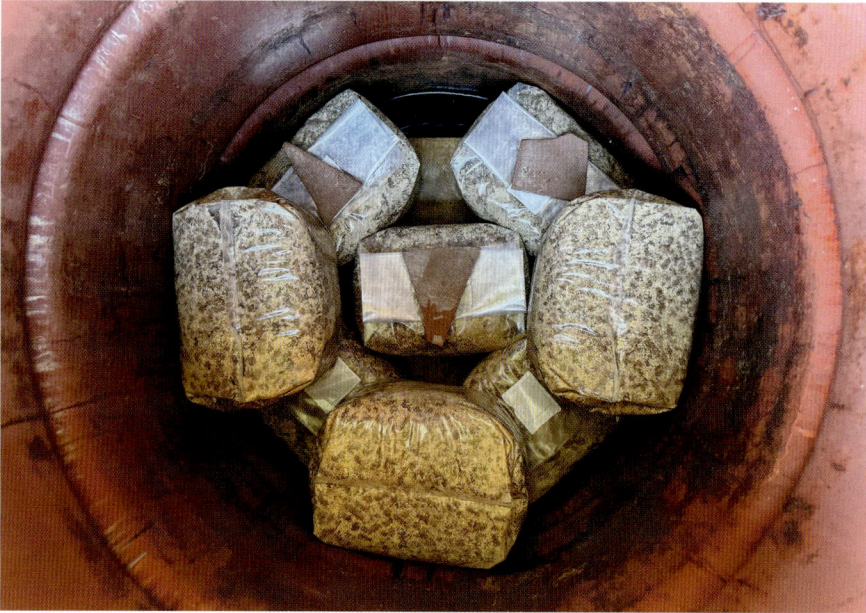

Figure 5.4. Loading pattern for substrate bags in the barrel.

the barrel and secure it with a locking lid ring or a ring with a bolt. The lid with the bolt is preferred but the locking-style lid will work if that is all you have available.

Next, we fire up the burners. The low-pressure steam sterilizers are fired with the burners at a medium setting and will operate for ten hours at 2–3 PSI. One 20-pound tank of propane will heat two low-pressure sterilizing barrels for around ten hours. We usually let this setup run overnight. If we used a bigger propane tank, we would need to manually turn off the burner after ten hours. We remove the bags from the sterilizers when the substrate has cooled sufficiently. Cooling often takes twenty-four hours after the end of the firing. Low-pressure steam sterilization of sawdust substrate has proven an effective way of sterilizing substrate on our farm. We can make one hundred 6-pound bags of substrate and sterilize them in a twenty-four-hour period. This is a small operation and can be scaled up or down to meet your needs.

We do *not* recommend attempting to sterilize grain in this manner. With prolonged heating, the grains end up turning into a bag of mush.

INOCULATING BULK SUBSTRATE BAGS

Whether you use a pressure cooker or an improvised setup to sterilize bulk substrate, once the bulk substrate bags are cool, you will transport them to a table or work area in front of a flow hood for inoculation. Open only one sterilizer barrel at a time. We recommend setting up a separate flow hood work area for inoculating substrate bags. For example, we do this work in front of a flow hood in our spawn room, not at the flow hood in our lab. Having a second hood in a separate location helps to prevent introducing contamination in your most aseptic environment, where you do the delicate work of cloning, petri plate and media tube preparation, and grain inoculation.

The size of the flow hood will determine the number of bags you can open to inoculate at one time. A simple 24 × 24-inch hood is only large enough to allow two to three bags to be processed at once. A 24 × 48-inch flow hood should allow for inoculating at least four substrate bags at once.

The first few times you try inoculating the substrate, use a heavier dose of grain

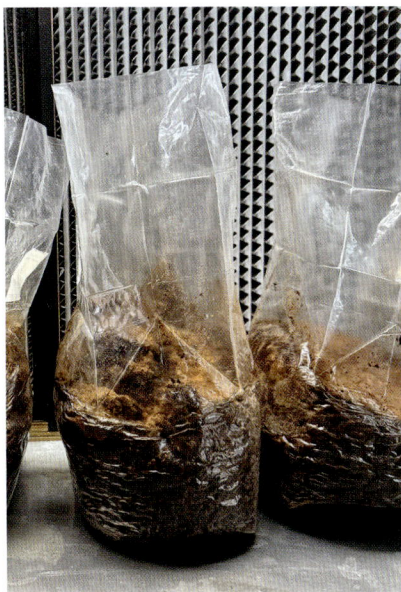

Figure 5.5. Bulk substrate prepared for inoculation.

spawn than the usual. Beginners usually start with approximately ¼ cup. Once you master the technique, it is possible to use just a tablespoon or less of grain spawn per bag and be successful with inoculating the bulk substrate. Cutting down the amount of grain spawn used per bulk substrate bag maximizes the number of bulk substrate bags you can inoculate from one bag of grain spawn. You will build confidence every time you do the process. Just as with any skill worth learning, it can take time to perfect your sterile technique.

If you plan to process a large number of bags of substrate at a time, a foot-operated impulse sealer is a labor saver and is better for the body. Spending hours pressing down repeatedly with your arms on a sealer will eventually wreak havoc on the wrists.

Procedure

EQUIPMENT NEEDED

Isopropyl alcohol, in a spray bottle
Paper towels
Bags of sterilized, cooled bulk
    substrate

Bag or jar of grain spawn
Impulse sealer
Permanent marker

1. Clean the table in front of the hood with isopropyl alcohol.
2. Bring in bags of bulk substrate (only two to four bags at a time, depending on hood size, as explained above) and place them on the table.

3. Open the bulk substrate bags directly in front of the hood.
4. Spray the bag or jar of grain spawn with isopropyl alcohol and wipe it down.
5. Open the grain spawn and then pour the desired amount of grain (between 1 tablespoon and ¼ cup, as noted above) directly into each open bag of substrate.
6. Set the grain spawn aside and seal the bags of substrate with an impulse sealer.
7. Shake each bag thoroughly to distribute the grain spawn evenly throughout the substrate. Shake until the spawn and substrate are well homogenized. It is worth the labor to spend a few extra seconds shaking each bag. Well-homogenized bulk substrate can become colonized in half the time as poorly shaken substrate.

As mentioned earlier in this chapter, if you are having problems with the contamination of bulk substrate as it incubates, there are tricks you can try to figure out the cause. If you suspect that the bulk substrate itself is the cause of contamination, then do not shake a few of the bags after inoculation. Set these bags aside to observe. If the grain spawn is the source of the contaminant, you will see the contamination beginning in the spot where the grain was added; then the contamination will spread through the bag. If you see contamination growing in various separate spots in the bag, this could be due to contamination in the nitrogen supplement that was added

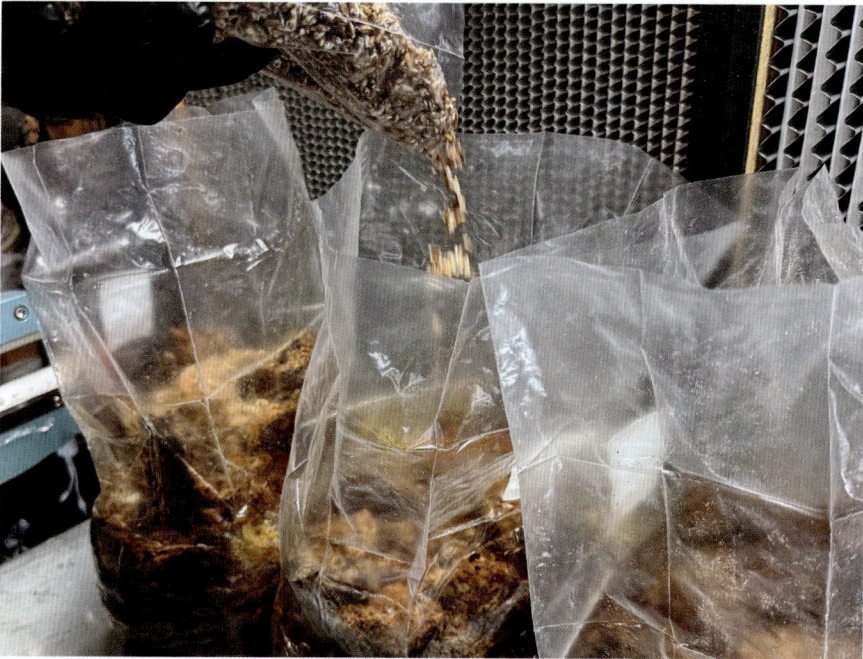

Figure 5.6. Progression of inoculation.

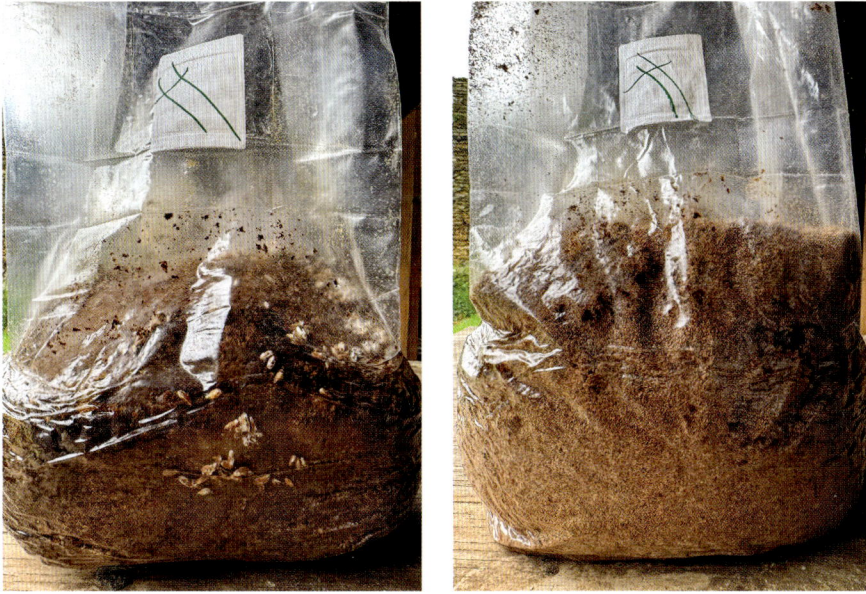

Figure 5.7. Bulk substrate that is not homogenized (left) and the substrate after homogenizing (right).

to the substrate. The supplement or the grain are the two usual suspects that we deal with.

If you are using a homemade low-pressure steam sterilizer, and you suspect it is the problem (because it may not be thoroughly sterilizing the bags of substrate), set aside one of the bags without inoculation and see whether contaminants eventually develop, and how long that takes.

SETTING UP A SPAWN ROOM

Bags of inoculated substrate should be placed on shelves in a climate-controlled spawn room. A spawn room can be simple as a closet or it can be a room large enough to house thousands of bags. Room-temperature storage is fine for most species. The main choice to make when setting up a spawn room is what type of shelving you want. Preconstructed shelves can be expensive if you are just starting up or if your operation could require hundreds or thousands of square feet of shelf space. We've come up with a simple yet effective shelving system that we constructed ourselves from metal hog panels (which can be purchased from a feed-and-seed supplier), some 2×4s, and metal conduit as supports for the panels. Since these shelves will not be in contact with water or moisture, the 2×4 lumber does not need to be treated. With a pair of bolt cutters and a couple of hours of work, we can create several shelves that allow air flow and will last for decades. Shelves that are 24 inches deep and 18 inches apart seem to be suitable for most

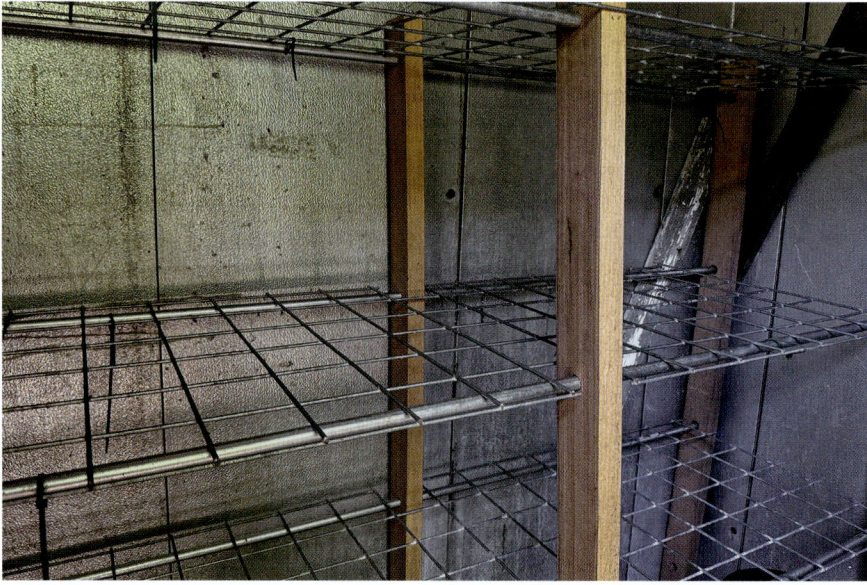

Figure 5.8. Spawn room shelving.

spawn room shelving. We leave 12 inches clearance below the bottom shelf to allow for cleaning beneath. Each rack of shelving will have four or five shelves.

Procedure

EQUIPMENT NEEDED

Bolt cutters

Hog panels: 4 × 16-foot panels with 4 × 4-inch squares

8-foot-long wood 2×4s

Drill

1-inch spade drill bit

¾-inch metal conduit

Fasteners

Cross supports

Zip ties

1. Use the bolt cutters to cut each hog panel in half lengthwise, and use the cut ends to face the wall.
2. Starting at one end of a 2×4, measure up to approximately 12 inches and mark the spot at the center. Continue marking spots 18 inches apart. Mark a second 2×4 in the same way. (Some folks position the bottom shelf higher than 12 inches off the floor so that they can use the floor as a bottom shelf, setting bags directly on the floor.)
3. Use the spade bit to drill a 1-inch hole through both 2×4s at each marked spot.
4. Insert conduit into each hole.
5. Anchor the 2×4s to the wall, positioning fasteners approximately 24 inches apart vertically. If not anchored properly, mistreatment of the shelving

106

could cause it to fall under the weight of hundreds of bags of substrate. Please take precautions and use discretion.

6. Use the bolt cutter to trim out parts of the panel as needed to accommodate the 2×4 supports. Then simply lay the panels in place.

7. Once the shelves are completed, place cross supports in between the 2×4 uprights to make them more stable and zip-tie the panels to the conduit, further securing the panels in place.

Of course, if one is not handy or able to construct shelving, it is possible to get friends to help with the promise of some freshly harvested culinary or medicinal mushrooms.

Incubating Bulk Substrate

Bags of inoculated substrate will incubate on shelves in your spawn room. Make sure the bags are not pressing against each other. They can touch, but barely. When they are pressed firmly against each other they will heat up at the contact points. It is common for these areas to heat up enough to kill the mycelium and lead to contamination that could ruin a lot of your hard work. We slide one bag against the next, then run a hand between the two bags. If necessary, adjust the bag to pull it away from the neighboring one.

Some species have a quicker spawn run than others. The average time for a bag of substrate to colonize can be upward of thirty days. This may seem like a long time, but it is faster than the turnaround time for the spawn run on inoculated logs to be ready to produce mushrooms. Watch your substrate bags for signs of contamination. Inspect every two days. Making a habit of looking every day is better.

This is especially important if you are creating sawdust spawn to use as an inoculate for logs or other outdoor substrates. It is not uncommon in the process of incubation to see a contaminant show up on sawdust substrates, only for the mycelium being cultivated to run over it. The mycelium completely covering this contamination is not a bad thing when left undisturbed in an indoor environment—it speaks to the power of the mycelium that is being grown. The issue ultimately arises when the spawn is not flagged as contaminated and is brought out to inoculate logs or other substrates outdoors; that is, wood chip beds, pasteurized straw, and so on. When these contaminated bags are used to inoculate, the mycelium is damaged in the process of crumbling the substrate to spread it as spawn. The mycelium will often never recover from this damage because the remaining contaminant will use the substrate and damaged mycelium as a food source, shifting the balance from the mycelium to the contaminant. In this situation, the risk of failing in the next cultivation step is great.

We identify contaminants in the spawn room by using a permanent marker to make circles on the bags around the contaminated spots. Sometimes, according to the aggressive nature of the contaminant, we may give up on a contaminated bag and dump the contents on the compost pile. When you cultivate mushrooms on sawdust blocks, you will inevitably have contamination. Depending on the extent of contamination, you may be able to use these blocks for mushroom production, but it may severely limit the normal output of the block.

The Grow Room

Grow rooms can be as complicated or as simple as your needs require. Something as simple as a greenhouse that is utilized seasonally might serve the purpose. Reishi (*Ganoderma* spp.) is often cultivated in greenhouses with shade cloth suspended above, depending on the climate. If you grow plants such as ginger or turmeric as a greenhouse crop in a temperate climate, mushrooms can be snuck into areas that remain shaded by the plant foliage. If you only want to grow Cordyceps, then a closet or spare room can work because Cordyceps cultivation is self-contained and does not require misting systems or lots of fresh air exchange.

From there you may scale up to a home or small commercial grow room that is built strictly as a mushroom growing operation. Factors to consider include proximity to your lab, the kind of mushrooms you plan to grow, lighting, fresh air exchange, and humidity. We have been growing commercially for decades in small purpose-built grow rooms. The first commercial grow rooms that we built had all of the bells and whistles; but this is not always necessary. Our goal in this discussion of grow rooms is to help make mushroom production more accessible.

PROXIMITY TO THE LAB

When the growth of mycelium reaches full colonization of supplemented bags or blocks, then it is time to move bags of bulk substrate into a grow space or room. One of the most important points is to place the grow room far away from the lab. On our farm, the grow room is nearly 100 meters away from our lab. When a grow room is located within the same building as a lab or other aseptic environment, it is not a question of *whether* spore loads will build up and create contamination in the lab, it is a question of *when*.

ENVIRONMENTAL RANGES

The basic function of a grow space is to provide ample humidity, light cycles, and fresh air exchange, and to maintain the desired temperature range. Some species do well with more moisture, and some will rot in moist environments before maturing. Each mushroom must be considered and treated according to the specific conditions needed.

One grow room can serve a variety of mushrooms that have the same fruiting conditions. For example, mushrooms that prefer cool weather can all be grown in one environment. These include cool-weather types of Oysters (*Pleurotus* spp.) as well as Shiitakes, Lion's Mane, Chestnut mushrooms (*Pholiota adiposa*), and Pioppini (*Agrocybe aegerita*). Some mushrooms, like Maitake (*Grifola frondosa*) and Enoki (*Flammulina velutipes*), that enjoy cooler temperatures will need their own grow room. If you drop the temperature of a grow space low enough for the Maitake, it would slow production for the species that grow much faster at a higher temperature range.

Hot weather species such as Reishi, Golden Oysters (*P. citrinopileatus*), or Pink Oysters (*P. djamor*) need higher fruiting temperatures. There are various ways to approach this. When living in a temperate rainforest such as the Southern Appalachians, it is better to grow, even when indoors, in harmony with the seasons. We don't try to grow hot-weather species during the winter, because we live in a climate that has cool-to-cold winters. Our grow rooms run cooler in the winter to save on electrical costs, and warmer during the summers for the same reason. We have provided information about fruiting temperatures for various species in appendix 1.

LOCATION EFFECTS

For beginners, a grow space can be as simple as a wire shelf tented with plastic to keep the humidity in. Place an ultrasonic humidifier on the shelf and attach to a mechanical timer. The amount of humidification needed depends on both the species and the location of the shelf. For example, if the shelf is set up in a basement, then the humidifier would likely be run less frequently because a basement typically remains more humid than other environments. We have a grow room in a barn located on the edge of the forest and down a slope. The humidity remains higher in this area than in another barn that is on top of the hill, which is south facing with no trees.

LIGHTING

Mushrooms do not need light in order to grow, but they do need light to initiate pinning. A 12-hour-on, 12-hour-off cycle of lights is sufficient for most medicinal mushrooms. Some mushrooms, such as Oysters, do not need as much light to produce well. A light intensity range of 500 to 1000 lux is sufficient for most mushrooms. However, we have found that using the higher end of this range generally produces firmer and denser mushrooms. If you are cultivating Maitake, we do not recommend anything less than 1000 lux. They will develop a much deeper, darker color with a higher lux.

FRESH AIR EXCHANGE

Fungi breathe in oxygen and, just like us, exhale carbon dioxide (CO_2). Carbon dioxide is heavy and will eventually sink to low-lying areas. We don't want too much carbon dioxide to build up in a grow room.

For a single-shelf operation, fresh air exchange is not that big of a deal. The carbon dioxide produced by the mushrooms will drain down and out from under the plastic tent over the shelf. In a larger grow operation, however, a fan to bring in fresh air is needed. How much fresh air, and how often to run the fan? This will depend. Observing the mushrooms in your grow room will tell you all that you need to know. If the mushrooms are becoming "leggy," then the CO_2 level is too high and fresh air should be increased until the balance is found. CO_2 monitors can be installed in tandem with a fan to bring in fresh air when the CO_2 reaches a certain ppm (parts per million). But this equipment is often unnecessary and can be costly for a hobbyist or start-up. It takes only a short period of time to bring in the amount of fresh air needed. A tip to save on energy costs: during the winter, set the fan to bring in more fresh air during the day rather than at night, when temperatures are coldest. This reduces excess strain on the heating and cooling system. In the summer months, do the opposite: run the fan mostly at night to avoid pulling in the high heat of day.

HUMIDITY

The humidity level in growing spaces ideally should mimic a mushroom's natural world. Humidity controllers are not required. In some cases, they can cause more problems than they solve. In fact, we have found that letting the humidity drop between 50 and 60 percent and then bringing it up to 100 percent every four to six hours works much better than trying to keep the humidity level constant. If you live in a climate with high humidity during the warm months, keeping humidity at 90 percent or above will result in contamination problems. A stable warm and wet environment is a recipe for disaster.

You can use an automatic programmable timer to control ultra-fine misters placed above grow shelves. These can help raise humidity without producing so much moisture that they soak the mushrooms. The timers are cheap, easy to acquire, and easy to program.

PREPARING SUBSTRATE FOR FRUITING

Some mushroom blocks can be brought directly from the spawn room to the grow room and start to produce mushrooms. Oysters are the perfect example.

Some of your species, however, will need special care, such as preparing the bags in specific ways, once they are in the appropriate temperature of the grow room, and again once pinning is initiated. For example, after we bring Chestnut mushrooms into the grow room and pins begin forming, reaching about

0.5 inches tall, we open the bags to expose the primordial Chestnuts to fresh air.

For some of the blocks that we produce in the bags, we will simply cut series of slits; for some we will open up the tops; and for some we will remove all but the base of the bag. Occasionally, we will cut many slits into the bags; upward of eighteen to twenty-four cuts for some species.

Oysters

Oysters are typically grown directly from substrate blocks by simply making a few cuts along the sides of the bag. Two to three equidistant cuts are made on the broad side of the block. These cuts allow fresh air to contact the mycelium, and the mycelium responds to this fresh air and produces a fruiting body. The tops of the bags are rolled down even with the top to create a solid block, and packing tape is applied to keep the top from unrolling. When placing these prepared blocks on the shelving, take care to allow space for the mushrooms to develop so that they do not crowd each other when coming to maturity. Most Oysters can be grown out for two to four flushes.

Oysters grown from straw and other agricultural waste products can be set up with poly tubing or in buckets. The tubes or "logs" are typically created to equal the depth of the shelf and placed accordingly. The beauty of buckets is that they are reusable and can be stacked nearly to the ceiling in a grow room, reducing the need for shelf space.

Lion's Mane

Lion's Mane is grown in a similar fashion to Oysters, but instead of making multiple slices on each bagged block, we make only

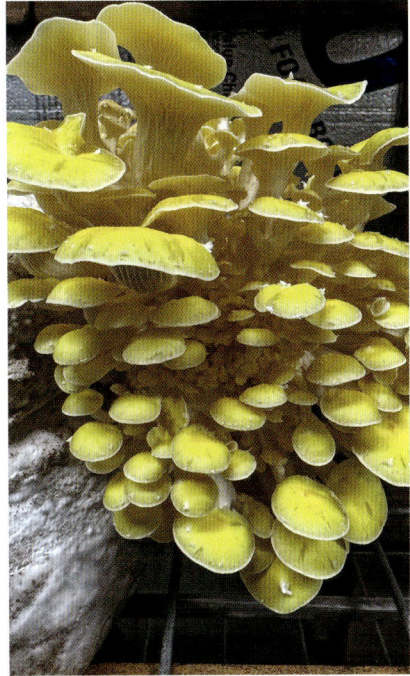

Figure 5.9. Golden Oysters fruiting indoors.

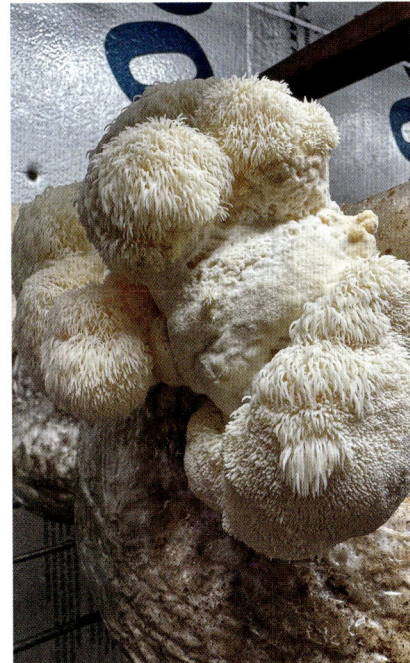

Figure 5.10. Lion's Mane fruiting indoors.

one cut, placed at the top of the block. This allows one big mushroom to form, and placing the cut at the top results in the mushroom growing with its spines cascading slightly downward. Giving this mushroom the space to expand downward keeps the fruitbody from growing into the shelves.

Most of the time, making more openings in a Lion's Mane block will not equal more mushrooms, and it will be more problematic than advantageous. The extra holes often invite the mycelium to create several primordial fruitbodies, but all but one will abort. The aborted fungi invite contamination. Take our advice and avoid this frustration.

Harvest Lion's Mane as soon as the very top of the fruiting body has started to change from pure white to off-white or yellow. This is an indication that the "spines" on the top of the mushroom are not going to continue growing. The energy has shifted and is being sent to the lower sections of the mushroom to the next stage of spore production.

Reishi

Reishi can be grown in many ways; it depends on which species of Reishi you are growing. This is one of many instances in mushroom production where

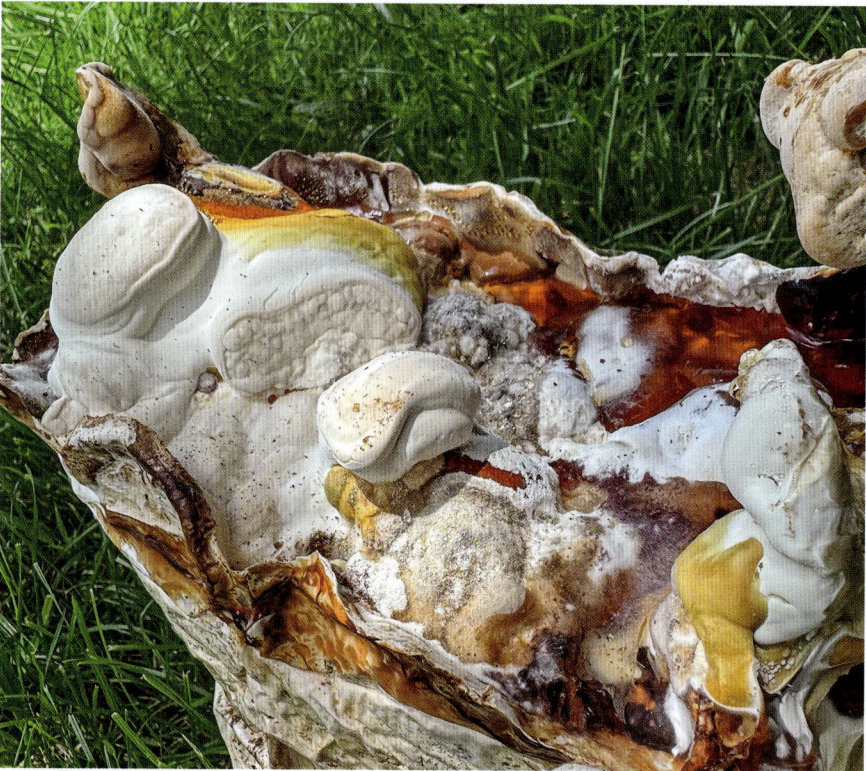

Figure 5.11. Reishi growing from a sawdust block.

genetics and strains are important. Once the Reishi substrate is fully colonized, grab the top of the bag and squeeze. This will cause the bag to separate from the now-solid block of mycelium and substrate, and allows air to reach all parts of the substrate block, even the areas that were stuck to the bag. This will initiate pinning quicker. We refer to these Reishi pins as "marshmallows" because of their soft, pure-white appearance.

Make cuts in the bag close to or on a primordial fruitbody. This method will allow the fruitbodies to escape the bag much quicker. Some strains will produce many mushrooms at once and some will produce only one or two. Often the one-cut method will produce one big fruiting body.

Another option is to leave the mushrooms to grow inside the bag without making any cuts. Be aware, though, that with this choice, it will take much longer to produce a harvest. The higher CO_2 level inside the sealed bag will cause the stems of the Reishi fruitbodies to grow longer, forming antlers. It often takes the antlers six weeks or longer to reach the top of the substrate bag. Once the top is removed from the bag, then proper conks will form on top of these antlers.

There is a third option: As soon as primordia are formed, strip the bag away from the top of the block. This allows the primordia to grow out, but not all of the primordia will come to maturity. It is important to allow the margins of the conks to finish growing out. If the margin of the cap is still white, then the mushroom is not mature yet.

Shiitakes

Shiitakes are relatively easy mushrooms to grow indoors. As stated earlier, the sawdust substrate should not be supplemented above 7 percent. The biggest drawback with growing Shiitake indoors is the prolonged waiting period required before production starts compared to outdoor production. The waiting time will be forty-five to sixty days. Once the substrate blocks of Shiitake have colonized, treat them similarly to Reishi. Squeeze the top of the bag to introduce air around the colonized block. This will speed up a process called *barking*, during which the outside of the substrate block turns brown and develops a thicker skin. Barking is essential to production of Shiitakes.

Once the barking is complete, a series of nodes will form under the bark. The nodes will swell and begin to crack. They resemble popcorn that has been slightly but not fully popped. When you observe a few of these swellings, it is a good idea to give the block a nice firm smack with an open palm. This stimulates the block to produce more "popcorn." As the popcorn starts to erupt, which typically takes only 24 to 48 hours, make a vertical cut through the bag from the top opening down to about 2 inches from the bottom. Then trim away the bag at that level, leaving only the base of the bag attached to the block.

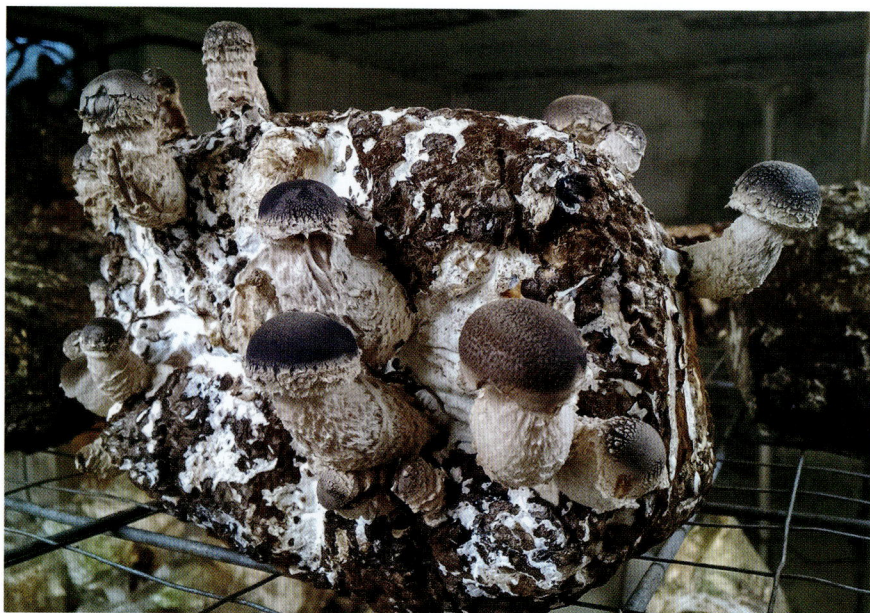

Figure 5.12. Shiitake block showing early fruiting.

Shiitakes do not respond to the presence of fresh air the way Oysters do. Shiitakes have a mind of their own.

Turkey Tail

Turkey Tail (*Trametes versicolor*) is a medicinal fungus that most people produce outdoors or wild harvest. For the mycophile who lives in a forested area of the planet, these options are fine, but for those who do not, indoor production may be the only option. The production of Turkey Tail is similar to Oysters. However, we have grown it several ways in bags of substrate.

One method we use is side fruiting. We make about two dozen cuts in a bag of substrate, which allows the Turkey Tail to grow out in thin fruiting bodies similar to how they grow in the wild. We make the cuts when the mycelium begins to thicken. We cut a series of three rows of four vertical cuts across the broad side of the block. The first row is at the top edge of the side; the next row of cuts will be directly below these. The final row of four cuts is 1 to 2 inches above the bottom of the block. This is mirrored on the other side of the block. The total amounts to sixteen to twenty-four holes. The top of the bag is rolled down and packing tape is used to secure the top in place. It's important to be mindful when taping so as not cover the cuts at the top edge of the side of the block. With this side-fruiting method, if you cut fewer than sixteen slits in the bag overall, the fruiting bodies that form will become thick—so thick and tenacious that they will be hard to process.

Another way to grow Turkey Tail is top fruiting. We allow the top of the block to develop strong, thick mycelium and then remove the top of the bag, cutting it away evenly with the top of the block. This method results in one big flush of mushrooms forming on the top of the block. We only get one good flush from this top-fruiting method, but with the side-fruiting method, it is possible to get upward of three flushes.

Split Gill

Split Gill (*Schizophyllum commune*) can be grown with the top-fruiting method as described for Turkey Tail. However, we do not grow this mushroom indoors, because the possibility that our lungs would become infected with Split Gill is a real danger. Split Gill grows abundantly in the wild here, and that supplies the needs we have here on our farm. It can be cultivated via log inoculation outdoors for those with little opportunity to wild harvest.

Cordyceps

Cordyceps is one of the easiest mushrooms to grow and it requires less space for production than other mushrooms. Cordyceps does not need a full grow room operation with misters and air exchange fans—a dedicated shelf or closet will do, making this a great genus for the beginning grower. Cordyceps mycelium can be grown on grain, but it will not produce fruiting bodies. We like the substrate recipe from Ryan Paul Gates and the company Terrestrial Fungi.[1] If you are looking for inspiration or liquid cultures, check out Ryan's work with Reishi and Cordyceps.

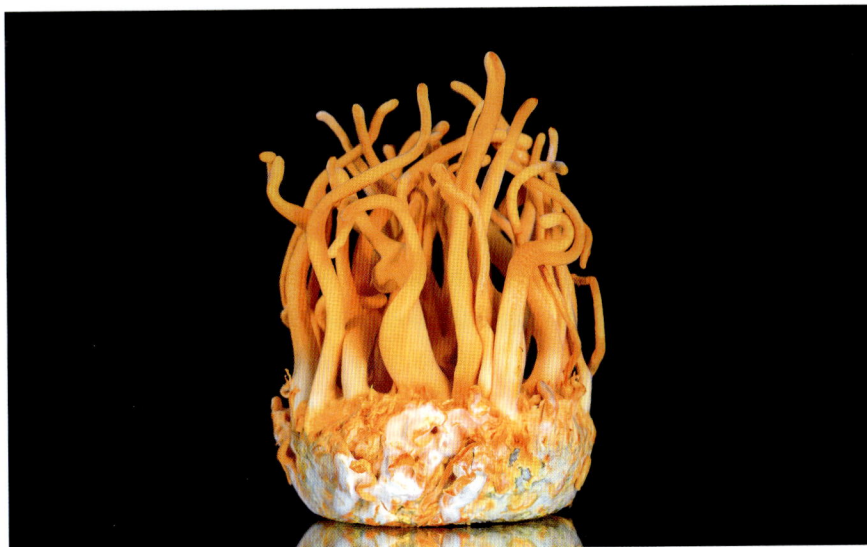

Figure 5.13. *Cordyceps militaris* on grain. Photo by gee1999 / Adobe Stock

Substrate Recipe for Growing Cordyceps

We wish to thank Ryan Paul Gates for giving permission to include his substrate recipe here.

1000 ml water
5 heaping cups (1000–1200 g) brown rice
1 tbsp (9 g) malt extract
1 tbsp (9 g) dextrose

1 tbsp (9 g) starch
3 tbsp (19 g) nutritional yeast
2 tsp (4.6 g) pea or soy protein powder
½ tsp (2.4 g) calcium carbonate
Optional additions:
¼ tsp (1.2 g) calcium sulfate
½ tsp (4 g) kelp meal

The calcium sulfate in Ryan's recipe can be replaced with more calcium carbonate if you are on a budget. You can also skip kelp.

If you are prepping your substrate in jars, use a grains-to-broth ratio of 1:1.6. A good amount for quart jars would be 35 g rice to 56 ml of broth sterilized for 60 minutes at 15 PSI.

Once the jars are cooled from sterilization, inoculate with agar or liquid culture, and put the lids back on. Incubation temperatures are between 70–72°F (21–22°C). The jars are incubated in complete darkness for two to five days until lightly colonized.

Place the tightly closed jars under lights (500–1500 lumens) at a temperature of 62–68°F (16–20°C) for a light cycle of 12 to 24 hours per day until growing is complete. Lower growing temperatures, down to 50°F (10°C), slow the fruiting time. The entire process, from inoculation to growing out fruitbodies, can take between fifty and sixty days at the standard temperature.

Maitake

Maitake mushrooms are one of the best culinary mushrooms as well as a fantastic medicinal that can be put into production. However, they are a difficult mushroom to cultivate indoors. It is best to have a room dedicated to Maitake production because the temperatures they prefer (55 to 60°F, or 13 to 16°C) are so much lower than the

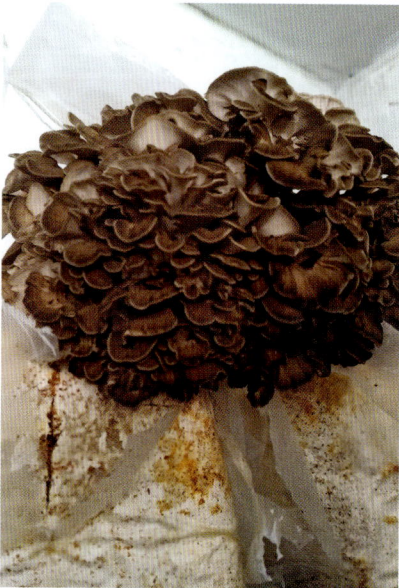

Figure 5.14. Maitake fruiting indoors. Photo by Vincent Taddeo

other cool-weather medicinal fungi. Maitake will form primordial fruitbodies on top of the blocks within thirty-five to forty-five days. It is important to watch for the primordia to form before opening the bag. Higher humidity and opening only the top, keeping the bag intact, will help to keep the fruitbodies from aborting. Keeping the humidity higher is important, especially if the mushrooms are to be grown from a single cut in the bag.

PESTS AND PROBLEMS

Pest problems and contaminants are the two biggest obstacles to success in growing mushrooms indoors. When first starting out with a grow room, all may go well for six months to a year. Then, all of a sudden, pests or contaminants will become a problem. There are a few possible reasons for the sudden change, but whatever the cause, it

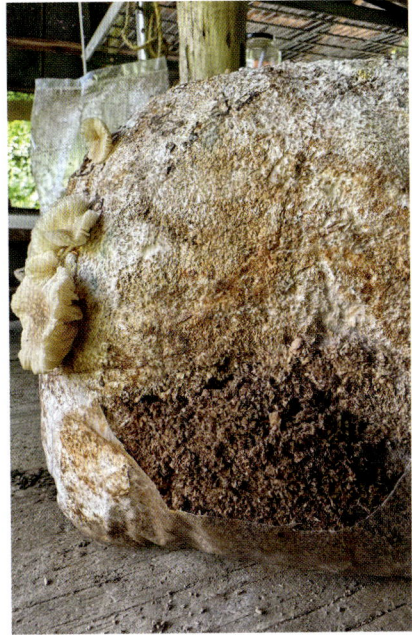

Figure 5.15. Insect damage on substrate block. Note brown grainy area devoid of mycelium.

can be a serious challenge to get pests or contaminants under control once these problems arise. The ideal situation is to stay observant and deal with any problem you notice as soon as it shows up. Mushroom farming is just like the intense cultivation of any type of crop. Ask any experienced farmer, and you will find that most of what they do is put out fires. Left alone, fires—and pest problems—will destroy everything we have worked for. Planting and tending crops are the easy parts of farming. We understand that cycle well. It is the unknowns that will kick you in the production.

The most problematic pests are fungus gnats and fruit flies. These pests do not attack the mushrooms themselves. Instead, they have a voracious appetite for the myceliated substrate. This is not to say that they will not eat your mushrooms. Adult gnats lay eggs at the base of mushrooms and consume the myceliated substrate until the mushroom reaches its growth peak. Fungus gnats have had this relationship with mushrooms for a very long time. The larvae have a tuned-in knowledge of the exact moment that the mushrooms are ripe. As the mushroom begins the descent from peak ripeness toward rotting, the larvae tunnel up the stems and into the caps. They enter the hymenium, consuming the spore-producing surface as well as the spores. Once the larvae crawl away from the substrate to a protected area, they will pupate, and the emerging adults fly away. Some spores will survive

117

in the insects' digestive system through the pupation process, and the adults deposit those spores somewhere else via their frass. This is one of many spore dispersal strategies. This coevolved spore-dispersal relationship is a problem for us indoor growers that can become a contamination problem as well. If fungus gnats are allowed to roam freely in the grow room, they can enter open cuts on a substrate block, then hop from block to block, spreading other contaminants.

Some fungal contaminants, such as penicillium, rhizopus, Trichoderma, and *Sporendonema* spp., pose different problems for the cultivator. If the contaminant is aggressive, such as Trichoderma or *Sporendonema*, the contaminated bags should be tossed immediately (we use it as compost in our gardens). Some contaminants such as penicillium are less serious, and the cultivated species of fungi can typically overcome or at least prevent the contaminant fungi from spreading to other parts of the substrate.

Toxic molds are another type of contaminant that should be taken out of the spawn room immediately. It is advisable to take them far away from the growing operation. We put them in our compost piles, which are about 165 feet (50 m) from our spawn room. Toxic molds are not to be taken lightly and can create very serious health concerns in humans if ignored.

Bacterial contamination is not a typical problem in a grow room or on bulk substrates for the simple fact that the substrates are higher in cellulose and lignin than carbohydrates and nitrogen. This combination is not favorable for the growth of most bacteria. Bacteria that produce cellulolytic enzymes can consume cellulose, but for the most part saprotrophic fungi will readily colonize over bacteria.

Harvesting and Post Growth Handling

Post-harvest handling of mushrooms is a very important aspect of working with medicinal mushrooms. Clean hands are essential, and clean tools, knives, trimmers, and so on, must be used. Boxes or bags for storing harvested mushrooms must be clean and new. It is the responsibility of the grower to make sure that medicinal mushrooms do not carry contaminants.

The mushrooms themselves should look vibrant and healthy. According to variety and species, fungi that are in good condition have a firm but yielding texture. Through experience, you will learn how each species of mushroom you grow should appear when it is at its peak. The mushroom's Latin name may provide clues of what to look for. For example, the genus *Ganoderma* for Reishi translates to "shiny skin." When these mushrooms are fully mature and medicinally charged, they have a vibrant, shiny, shellacked appearance that seems almost unnatural. You then know that mushrooms are ready for harvest.

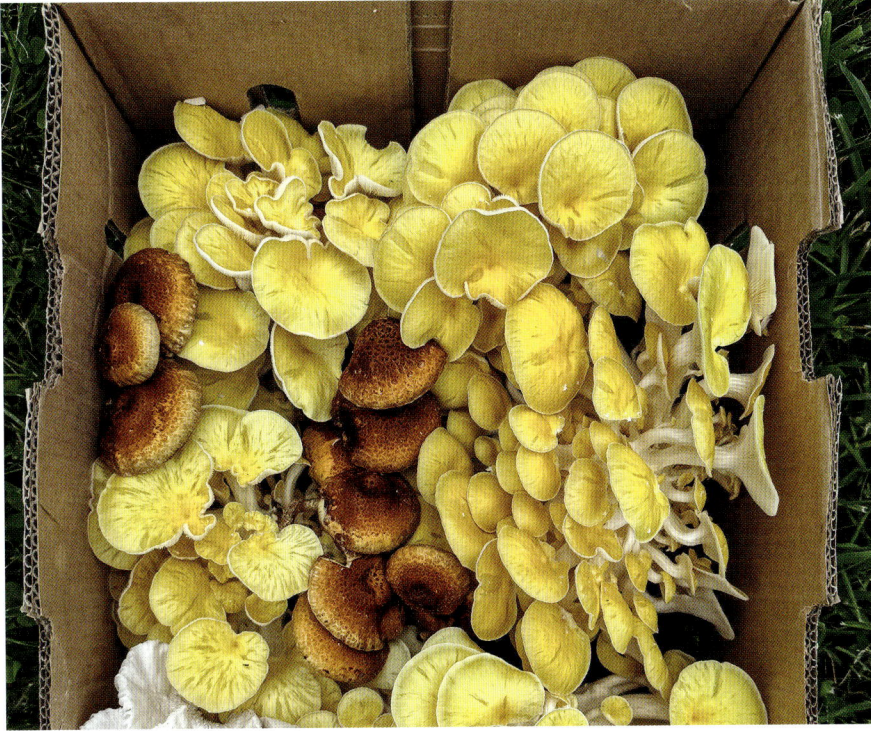

Figure 5.16. Boxed mushrooms heading for storage.

Watch out for signs of post-harvest problems, too. One sign of a potential problem is oily or greasy spots on the mushroom. If this occurs, it is almost certainly bacterial contamination, and the mushrooms should be disposed of. This can happen because the mushrooms have been oversaturated in the growing process, or because growing conditions have become too warm at some point.

Often, the biggest problem results from delaying harvesting in an attempt to allow the mushrooms to gain as much mass as possible. The early stages of decomposition may have been initiated. It can show up as a greasy surface, which is consistent with bacterial contamination, and the fungi may lose the usual strong, vibrant look that they possess when healthy. Do not utilize these mushrooms as medicine or food. They are to be tossed into the compost. Dark spots or fuzzy growth are also signs that mushrooms are past their prime. Concerning different species, the seasoned mycologist will be able to quickly identify potential problems. With Turkey Tail, dark spots on the hymenium are a sign that these specimens are not to be used. Reishi that are past prime lose the color on the spore-producing surface and mold will quickly begin to grow. Maitake has a habit of growing a fuzzy, thick, white mycelium starting at the base after the normal white hymenium has turned brown. This fuzzy growth is not the mycelium of Maitake; it is a contaminant there to consume the mushroom that is past its prime.

The best time to process mushrooms to make medicine is on the day of harvest, because the goal is to capture volatile medicinal compounds. It is possible to hold the mushrooms for a few days post-harvest before processing. Most types of mushrooms harvested for food can be held for several days up to a week before being eaten. But for both medicinal and culinary mushrooms, care must be taken to guarantee freshness and safety. Place the mushrooms in a walk-in cooler (for large operations) or a refrigerator. Ideally, store them in waxed produce boxes with butcher paper placed in the bottom of the box and a layer of wax paper over the top of the mushrooms. Storage at temperatures between 35 and 38°F (2 to 3°C) is best. Even soft-bodied Oyster mushrooms will remain fresh for five to seven days in cool storage. It is not advisable to place fresh fungi into sealed plastic bags. This asphyxiates the fungi, and they quickly rot. If smaller batches of mushrooms are harvested and cannot be immediately processed, they can be stored in a partially closed, large zipper-locking plastic bag with butcher paper inside.

— CHAPTER SIX —

Mushrooms as Food and Medicine

W e call mushrooms our daily dose of health. We add them to home-made broths, we brew mushroom tea, and we cook with mushrooms. We also use some special methods to increase the potency of the medicinal mushrooms we grow, including sun treating them. We make double extractions—a long alcohol extraction followed by a hot-water extraction—to harvest as much of the medicinal goodness as possible.

Increasing the potency of our medicinal mushrooms may seem like a new concept. However, people have been doing this for a long time. It is slow a form of medicine-making that results in very potent medicine. We live in a world where everything has been bigger, faster, and more. Not only does this reduce the quality of our life, but it also reduces the quality of the food we eat, and it creates a sense that the slow process is unsatisfactory, not worth the effort. Deep within, though, we know that when something takes time and energy to create, we will be more satisfied when our efforts come to fruition. Making an alcohol extract takes eight weeks, and even the hot-water extraction for mush-rooms can take up to two hours, much longer than what is required to brew a medicinal plant tea or decoction.

The surge in popularity of medicinal mushrooms has resulted in the arrival of many brands and formulations of mushroom supplements in the market-place. A lot of the mushroom coffee products are made with myceliated rice that has been ground and added to coffee. But for the majority of medicinal mushrooms, the fruiting body is the part that contains the highest amount of medicinal compounds. (We discuss other issues with mushroom coffee prod-ucts in "Role in Holistic Healing" on page 189, in the Lion's Mane profile.) Some supplement labels will list the ingredients as simply the name of the mushroom, e.g., "Lion's Mane," and others will say something more specific like "Lion's Mane extract." It is likely that the "extract" contains compounds that have been extracted from the mushroom rather than simply dried and ground mushroom parts, which our bodies cannot absorb. It is best to thoroughly research the company and learn about their extraction methods before you buy. In this chapter, we will dive deeper into how to process mushrooms for maximum benefits so you can take charge of this process for yourself.

What Makes Mushrooms Medicinal?

Fungi have been on this planet for nearly one billion years. They have become the masters of their environments, and along the way have performed some amazing life-supporting tasks.

We know that fungi can adapt to changes in their environment very quickly. One amazing example arose after the Chernobyl nuclear reactor meltdown, which was one of the worst environmental catastrophes in modern human history. Two species of fungi, *Cryptococcus neoformans* and *Cladosporium sphaerospermum*, were found growing toward the core of the reactor and thriving deep in this extremely radioactive environment.[1] A tendency to grow toward ionizing radiation is seen as a rarity and is called *radiotropism*. This ability to grow and thrive in this extreme environment is a testament to how quickly fungi can adapt. For a quick response like this, organisms need to rapidly assess what is happening and execute actions. The highly adaptable nature of fungi is a characteristic that makes them one of the most prevalent forms of life on our planet. Fungi have even adapted to be able to consume some plastics humans have discarded. Numerous studies have found unique communities of microorganisms, with a high concentration of fungal species, on plastics buried in landfills.[2]

Not only do fungi have the ability to be highly adaptive to their environment, but they also know how to protect themselves from toxins when necessary. We are fortunate to have many dermal layers to protect us from pathogens. Fungi do not have this luxury. They have only a single-layer cell wall to protect themselves. This thin layer between fungal cytoplasm and the outside world is not as robust as an animal's thick skin or the substantial bark layer of a tree. Fungal cell walls are made of chitin and other polysaccharides, and chitin is a considerably tough polysaccharide. Fungi also have the ability to produce biocompounds such as polysaccharides, enzymes, and even toxins that help them neutralize potentially harmful organisms. This is a superpower we can benefit from. For example, chitin acts as a prebiotic to help feed good gut flora, such as bifidobacterium, and suppress flora that are out of balance, such as candida. It is also an immune stimulator (for animals and plants), has anti-inflammatory and anticancer actions, and is used in wound healing.[3]

Chitinase, an enzyme produced by some types of fungi, breaks down chitin in the cell walls of other fungi. Soil-dwelling Trichoderma species fungi are known for producing this enzyme, which is useful for keeping fungal pathogens in check. Vegetable gardens are a place where Trichoderma could be used to fight fungal pathogens. Consider the fungal problems that farmers face every year. It is estimated that, worldwide, fungal pathogens are responsible for losses of crops in the field of upward of 25 percent and another 10 to 20 percent post-harvest. This translates to at least 100 billion dollars in crop losses per year. Why not use fungi to fight fungi? This could be an untapped potential to save crops and money.

Chitinase and another enzyme, glucanase, can act to weaken or break down the cell walls of bacteria and fungi. The weakened cell walls rupture, and the enzyme-producing fungus can then absorb nutrients from the damaged bacterial or fungal cells. This is the main mechanism by which some fungal hyphae feed.

Wood is composed mostly of cellulose, along with structural compounds called lignin and hemicellulose. Wood-decaying, or saprotrophic, species of fungi use various enzymes, such as cellulase, to break down lignin and cellulose into smaller compounds, such as glucose, that can be more easily transported and absorbed. It makes sense that most wood-loving fungi would produce cellulase, given that cellulose is a major component of wood.

Producing enzymes that break down compounds into smaller parts, such as glucose, allows a fungus to more easily transport the compounds into the hyphae. Once these sugars are in the mycelium, the fungus can then start building complex saccharide structures that are known to have human-healing properties, such as the polysaccharide krestin (PSK), polysaccharide peptide (PSP), chitin, pleuran, lentinan, and others, many of which are listed in appendix 2 on page 260.

Why do fungi build these polysaccharides? First, we have to talk about the building blocks. The simple sugars that fungi have previously broken down

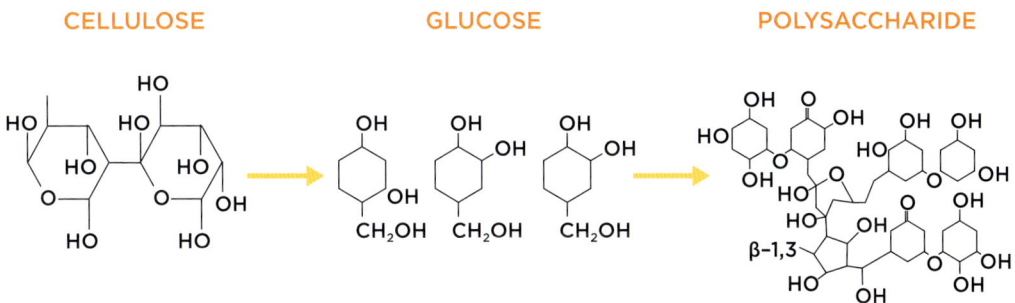

Figure 6.1. Mushrooms break down cellulose into glucose and then use it to build complex saccharides.

can be assembled and used as the building blocks for structural supports, cell walls, immune response, and protection. The simple sugars are joined together with glycosidic bonds into more complex polysaccharides. These strong chemical bonds form a chain-like structure that is hard to break down. This is why even when we simmer medicinal mushrooms in water for hours, they retain their polysaccharide content, and the important medicinal compounds are not destroyed.

In general, polysaccharides tend to have antitumor, immunomodulatory, antioxidant, anti-inflammatory, antimicrobial, and antidiabetic activity. The best-known polysaccharides are α-glucans and β-glucans, which are responsible for much of the immunomodulatory effects by binding to cell walls and stimulating specific immune responses.

Terpenes are another category of important fungal medicinal compounds that result from the processes of metabolism. Terpenes are known as secondary metabolites; they provide many functions outside of the fungal cells and have evolved to fill niche roles. These compounds can be used by the fungus for defense or chemical signaling to other organisms, drawing in organisms, or repelling others. They have antiviral, antiparasitic, antimicrobial, anti-inflammatory, and other effects on animals. They modulate the human immune system by stimulating the expression of genes that code for immune related proteins. Terpenoids are the most common secondary metabolites; the leading ones are sesquiterpenes and triterpenoids.

Fungi use specialized hyphae to capture excess nutrients and minerals as a storehouse for their community partners when needed. This is a microscopic habit that we can see in the macro world. For example, we harvest and use the sclerotia of certain mushrooms. A sclerotium is made from specialized hyphae that accumulate nutrients and contain medicinal compounds that are important to the fungal growth and the production of fruitbodies and eventually spore dispersal. Chaga sclerotia (*Inonotus obliquus*) are one example (more about this in the Chaga profile on page 193).

Some of the medicinal compounds that fungi produce are generated from the substrate they find themselves growing on or in. These can be essential nutrients such as amino acids, minerals, and polysaccharides. Some fungi uptake minerals such as magnesium, copper, sodium, and zinc. Morels (*Morchella* spp.) can hyperaccumulate lead up to one hundred times the background level. This is extremely dangerous, and yet, it can also serve a medicinal function in the environment. Wait, what?

The fungus both sequesters the toxic metal and makes it digestible to animals, who eat just a little then spread it more widely around the area through their feces, effectively reducing the concentration down to less harmful levels. Yes, the fungi remove these dangerous heavy metals from a polluted environment and hyperaccumulate them. Then they offer the metals in a form that can be safely consumed by turtles, deer, squirrels, or insects. All of the morel damage I have ever seen from any creatures besides humans is small nibbles. The adage "The solution to pollution is dilution" is true here. It is best to reduce the concentration of these toxic metals. So the fungi by their very existence are medicinal for the ecosystem. They have a vested interest in keeping the ecosystems in which they are embedded in balanced, healthy condition. In this way, they are a teacher for us humans.

Methods for Increasing Medicinal Compounds

Years ago, when I first started growing Reishi, the common wisdom was that the antler (or stem) form of Reishi was the most highly medicinal. This was based on stories about the royalty of ancient China, who highly treasured the antler forms of this medicinal mushroom. It takes antlers two to four times as long to form and grow as it does for a conk to grow. Some varieties and species take two weeks to produce a conk to maturity. It is not uncommon for antlers to take eight to ten weeks to mature. These antlers are indeed higher in certain medicinal compounds and lower in others.

One study of the medicinal compounds in the antler (called stipe or stem in the study) compared to the cap showed that the antler produced a higher quantity of phenolics and flavonoids. The polysaccharides are concentrated in the skin on the cap. The study also found that levels of some ganoderic acids (which are triterpenoids) were higher in the elongating bud (antler), and certain ganoderic acids were produced in higher amounts in the mature stage of the cap (pileus). The lion's share of the ganoderic acids were located in the mature pileus.[4]

Another study provided data suggesting that phenolics, polysaccharides, and ganoderic acids have a two-fold increase in the antlers as compared to the cap.[5] This study did not mention the maturity level of the caps nor the level of growth at which the samples were taken, which are important aspects to the cultivator attempting to increase the potency of a medicinal mushroom. These research results seem to suggest that we should use a combination of types of fruiting bodies when making medicine. It would make sense to use a one-to-one ratio of mature antlers to mature conks. This research helped us to improve our medicine making.

SUN TREATING MUSHROOMS

Ergosterol, a precursor to vitamin D_2 for humans, is one of the potent medicinal compounds found in medicinal mushrooms. It is the most prolific compound in fungi and serves many functions, ranging from maintaining functions of cells to

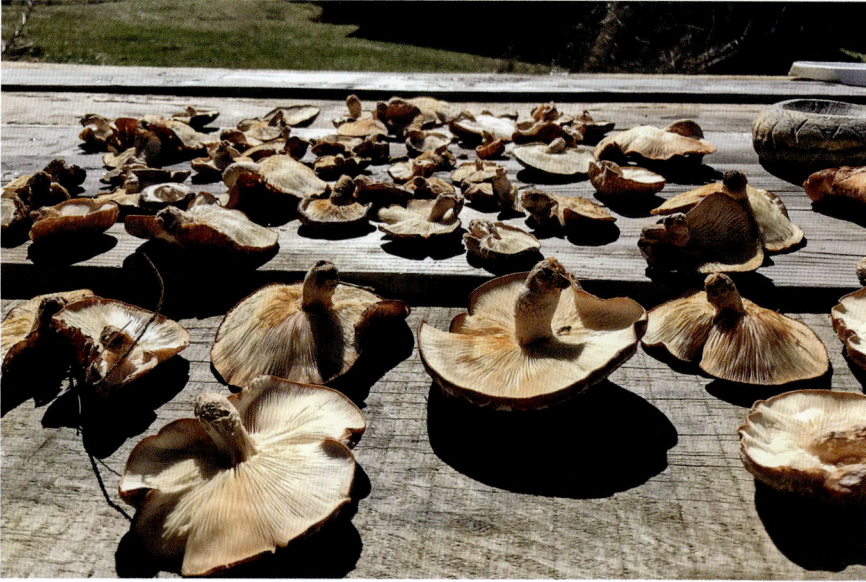

Figure 6.2. Shiitakes in the sun.

regulating proteins and enzymes. Upon exposure to ultraviolet light, ergosterol is converted to vitamin D_2. Some studies have shown a ten-fold increase in vitamin D_2 production when mushrooms are exposed to sunlight.

Many of us do not get outdoors into the sunlight enough to allow our bodies to naturally create sufficient vitamin D. This is especially challenging during the winter and at higher latitudes.

Shiitakes are one of the best responders to sun treatment. After picking Shiitakes, we turn them gill side up and leave them in the sun for 60 to 90 minutes. After 90 minutes, the mushrooms will start to lose some D_2, so it is advisable to move them to a dehydrator to finish drying, or to put them in the fridge. Fortunately, Shiitakes, one of our top-five favorite mushrooms to eat, are prolific in the mid- to late fall when our region tends to have plenty of sunshine. We sun treat them and usually eat them that evening. We dehydrate the mushrooms we don't eat right away and add them to soups and stews, or we rehydrate them for stir-fries or mushroom pies during the winter. We like to ebb and flow with the natural cycle, seizing the opportunity right before winter sets in to harvest, process, and store mushrooms that will give us high doses of D_2 all winter. We encourage you to pay attention to these types of cycles that our ancestors participated in. They likely dried mushrooms in the sun, as well as close to the fire inside, and then stored them to use over time. Fire produces some ultraviolet light—not nearly as much as the sun produces, but on a cloudy day it will help. There is deep wisdom for us to learn from such practices—we just need to listen.

SUBSTRATE SELECTION

What mushrooms eat affects who they are and the medicine they carry. Many of the medicinal fungi we grow are saprotrophic, typically wood decomposers. They are not known to hyperaccumulate lead, mercury, and other heavy metals as the ectomycorrhizals can—that is, *Lactarius* spp., morels, boletes (*Boletus* spp.), and so on. However, some do take up medicinal compounds from the materials they grow on, including Amadou (*Fomes fomentarius*) and Chaga (*Inonotus obliquus*). Birch Polypore (*Fomitopsis betulina*) accumulates betulinic acid from birch trees (*Betula* spp.), or trace minerals from a substrate. Thus, the choice of substrate can be a way to increase the nutrient density and medicinal value of saprotrophs.

A study from 2015 comparing two species of Oyster mushroom against substrate variations found that the size of the mushrooms, the protein content, and mineral accumulation were dictated by the type of substrate that the mushrooms were grown on. Corn cobs and sugarcane bagasse were the two substrates that tested best. When grown on 100 percent corn cob or sugarcane bagasse, the mineral content (Ca, K, Mg, Mn, and Zn) of both species was higher than when grown on other substrate groups. The biggest drawback with these substrates was that the colonization times were often doubled or severely slowed.[6] When growing medicinal mushrooms, you are looking for a higher-quality product, so you need to accommodate the slower growing times into your production schedule.

A study from 2021 on growing mycelium on media supplements with cow's milk looked for an increase in medicinal compounds. The analysis showed compounds such as polysaccharides and proteins increased from 3.5- to 4.5-fold. A 10-fold decrease in free radicals was also observed, which contributed to the increased activity of two enzymes: catalase and superoxide dismutase. The study authors suggest that Funnel Woodcap (*Lentinus sajor-caju*) cultivated with milk supplement can be used as a healthy source of nutritional and anti-cancer compounds.[7]

How does this translate to other medicinal mushrooms? This could have some application with growing *Cordyceps militaris*. We use a nutrient broth to grow Cordyceps on organic brown rice, but it may be possible to use a milk supplement when growing out Cordyceps mycelium on grains or beans that will be eaten (this process is described in "Incorporating Myceliated Grains and Beans" on page 134).

C. militaris production has become widespread in the last fifteen years. Many cultivators have been experimenting with methods of cultivation to maximize efficiency of cultures by breeding and experimenting with substrate recipes. Twenty years ago, trying to grow Cordyceps on a home or commercial scale was still unfamiliar for people in the United States. But at that time, Asian cultivators were refining techniques. Most of these growers have followed a process using some version of rice with a nutrient broth. Several papers have been written about

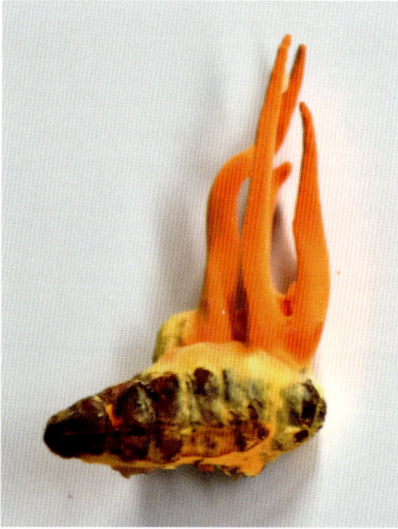

Figure 6.3. *Cordyceps militaris* on a pupa. Photo by Kornwipa Ponganan / iStock

various substrates and cultivation methods with the focus on increasing levels of the medicinal compounds cordycepin, cordycepic acid, ergosterol, and mannitol. The indoor cultivation of Cordyceps is an exciting prospect that relieves the pressure on wild populations, driving wild crafters and cultivators to cherish the few Cordyceps we find in the wild.

A study from the early 2000s focused on the improved production of cordycepin by introducing carbon sources in the substrate for Cordyceps. Glucose, sucrose, lactose, galactose, xylose, fructose, and maltose all increased cordycepin production. They found the highest levels of cordycepin production when the substrate contained a combination of glucose and peptone.[8]

Another study, from 2024, found that some common substrates may contribute to a lower quality of medicinal compounds in Cordyceps. Rice is the most commonly used base substrate in the United States. The lower quality bioactive compounds in Cordyceps grown from rice are attributed to the lower nutrient density. This same study showed that silkworm pupae are a preferred substrate for cultivation because of their rich nutrient density and nutrient profile. That substrate enhances the production of polysaccharides and cordycepin. Cicadas and beetles were also used as substrates: cicada provided a high-quality product; beetles, because of their tough exoskeleton, resulted in lower levels of cordycepin. The Lepidoptera order (moths and butterflies) is rich in lipids and proteins. They also provide the raw ingredients and precursors for Cordyceps to synthesize bioactive compounds. This nutrient-dense moth/butterfly environment allows for higher metabolism for Cordyceps, resulting in higher cordycepin levels. The immune response of the host species to fungal infection can also trigger secondary metabolites in Cordyceps, resulting in higher cordycepin production.[9]

There are many challenges and rewards when it comes to cultivating *C. militaris*. The fungal diversity with this species, as with other medicinal mushrooms, will determine the quality of medicinal compounds, and as we have seen by this research, many factors are at play.

GROWING ENVIRONMENT

The third factor to consider when looking at how to increase medicinal compounds in mushrooms is, of course, the environment in which the mushrooms are grown. Very little research has been done on this. The aforementioned paper from 2024 reports that many aspects of the cultivation environment will increase the production of *Cordyceps militaris* and the production of the prominent medicinal compounds. Selection of strains or genetics through cloning and breeding is important. Growth medium and environmental factors such as humidity or light all have an impact on the quality of final medicinal compounds. Maintaining temperatures is key in producing a consistent medicinal mushroom. It was found that at temperatures of 68 to 77°F (20 to 25°C), the fungi produce the optimum growth and production of medicinal compounds, including cordycepin. Temperatures above or below this range may slow or inhibit growth.[10]

Optimal humidity levels are important for mycelial growth and the production of important medicinal compounds. Low levels of humidity are a stressor for the fungi and have been shown to inhibit growth of fruitbodies and mycelium. On the other hand, excessively high humidity will often lead to contamination problems. Optimum humidity levels for Cordyceps were found to be between 60 and 80 percent.

Light is an important environmental factor. It affects cordycepin and carotenoid production. Exposure to certain light conditions optimizes concentration and yield of medicinal and other biological compounds. Using blue-light LEDs for eight hours a day has been shown to increase biomass production and cordycepin in liquid culture. Short wavelength light has shown to increase carotenoid content in *C. militaris* fruitbodies.

The idea that the growing environment plays a big part in the ability of fungi to properly metabolize the host substrate and reach their full potential is not a new concept. For example, vegetable growers have come to realize that, to produce better vegetables with higher nutrient profiles, it's important to support proper microbial activity in the soil environment. It is no different with fungi: if you want higher-quality medicinal and culinary mushrooms, you have to be sure you meet the fungi's needs.

Making Mushroom Double Extractions

Double extractions deliver one of the most shelf-stable medicines possible. Double extracts of medicinal mushrooms include both an alcohol and a hot-water extract successively, which are then combined. The end product is convenient: it fits in your hand, luggage, or pocket; and it doesn't weigh much because double extractions are so concentrated. When double extractions are done properly, the resulting liquid contains the full range of compounds offered by the mushrooms, everything from volatiles to heavy molecular weight compounds.

One disadvantage of double extractions is the long wait time before the final extract is ready. Another is that people in recovery from alcohol addiction may not be able to use double extractions because of the ethanol alcohol content.

Let's go through the full process of making the alcohol extract, then the hot-water extract, and then the combination of the two extracts. Once you have mastered this process, you can make shelf-stable medicine using any of the mushrooms discussed in this book.

If you or the people that will be taking the finished double extraction have celiac disease or gluten intolerance, please make sure to acquire alcohol that is not made with grains. We use organic cane alcohol, which is made from organic cane sugar.

THE ALCOHOL EXTRACTION

You can make an alcohol extract with any fresh mushrooms that you have grown, wild harvested, or purchased. Before extracting them, though, you must dry them. Because the water content of fresh mushrooms is an unknown, using them fresh would upset the alcohol percentage of the finished product.

You may come across recipes that suggest using less mushroom with more alcohol than in our instructions below. Doing so will create an insubstantial extract, and we don't recommend it. These are medicinal mushroom extractions to help with healing or maintaining health. They are worthy of being potent and powerful.

Procedure

EQUIPMENT NEEDED

Medicinal mushrooms
Dehydrator
Ethanol alcohol, 100 proof

Glass jars, preferably graduated,
  with lids
Parchment paper
Permanent marker

1. Slice the mushrooms as thinly as possible to speed drying time and expose more cells to the solvents.
2. Dry the sliced mushrooms in the dehydrator until they "snap" when bent. This guarantees they are ready to process.
3. Put the dry mushrooms in a glass jar and add enough alcohol to almost cover them. Do not cover them completely. For example, if you are using a 1-gallon jar, fill it with dried mushroom slices up to the shoulder. Then add alcohol up to 1.5 inches below the shoulder. Some mushrooms should stick up above the liquid.
4. Fold a piece of parchment paper to make a double layer of paper. Put the paper across the mouth of the jar and then put on the lid and screw it

tightly in place. (The parchment paper prevents the alcohol from interacting with the metal in the lid.)

5. Put a blank label on the lid and use the marker to write the date, alcohol content, type of mushroom, and any other information you need.

Extraction will progress over the course of eight weeks. Store the jar out of direct sunlight, preferably in the dark, at room temperature. During that time shake the jar daily, if you can, or as many times as possible, at least once every few days.

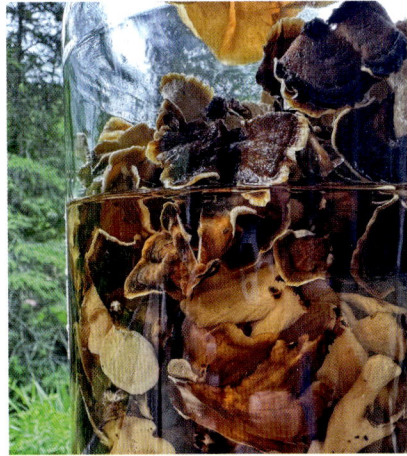

Figure 6.4. Turkey Tail (*Trametes versicolor*) being extracted in alcohol.

THE HOT-WATER EXTRACT

When the date of the finished alcohol extract arrives, it is time to complete the hot-water extraction. Many instructions for this method call for double the amount of water as alcohol. If this is the case, 4 liters of alcohol extract should warrant starting the hot-water extract with 8 liters of water. But we do not find this to be a requirement. We use about one and a half times the amount of water as alcohol. So, for 4 liters of alcohol extract, we start with 6 liters of water. In the water-extraction process, some of the water will evaporate, ultimately leaving us with a one-to-one ratio of alcohol extract to water extract.

For this double-extraction recipe using 4 liters of alcohol extract made with 100-proof alcohol, we will use 4 liters of hot-water extract cooled to room temperature. This is as simple as it can be made.

Procedure

EQUIPMENT NEEDED

Alcohol extract
Glass jars, preferably graduated, with lids

Tincture press or a new, undyed linen cloth or cheesecloth
Large pot with tight-fitting lid
Water

1. Drain off the liquid from the alcohol extraction and then transfer the liquid to a jar with a tight-fitting lid. This liquid is precious; don't let anything contaminate it.
2. Using a tincture press, or cheesecloth, press as much of the alcohol out of the mushroom material as possible, and add it to the liquid in the jar. Close the lid tightly.

3. Place the leftover mushroom material in a pot and add water, 1.5 times the volume of the alcohol extraction liquid.
4. Gently heat the mushrooms and water in a covered pot until it begins to simmer. Keep it simmering for 90 to 120 minutes. Ideally, enough water will evaporate to result in the same amount of water as you have alcohol in the jar. If you end up with more water than needed, simply remove the lid and allow the water to evaporate to the correct volume. Conversely, if there is not enough water in the pot to make a one-to-one ratio, simply add a bit more water to get to the volume needed.
5. Let the water cool to room temperature.

MIXING THE ALCOHOL AND WATER EXTRACTIONS

Combining the alcohol and hot-water extracts results in a finished double extraction of 25 percent alcohol, or 50 proof. This is plenty of alcohol to make the double extraction shelf stable. Many beginners make a double extraction with a higher alcohol content, but this is not a good idea. If the alcohol content of the finished product is higher than 37 percent, the alcohol will degrade the valuable polysaccharides in the extract over time. Pay attention to this. We do not want you to invest your time growing, harvesting, and processing your medicinal mushrooms, only to only ruin the medicine at the final stage.

Keep in mind that the hot-water extraction is what breaks apart the chitin in the mushroom cell walls, releasing other polysaccharides. The alcohol is a

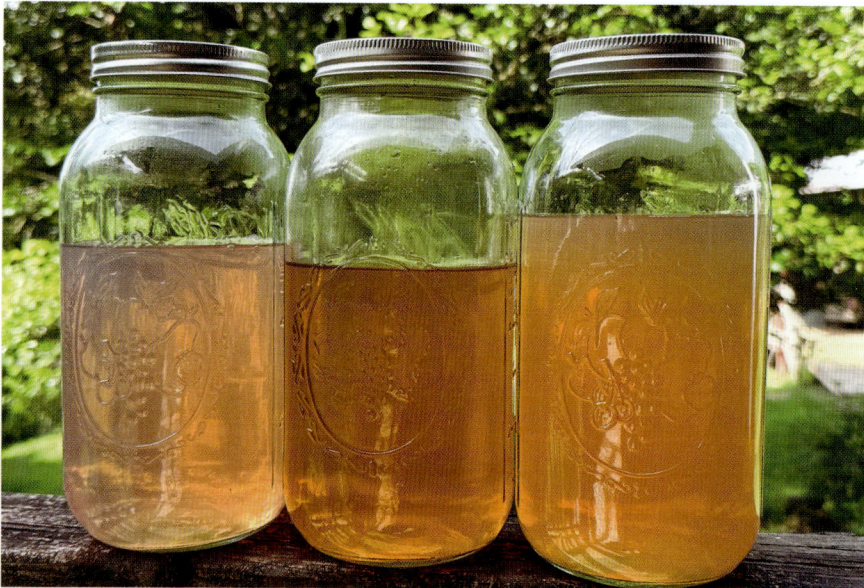

Figure 6.5. Alcohol extraction, water extraction, and double extraction. Note the color difference after extracts are mixed together.

solvent and preservative, but it does not break apart the cell walls. Alcohol does have the ability to pull out the volatiles, terpenes, triterpenes, sesquiterpenes, and other medicinal compounds through the intact cell walls.

Some people practice the double-extraction method by making the hot-water extract first and the alcohol extract second. To us this makes no sense because the water extraction must be stored, perhaps in a freezer, until the alcohol extract is done. It also puts the medicine maker in the possible position of having not enough or too much water extract in proportion to the alcohol extract created. Additionally, if the hot-water extraction is done first, then the mushrooms have to be dehydrated afterward to make sure the alcohol is within the correct proportions. All of this makes things way too complicated and adds more steps than are necessary. Let's keep this as simple as possible.

STORING THE DOUBLE EXTRACT

When your double extract is finished, place it in a large glass jar. Since the alcohol is acidic, place parchment paper between the lid and the rim of the jar, especially if your jar has a metal lid. Label the jar with the finished date, type of mushroom, and alcohol content. The finished dual extract can be decanted into amber glass bottles with droppers for ease of dispensing. Place the rest of the extract in a dark, cool place, where it will keep for up to a year.

Medicinal Mushrooms as Food

The medicinal mushrooms we discuss in chapter 7 are, by a large portion, not only medicinal but also great culinary mushrooms. The top two, in my opinion, are Wishi (*Grifola frondosa,* also called Maitake) and Milky mushrooms (*Lactarius* and *Lactifluus* spp.).

You may have loved ones who are in need of medicinal mushrooms but do not want to ingest them on a frequent basis, even though doing so could improve their physical and mental health and well-being, or help cure a disease. Many children have not yet developed a palate for mushrooms. We know that caretakers or parents can struggle with getting their children to eat well.

The easiest way to consume the medicinal properties of mushrooms is to incorporate them into the diet a few times a week or month. There are pros and cons to just simply cooking with mushrooms. When mushrooms are cooked in a meal, they may not be fully cooked so as to break the cell walls down, which is necessary to free up some of the beneficial heavy molecular weight compounds. Additionally, some of the volatile medicinal compounds can be driven off, which is a loss. So we want to share with you the basics of cooking with mushrooms to make the medicinal properties as available as possible.

INCORPORATING MYCELIATED GRAINS AND BEANS

An idea came to me years ago when making grain spawn. Why not utilize the grain that is covered in mycelium to cook and eat? This turned out to be an excellent idea and a horrible one at the same time. There are some mushrooms that work with this method and some that do not. It's important to consider whether the mushroom mycelium grown on the grain is a mushroom that tastes good, such as Oysters, Lion's Mane, or Shiitake. Some medicinal mushrooms do not have a good flavor at all. For example, Reishi mycelium contains too many bitter compounds to make for a palatable food. The Almond Portobello (*Agaricus blazei*) has a great flavor—however, the mycelium, even though reminiscent of the fruitbody, makes the grains bitter.

We can apply some of the techniques we learned in previous chapters to create supercharged grains or legumes. For example, we can use a liquid culture to inoculate jars of grains or beans. (When we do this, we usually use black beans. We cook the beans until they are still firm but yield under a little pressure. If we use grains, we cook them as described starting on page 85.)

After cooking grain or beans, load them into jars approximately three-quarters full, and put DIY manufactured lids on the jars (the method for making these lids is described on page 47). You'll recall that these lids have one hole for fresh air exchange and a second hole with an injection port. Put foil over the top of the lids to keep out excess moisture, then sterilize the beans or grains at 15 PSI for 90 minutes. When they are fully cooled, inject liquid culture of the desired mushroom species into the jar using the sterile technique as described starting on page 91. Since you will be consuming the grain or beans as food, it is more important than ever to watch the colonization of the beans or grain very closely. If you see *any* contamination, discard the entire jar and start over.

Fully colonized beans or grain can be treated a few different ways. Our preferred method is to immediately use them in cooking, or to simply freeze them until we are ready to use them. You can also dehydrate them and turn the dried material into a powder. This is a shelf stable food product; the grains can be a great soup thickener or

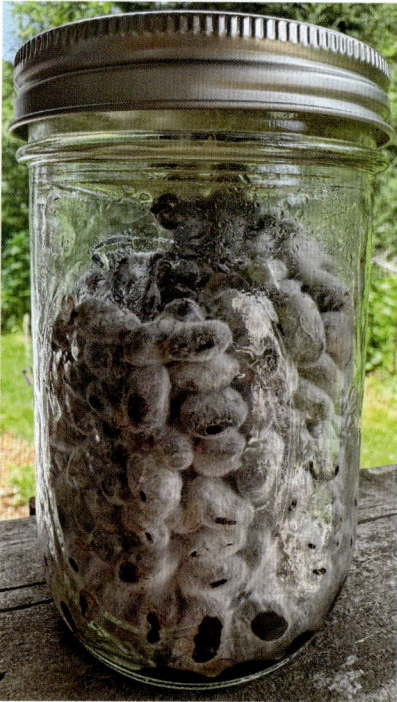

Figure 6.6. Black beans being colonized by Lion's Mane mycelium.

utilized as the base for gravies and sauces. Beans and grains can also be cooked in soups and stews. Cooking mushrooms in soups or stews is the best method of using mushrooms as medicine in food. The low-and-slow cooking exposes the mushroom cell walls to a longer cook time, breaking them apart and releasing more of the beneficial polysaccharides into the food.

TEAS AND BROTHS

Tea is an obvious choice for using medicinal mushrooms. Not only does making tea bring out the compounds that are healing, but the act of making tea is also good for the spirit in and of itself. Humans have used teas and broths as medicine ever since the art of cookery began. Preparing mushrooms with a long exposure to hot water makes the nutrients and medicinal compounds available to be digested easily. When we make tea, we do not simply steep mushrooms in hot water as we would with plant medicines, because of the higher chitin content of mushroom cell walls. As noted previously, their cell walls are usually around 20 percent chitin, and this chitin needs to be broken down in order to release the other medicinal polysaccharides, including PSK, PSP, and α-glucans. Instead, we simmer mushrooms in water for 90 to 120 minutes. It is the same method as making a hot-water extraction. We usually do this in a large batch and save the tea for several days to a week in the fridge. Compared to making tea with plant material, this is a long process that requires a lot of energy, and it isn't necessary to do it every day.

An alternative way to store mushroom tea or hot-water extract is to turn it into ice cubes. This is a good strategy when treating a long-term illness that requires a daily dose. Simply cool the water extract, pour it into ice cube trays, and freeze. Then pop out the frozen cubes and store them in large freezer bags. This makes for convenient doses that can be dealt out as needed. If you like adding mushroom extracts to your coffee, then try tossing an ice cube on top of the coffee grounds in a programmable coffee maker the night before. When the coffee is ready in the morning, so is the mushroom extract. This is a way to avoid the expensive and inferior coffee additives that are flooding the market, not to mention the packaging waste. You are in control of the dosage, sourcing your mushrooms, and hopefully even growing them yourself!

Using the water-extraction method for mushrooms is not limited to tea. On our farm we save vegetable trimmings to make broths as described on page 138, and we include medicinal mushrooms with the trimmings.

Cooking with Mushrooms

Unfortunately, many people are not aware that eating mushrooms raw is not good for the digestive system. We have been trying to educate people about this for decades. Yes, even the White Button mushrooms (*Agaricus bisporus*) topping a salad are not something the human digestive system wants to participate in. The chitin in their cell walls cannot be broken down by our digestive system. Eating raw mushrooms gives us no nutritional or medicinal benefits, and eating too many raw mushrooms might even lead to red blood cell damage.[11] Uncooked White Button mushrooms have been found to cause cancer in mice, and some people may develop skin irritations from uncooked Shiitakes.[12] Please, cook all of your mushrooms.

The easiest place to start when cooking mushrooms is to cut, slice, dice, or tear the mushrooms. Cook the mushrooms in some type of fat; we prefer butter or avocado oil. Some people may prefer coconut oil according to the dish being made. Animal fats can also be used. (Please avoid using seed oils in cooking. Especially if you or someone you know is trying to heal. The seed oil industry uses practices that are aligned with the profit motive, not human health. Some manufacturers use hexanes, which are known as neurotoxins, in processing seed oils. Hexanes are not used, however, in processing of certified-organic seed oils.)

One of the first things that you will notice when you cook mushrooms is that excess water will show up in the pan. This leads to longer cooking time because the water has to be driven off before the mushrooms start to brown. The extra time means you get better extraction of beneficial compounds. Move the mushrooms around occasionally to cook them evenly. At some point, the moisture will dissipate, and the mushrooms will begin to brown. This is the moment to add some type of sauce, to incorporate the flavor of the dish you will make. We recommend a sauce that contains a fair amount of water, which will help to extend the cooking time overall. The possibilities are endless depending on your taste—barbeque sauce, Asian sauces, Italian sauces, taco seasoning, and so on.

The simplest choice is a sauce that we make for a noodle bowl. We use at least 50 percent water, and then add mirin, tamari, certified-organic toasted sesame oil, powdered ginger, and garlic to taste. Toss this mix into the pan with the mushrooms and immediately cover with a lid. The idea behind this cooking method is that the mushrooms will absorb the water along with the spices and flavors. As they continue to cook in this spice broth and absorb the flavors, the chitin in the cell walls is broken down further to release more of the medicinal polysaccharides. After the mushrooms have plumped back up, we remove the lid and stir the mushrooms occasionally. Once most of the water has dissipated again, you will notice that the size of the bubbles in the sauce will become bigger. This is because the mushrooms have started releasing polysaccharides, which creates more surface tension in the liquid, allowing the bubbles to grow bigger before they break. When the mushrooms begin to brown for the second time, we remove them from the heat and add them to the noodles in the noodle bowl.

MEDICINAL MUSHROOM CRACKERS

Adding mushrooms to dough for homemade crackers is a simple way of incorporating medicinal mushrooms into the diet, especially if you have fussy eaters in your household. You can start with your favorite cracker recipe. If you make substantially more hot-water mushroom extract than you can use for one batch, it will freeze well until ready for next time.

We like to make crackers using Oyster mushrooms, but any mild-flavored mushroom works well. Lion's Mane is a good substitute.

For a recipe calling for 2 cups flour, we add 1 cup hot-water-extracted mushrooms. We start with ½ pound of Oyster mushrooms, chop them fine, and simmer them for 90 minutes in 2 to 3 cups of water. After they cool, we blend them in a blender until thoroughly homogenized. Take 1 cup of the blended mushrooms and mix it into 2 cups of flour. At this point, we also like to add 1 tablespoon of chopped fresh rosemary or ¾ tablespoon dried rosemary.

If you've never made crackers, there are plenty of good recipes and instructional videos available online. Once you've mixed the dough and adjusted it for the right level of moistness, roll it out and cut it, slide it onto parchment paper and then onto a baking sheet, and bake them. We use a 400°F (204°C) oven and bake for 12 to 17 minutes.

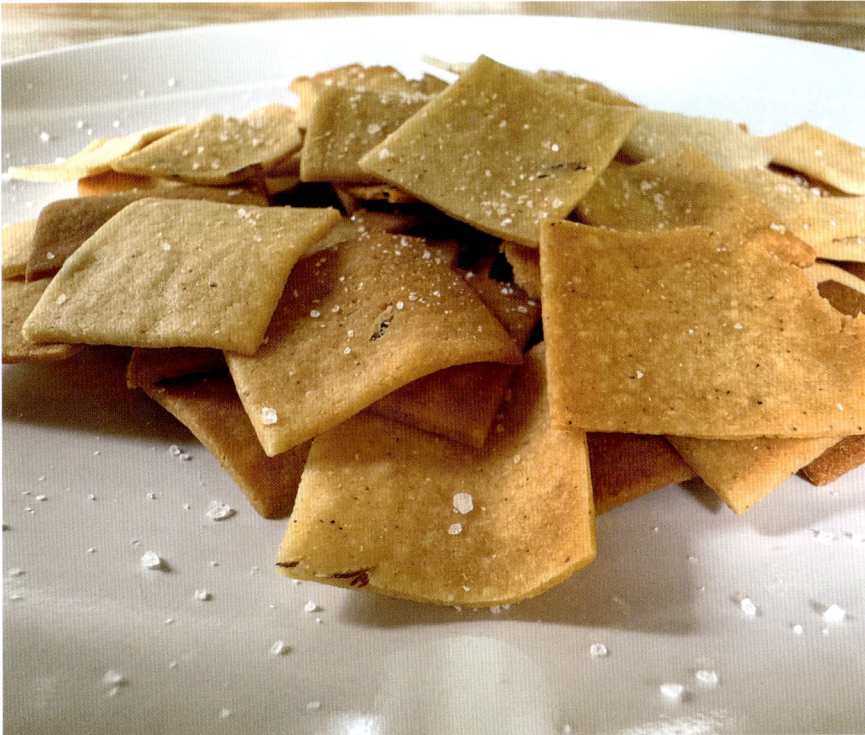

Figure 6.7. Rustic rosemary–mushroom crackers.

Don't get busy and forget about your crackers! They can overcook quickly. The edge crackers may brown a bit more than the center ones. Remove the whole sheet from the oven and allow them to cool before snapping the crackers apart. They will become crispier as they cool. Store in an airtight container and enjoy.

MEDICINAL MUSHROOM AND VEGETABLE BROTH

We save onion skins, carrot tops and tips, parsnip trimmings, celery, and other vegetable trimmings whenever we are prepping vegetables for a meal. We toss the trimmings in the freezer, and when we have collected enough, we put them a slow cooker with water, add in medicinal and culinary mushrooms, then set the cooker on simmer overnight. You can then use this broth for making soup, or you can add sea salt and run the broth through the pressure canner to have on hand whenever needed.

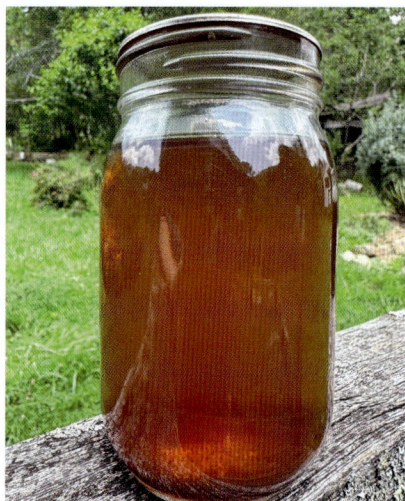

Figure 6.8. Medicinal mushroom–vegetable stock.

Broths have seen a resurgence in recent years. This is part of us taking back the power to give our bodies the healthy nourishing components they need to heal or maintain health. We also make a supercharged bone broth from scrappy mushrooms, mushroom stems, perfect mushrooms, vegetable scraps, wild herbs, and bones from animals we have hunted. This broth can be made vegan if you do not consume animal parts.

We usually wait until we have about 12 cups of mushroom and vegetables scraps, which is enough to produce 1.5 gallons of stock. We like to have about a one-to-one ratio of veggie material to mushrooms. We simmer this broth in a large stockpot on the stove for 90 minutes for best flavor and to process the mushrooms for ultimate extraction. We store the broth in pint jars; 1.5 gallons of stock will produce 12 pints of stock. This is simply what works for us, but you can adjust and make broth at the scale that works for you.

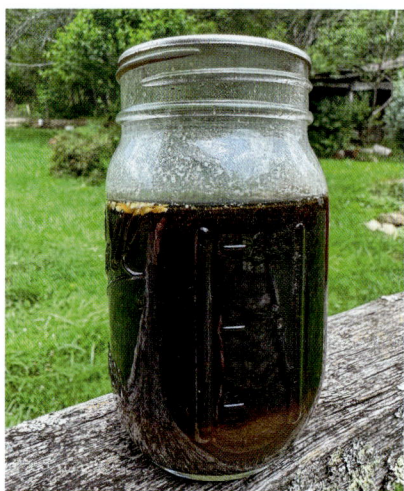

Figure 6.9. Home-canned medicinal bone broth.

For the mushrooms, we like to use Oysters, Shiitake (especially the stems), Turkey Tail, and Birch Polypore. Use any soup bones you have available. Another option is to add a couple of venison bones, or a front shank with the bone cut into two so that the marrow can be extracted. If you are not using bones, some type of fat will be needed to improve the flavor of the broth. Avocado oil is a great high-heat oil that adds a mild buttery flavor.

Add some wild herbs too, such as Queen Anne's Lace (*Daucus carota*), Wild Violet (*Viola sororia*) greens, or mallow leaves. We advise against using brassicas (such as kale, cabbage, or Brussels sprouts). They will impart bitterness to the finished stock.

Just like the ceremony of making tea, this ceremony of tending to all of the vegetables, picking wild greens, and even processing the bones of the animals from your local farms can be very beneficial for your mental and spiritual health. You are closing the nutrient cycle and winding the circle of life a bit closer to you.

CHAGA-REISHI CHAI

Our Chaga-Reishi Chai is not only delicious and soothing for the body, but it is a heavy-hitting medicinal as well. Feel free to experiment with other combinations of ingredients to find what works best for you. We use a 1-gallon slow cooker. Making this chai is a long process, so we like to prepare a large batch, which we keep in the fridge to heat up whenever we want to enjoy it. If you don't have a slow cooker, you can use a stock pot with a capacity of 1 gallon or more. You can leave it cooking for several hours. This is a good project to start in the evening—you'll have chai in the morning.

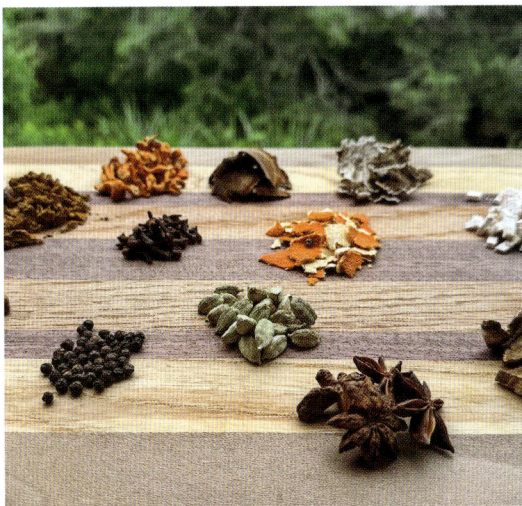

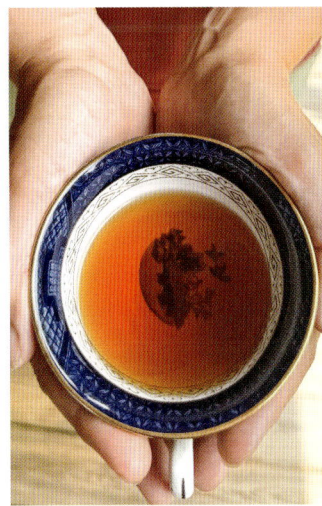

Figure 6.10. Dried medicinal mushrooms and chai ingredients and a cup of chai ready to drink.

Ingredients for Chaga-Reishi Chai

All of the mushrooms in the ingredients list can be used, but not all of them must be used. The first three are highly recommended.

¾ cup sliced Reishi

⅓ cup ground or pea-sized pieces of Chaga

¾ cup packed Turkey Tail

⅓ cup Cordyceps

¼ cup sliced Amadou

¼ cup sliced Birch Polypore

4 to 6 cinnamon sticks

2 tablespoons whole allspice

5 to 10 cardamom pods

2 tablespoons whole cloves

½ orange

3 tablespoons fresh or dried orange peel (more or less to taste)

1 teaspoon black peppercorns

1.5-inch-long fresh ginger root, sliced

1 tablespoon fennel seeds

We first put the medicinal mushrooms into the cooker and add water up to about an inch from the top. We set the cooker on high, and once the water reaches a simmering point, we reduce the heat to low.

After the mushrooms have cooked for several hours or overnight, they can be removed from the water extract in the cooker, or left in the extract. Either way, at this point we add the spices. We use a mortar and pestle to crush the whole spices, but we don't pulverize the spices into a powder. We partially crush them just until they are open, which releases the flavors better. (The orange peel and sliced ginger do not need to be crushed.) Once we have added the spices, we turn the heat back up to high for 30 minutes, or until the chai becomes fragrant, then strain. We enjoy this chai with honey and whole milk or half-and-half. The choice is up to you. We find it will last for at least five to seven days in the refrigerator.

Sometimes the bitter compounds from Reishi can still come through all of these different flavors. The peppercorns add a bit of sharpness to take the edge off of the Reishi flavor. Most of the time, we opt to make this chai without black tea. If we want black tea, we add a mix of Assam, Darjeeling, and Ceylon to a tea ball or strainer and pour the hot chai over it into a cup. In this case, cover and let steep for 5 to 10 minutes. Remove the tea strainer, add the milk and honey, and enjoy.

CHAPTER SEVEN

Medicinal Mushroom Profiles

As interest in medicinal mushrooms increases, knowledge about their uses and benefits is also increasing. It's become clear how much is still to be learned about these fungi, and how much past knowledge about traditional uses of fungi has already been lost.

Every time we meet someone who has not tried a certain species of mushroom, we encourage them to try it and listen to what their body is telling them about that mushroom. Once they are able to slow down and listen to that voice, they move a little closer to understanding holistic health and how these mushrooms can be incorporated into their lifestyle.

One of the great benefits that medicinal mushrooms offer in our stress-filled lives is resilience. So many of us seem to move incessantly. We battle morning traffic to fulfill our obligations of getting ourselves and our children where we need to be on time. We come in contact with more strangers in one year than most of our ancestors encountered in their whole lives. The list of daily stressors speaks to the troubles of the postmodern society we have built and the problems we have created in so doing.

In this chapter, we celebrate in depth the beneficial gifts of some of the mushrooms we have come to know best through years of hunting them, growing them, and using them as food and medicine. You can read this chapter from start to finish, or dip into any profiles that you are curious about in the order of your choice.

In each of the profiles that follows, we introduce these mushrooms by name and explain some aspects of how they live—where they are native to, their host plants, and their way of reproducing. Some are saprotrophs, which feed on decaying wood, and others are parasitic fungi, which feed on living plant or insect tissue; they are all medicinal.

The Importance of Folk Wisdom

We also discuss the long history these mushrooms have of being in relationship with humans of various cultures. Traditional uses of fungi have been documented for centuries, and some species have been used medicinally for thousands of years.

In recent decades, many of the folk uses and traditional healing ways have been corroborated and confirmed by research, which is driving the revival and advancement of holistic medicine. Some of us are intuitive healers who use the old systems that have been around for thousands of years. But others question these ways of healing because until recently, such methods have had no scientific backing. Our question has always been, if they do not work, why have they been used successfully for thousands of years?

There are many inaccuracies in the historical record about medicinal mushrooms. For example, it is often stated that Hen-of-the-Woods (*Grifola frondosa*, also called Maitake) was first described in 1785 by a Scottish mycologist, James J. Dickson. This is simply false. Indigenous peoples in North America, east of the Rockies, knew and used this mushroom long before European scientists or naturalists arrived on the continent. This is another way in which history has been colonized and the wisdom of the Indigenous peoples' either outright ignored or not sought out. It is clear that different ways of thinking carry power. Science is helpful but we cannot dismiss native ways of thinking, ways that have been passed down the generations in relation to the place from which they emerged.

Modern research related to folk uses of mushrooms is far behind that on medicinal plants. It is likely that many folk uses of mushrooms have been lost entirely as elders and entire Indigenous languages die. This loss of knowledge should be waking us up to the need to seek out and listen to older people. Our smartphones and the internet cannot supply the wisdom that our elders can give us. Acknowledging this is more important than ever as generations are growing up immersed in the internet and separated from interaction with people and with nature.

People are overloaded with random information, and in response, they are craving wisdom—the ability to know when and how to *apply* information. Functional mushrooms can also support this transfer of experience and wisdom, and this is an opportunity that should not be wasted.

We have included as many scientific references to folk uses of these fourteen mushrooms from around the world as we could find. Asian cultures, especially the Chinese, are way ahead of most of the rest of the world in terms of using and cultivating medicinal mushrooms. We have included much wisdom from Traditional Chinese Medicine (TCM), a complex system of healthcare that has

Fungal Pathogens

Although our focus in this book is on mushrooms that benefit human health, we would be remiss to not acknowledge that fungi can also cause infections, some of which can be treated easily, and others that can be serious.

Tinea pedis, better known as athlete's foot, can be treated with over-the-counter medications, but treatment can take over a year to be effective. There are also prescription medications that can successfully treat this fungus, but they are more costly and can have serious side effects.

Madura foot (also called eumycetoma or fungal mycetoma) is a fungal infection that can spread to muscle and bone, and left untreated can eventually cause death or severe disabilities. It is known as a fungal infection of the poor; it usually enters the body through cuts. Treatment options are often antifungal medications and surgeries, and sometimes amputation.

Spelunkers' lung is a fungal infection caused by *Histoplasma capsulatum.* This fungal infection comes from contact with bird or bat droppings in dry areas such as caves. It can also be contracted by working in old buildings infested with dry bat or bird droppings. Farmers and landscapers are at risk of acquiring this infectious fungus as well. This infection can be deadly, especially in those with weakened immune systems.

One reason it can be difficult to treat fungal infections is the similarities between we humans and fungi. We share about 50 percent of our genes. This makes it particularly diffi-cult for drug manufacturers to develop drugs that can treat the fungal infection without harming human cells. We also know that fungi love a curveball. Remember that fungi are master chemists, and they can develop resistance to drugs at a much quicker pace than bacteria.

Most fungi thrive at temperatures between 77 and 86°F (25 and 30°C). There are also species that thrive at temperatures below 32°F (0°C) as well as at temperatures of 104°F (40°C) and even higher. That leaves our bodies, with a standard temperature of approximately 98°F (37°C), situated in the middle of a zone to which the majority of fungi have not adapted. Was this a driver in how we evolved to circumvent the need to fight off incessant fungal pathogens? A paper from 2010 describing a study conducted by researchers at Albert Einstein College of Medicine at Yeshiva University supports this idea. The researchers noted that cold-blooded reptiles and amphibians are affected by thousands of fungal pathogens, while warm-blooded mammals are only affected by a few hundred. The researchers developed a mathematical model showing that the optimal temperature for fighting off pathogenic fungi and minimizing the costs of doing so (in terms of needing to increase food consumption) fell in the 98°F range.[1]

There are many parallels to fungi and the human experience. We have evolved from a common ancestor and the more deeply we look, the more overlaps will be found. Fungi essentially are helping us to better understand ourselves.

been evolving for about five thousand years. This living tradition uses some terms that, if you are not familiar with TCM, you likely will not understand fully. We include this work because it is some of the most informative in the world and we are committed to including the voices of those beyond the

Eurocentric world in which we find ourselves. There are many excellent resources on TCM should you want to dive in further.

The Role and Risks of Research

Each year more and more studies on the healing properties and health benefits of mushrooms are published in peer-reviewed journals. It can be dizzying to keep up with, but we think it is important to people interested in using mushrooms for their health to know about this research so they can make an informed decision. To our knowledge, information on medicinal mushrooms is not included in any American medical doctor training, so we must educate ourselves. Paul Stamets's seminal *Growing Gourmet and Medicinal Mushrooms* published in 1993 included information on the science at that time, but much more research has been done since then.

When possible, we have included in our summaries of the published research the doses used in the studies, because your doctor likely will not be able to guide you. These doses may be a good place to start but we recommend you always listen to what your body is telling you when trying a new mushroom. We also report as best we can on the way the mushrooms were prepared for the study participants. Often this is not described in much detail because they are using a commercial product. Other preparations are not possible to replicate at home. In chapter 6 we explained how to make water and alcohol extracts that will allow you to experience the medicinal benefits of these fourteen mushrooms and can easily be prepared in your kitchen.

Like all areas of scientific investigation, the focus is biased to some degree by what funding is available to researchers. For the most part, pharmaceutical companies are not interested in funding research into mushrooms that people can easily grow for themselves, because there is no potential profit in it, unless they can come up with some complicated extraction process that no one else can replicate. The rate of scientific investigation into most mushrooms is slow. Nonetheless, the field of inquiry into medicinal mushrooms pushes forward, especially in Japan and China where there are millennia-old traditions of working with these fungi.

The pharmaceutical giants still have the lion's share of medicine sales. Recently many websites have arisen that are funded by these giants and will advise people to be careful with medicinal mushrooms such as Shiitakes, stating that these mushrooms are "Likely Safe" to eat and "Possibly Unsafe" when used as medicinals. We argue again that medicines that have withstood the test of thousands of years, that are still in use and effective, should be taken seriously. Meanwhile, these supplies of information are loaded with ads for pharmaceuticals that make navigating the information dizzying. We encourage people to use their understanding of what humans have been doing for long periods of time; those things are often healthy for the mind and body.

A lot of medicinal mushrooms have been studied around the world in the last fifty years, and the popularity of these mushrooms has led to more studies. This is encouraging, but we need to balance the attention paid to the effects of isolated chemical compounds with studies of the effects of utilizing the whole mushroom. The connection between our food, community, and medicine is crucial. If these connections are unhealthy, then we are unhealthy.

Just as "no man is an island," no medicine is an island, nor is one plant, tree, animal, microbe or fungus. Researchers attempt to remove all variables and focus on one aspect of a system, but the variables are sometimes just as important as the individual parts. When we isolate one aspect of a system to study it, we can only hope to learn about that one aspect. If we do not study how a whole system works in concert, we are liable to miss out on important insights. In an Indigenous world, the mushroom is embedded in a deep context that includes stories, spirits, history, and direct human experience. The whole complex is the medicine, not just the mushroom, and certainly not an isolated compound.

The research is at different phases for the fourteen types of medicinal mushrooms we cover in this chapter. Multiple human clinical trials have been conducted for some mushrooms such as Reishi, Lion's Mane, and psychoactive mushrooms (*Psilocybe* species). Meta-analyses of these trials have been published that are comparable to analyses of plant-based or pharmaceutical medicines in terms of scientific rigor. Other species of mushrooms that have a long folk tradition of human use, such as Split Gill (*Schizophyllum commune*), Chaga, and Milky Caps have been studied only at the cellular level in the lab or in trials with mice.

Holistic Healing

We believe that health and healing is a much bigger concept than usually accepted by Western medicine, and thus in each profile we include a section called "Role in Holistic Healing." In this section, we discuss ways in which these specific mushrooms are part of the health of ecosystems or are used in ways other than healing the human body. When we learn about these gentle ways to get what we need, we realize that we do not have to destroy, wreck, or displace people and animals. Then we can start to live our lives in a more balanced way. Fungi can give us many of the tools we need to bring this full circle.

We have only begun to understand how important these fungal beings are and how they can be employed in many ways in the industrial sector. It should come as no surprise to see this common thread of the modern uses of these fungi to help clean up our planet.

Other Notes

Each profile also includes information on ethical wild harvesting techniques specific to each mushroom. Each time you harvest mushrooms from the wild, you have an opportunity to participate in the cycle of reciprocity that has sustained us all for thousands of years. We see these actions as a way to heal damaged ecosystems and our fragmented human-fungi relationships. This is wild co-tending—participating in a cycle of care in which both forest and humans receive nourishment.

We conclude each profile with brief cultivation notes. Here we orient you to which cultivation methods are most beneficial for each specific mushroom and any species-specific information you might need to get started with growing. These notes refer to earlier chapters in the book for additional details on particular species.

Cordyceps species
CORDYCEPS

Cordyceps are a complicated group of fungi that have been misunderstood across the centuries. Although current technology allows scientists to identify species genetically, rather than simply by their morphological characteristics, the waters are still muddy when it comes to Cordyceps identification.

The deep history of this mushroom arises from peoples from the Far East, who have used Cordyceps for thousands of years and were ahead of the West in understanding the properties and uses of Cordyceps. Cordyceps have become wildly popular in the United States, and use increases each year in the United States and Europe as information on how this mushroom can be supportive to the human body reaches more people. Of this I am glad, for the simple reason that Cordyceps can be cultivated with relative ease using simple equipment. In particular, *Cordyceps militaris* can be cultivated worldwide to produce quality medicine.

Cordyceps are part of the class Ascomycetes: they are part of a phylum of mushrooms that develop a club or a cup rather than a cap as their reproductive structure. The name Cordyceps comes from ancient Greek *kordyle,* meaning "club," and Latin *-ceps,* meaning "head" or "headed." About 1,300 species have been identified in the family Cordycipitaceae, and *C. militaris* is the most popular fungus cultivated in this family. Oh, what a wonderful little creature! This parasitic fungus captured my fascination over two decades ago. *C. militaris* is a small, bright orange fungus with a club-shape fruitbody that stands out in vivid contrast to the forest floor. *C. militaris* is known variously as the Caterpillar Fungus and Scarlet

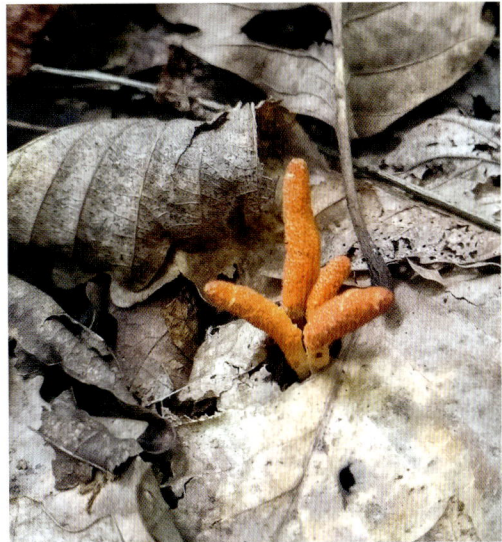

Figure 7.1. *Cordyceps militaris* in the forest.

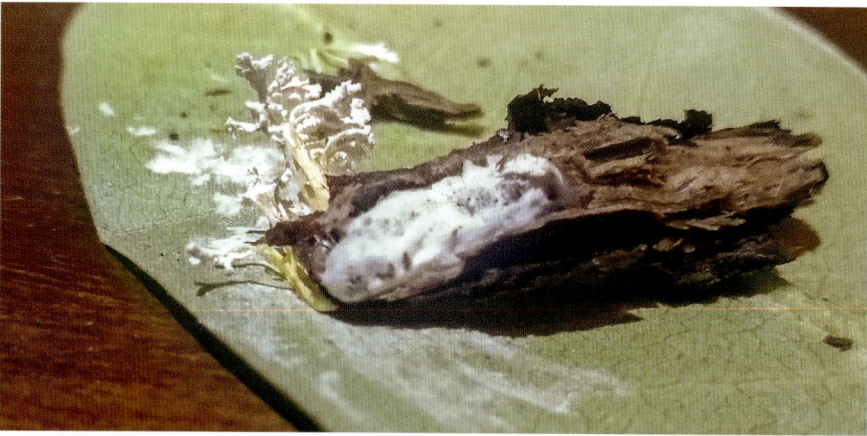

Figure 7.2. *Isaria tenuipes* fruiting from an insect body that it has turned into a sclerotium.

Caterpillar Fungus and lesser known as Cordyceps Flower. It can parasitize every species in the Lepidoptera order, which includes moths and butterflies. Other species in the Cordycipitaceae family parasitize only individual species of insects, including ants and even cicada grubs. Some Cordyceps are parasites of spiders, and others parasitize other types of mushrooms—truffles and false truffles.

In 1993, the species *Ophiocordyceps sinensis* (also called Caterpillar Fungus) gained worldwide attention when three Chinese runners broke multiple world records, a feat that their coach attributed to their ingestion of Cordyceps.[2] This species is native to high elevations in the mountains of China, Nepal, and Tibet. The name in Japanese for this mushroom is *Tochukaso*. The name in Chinese is *Dong Chong Xia Cao* or *Chongcao*, which means "Winter Worm—Summer Grass." In Tibetan, the name is *Yartsa Gunbu*. The "worm" is a reference to the larval stage of the Ghost Moth (*Gazoryctra novigannus*), the insect that this fungus parasitizes. The "grass" is a reference to the fruiting body of *O. sinensis*. It used to be believed that the "worm" became the "grass" in the spring and summer and then turned back into an insect during the winter, but it's now understood that this is not the case. Taken at face value, traditional stories may not make sense from an outsider's perspective. Often, though, these stories have a much deeper meaning that has been lost or is not easy to interpret.

British doctor William Watson, MD, wrote an account of finding Cordyceps in the West Indies in 1763. The mushroom was described by his colleague Dr. Huxham in this way:

> *The* vegetable fly *is found on the island of Dominica, and (excepting that it has no wings) resembles the drone in both size and colour more than any other English insect. The month of May it buries itself in the earth*

and begins to vegetate. By the latter end of July the tree is arrived at its full growth, and resembles a coral branch; and is about 3 inches high, and bears several little pods, which dropping become worms, and from thence flies, like the English caterpillar.[3]

This quote illustrates the limited knowledge 240 years ago about the Cordyceps fungi. We see that the two doctors did not realize they were observing a parasitization process.

If you live in an area where deer truffles (*Elaphomyces* spp.) grow, you might find Drumstick Truffleclub (*Elaphocordyceps capitata*) or Goldenthread Cordyceps (*Tolypocladium ophioglossoides*, but also called *Cordyceps ophioglossoides* and *Elaphocordyceps ophioglossoides*) which parasitize deer truffles.

Ant Eater (*Ophiocordyceps myrmecophila*) parasitizes ants. An infected ant is driven by an impulse to lock down its jaws onto a twig and exhibit zombie-like behavior. The fungal mycelium then secretes a cocktail of acids and enzymes that dissolve the muscle tissue in the mandible so that the ant cannot release its hold on the twig. The *O. myrmecophila* fungus essentially turns the insect body into a sclerotium, a hardened mass of mycelium used as an energy store. When conditions are right, the fruitbody grows and the spore-producing area (which is called the *perithecium*) releases spores to contact the next victim. *Isaria tenuipes* goes through a similar cycle, but with moths or butterflies as the host insect. Figure 7.2 shows an insect that has become a sclerotium.

In the mountains of the Southern Appalachians, we typically find about ten wild *C. militaris* mushrooms each year, usually by happenstance, not because we hunt for them. They just happen to "show up" in front of us. The location varies from year to year. My

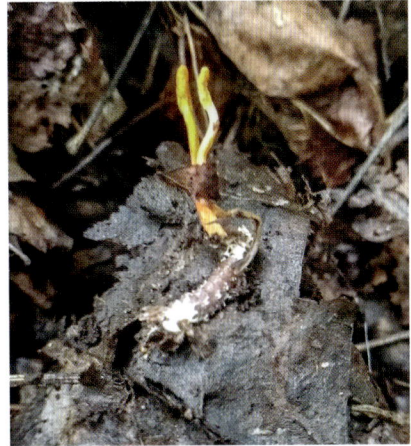

Figure 7.3. *Cordyceps militaris* fruiting from larvae.

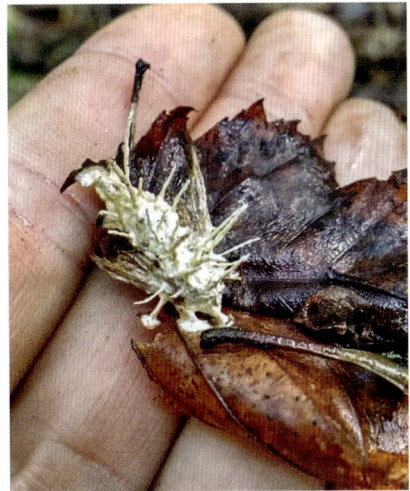

Figure 7.4. *Akanthomyces* mycelium infesting the body of an adult moth and running out onto a leaf.

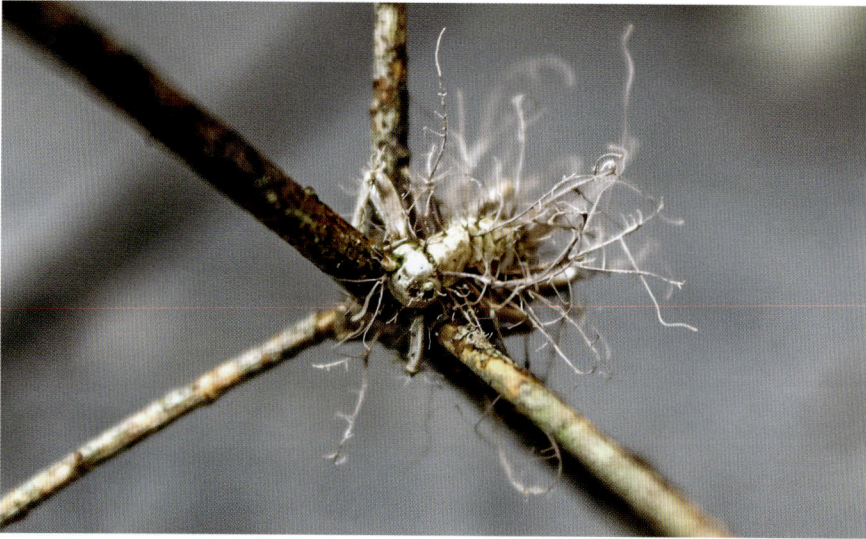

Figure 7.5. Cordyceps growing on a Carolina Leaf Roller (a type of cricket).

oldest daughter called to my attention that one year there will be plenty of Cordyceps in a particular cove or close to a creek, but then they will not show up again in that spot for a few years, sometimes many years. Could we simply be missing them? It's possible, but my daughter and I both have sharp, well-trained eyes, and these mushrooms are vivid little orange clubs that stick out like miniature Cheetos from moss-covered rocks and logs. It's my theory that the host insects make themselves scarce in the area that the fruiting bodies are inhabiting, which leads to the cycle of appearance and disappearance over time.

Paul Stamets has studied fungi in the genus *Metarhizium*. This type of Cordyceps infects termites and carpenter ants. Stamets found that there are certain stages in which insects infected by *Metarhizium* fungi will be ferreted out by the rest of the colony. They quickly dispose of infected colony members. My suspicion is that something comparable is happening among the moths and butterflies in our woods. They can detect that an area is ripe with Cordyceps fruiting bodies and will avoid it for a period of time until it becomes safe again: another example of how a forest is able to balance itself.

Traditional Uses

Along with Reishi, Cordyceps is one of the most important fungi to TCM practitioners. It has been used to treat infertility and erectile dysfunction, to increase stamina, to support kidney and lung health, and as an aphrodisiac. Cordyceps is mentioned in the *Shen Nong Ben Cao Jing,* a classic text of Chinese medicine from 220 to 280 CE. Through the lens of TCM, the kidneys

150

are responsible for pulling the *qi,* or life force, into the lungs from the air. Cordyceps tonifies both yin and yang in Chinese Medicine.

In *The Fungal Pharmacy,* mycologist and herbalist Robert Rogers concludes: "Cordyceps strengthen both the mind and body at a very basic level, replenishing yin jing and restoring the deep energy depleted by excessive stress."[4]

Research on Human Health Effects

Modern science is catching up to the idea that Cordyceps can be a powerful medicinal mushroom, and as traditional uses have been brought to light, they have guided scientific investigations. For example, in a recent meta-analysis looking at 31 randomized controlled clinical trials of Cordyceps, a group of researchers found the fungus to have at least 190 possible biological mechanisms through which it improves kidney health, including reducing inflammation and boosting immune function.[5]

CANCER

A meta-analysis of 12 randomized controlled trials with a total of 928 patients who received Cordyceps in addition to standard cancer treatments concluded that *C. sinensis* tends to result in improved tumor response rate, immune function, and quality of life while simultaneously reducing the likelihood of adverse reactions to the standard treatments.[6]

KIDNEY FUNCTION

Improving kidney function is one of the key uses of Cordyceps in TCM. A recent meta-analysis of seventeen studies with *Jinshuibao*, a powdered extract from *C. sinensis*, concluded that it has a positive benefit on patients with chronic renal failure.[7] Diabetic-related kidney failure is often treated by reducing blood sugar levels but without support for the kidneys. Patients with this condition have often already sustained kidney damage, and some researchers suggest Cordyceps could be added to diabetes treatments to reduce the impact on the kidneys.[8]

A 2019 study looked at another form of Cordyceps-derived medicine in those with diabetes before renal failure sets in. They found that when standard treatment was supplemented with Cordyceps, kidney function was improved more than when the standard treatment was used alone. This offers some hope for future prevention of diabetic-related kidney failure.[9]

LUNG FUNCTION

In TCM, the lungs are closely linked with the kidneys, and Cordyceps has also been investigated for its benefits in lung disorders. A 2019 review of studies of

Cordyceps on chronic obstructive pulmonary disease (COPD) found fifteen studies that, under meta-analysis, showed Cordyceps to improve lung functions and reduce symptoms, while increasing exercise endurance and quality of life.[10] A placebo-controlled study of treatment of tuberculosis patients (which affects about 14 million people globally) found a significant improvement rate of clinical symptoms in those that received Cordyceps in addition to chemotherapy.[11]

ATHLETIC PERFORMANCE AND ENERGY

Since the effects of Cordyceps were mistaken for those of steroids in the infamous 1993 event, many have sought out Cordyceps to improve athletic performance. There has been less research done in this area. One study was designed to see if daily supplementation with *C. sinensis* (2 g per day) improved athletic performance in thirty physically active people over a period of twelve weeks. Researchers found a significant improvement of athletic performance and called for more work to be done.[12]

One subsequent study looked at the effects of taking Cordyceps (1 g) immediately before high-intensity exercise in healthy volunteers. Muscle biopsies taken before and after exercise for two days showed significantly faster muscle repair in the group taking Cordyceps. This rapid muscle-damage resolution seemed to be an effect of stem-cells being recruited to the muscles, but more work is needed to fully understand the biochemical mechanism of Cordyceps's beneficial effect on muscle repair.[13]

IMMUNE FUNCTION

Research on the immune modulation effects of *Ophiocordyceps sinensis* and *C. militaris* is still at the lab- and animal-testing phase, but a 2024 review concludes that Cordyceps have the potential to be effective immune modulators.[14] And a clinical trial with forty healthy adults showed that drinking a functional beverage from the mycelium of *C. militaris* daily for eight weeks led to a significant increase in various biomarkers that indicate more healthy immune system activity in those taking the beverage than in the control group.[15]

PROSTATE HEALTH

In a study designed to investigate if *C. militaris* could be used to treat sexual dysfunction and benign prostate hyperplasia (enlargement), or BPH, in older men, subjects received two daily capsules containing 6 mg of cordycepin along with supporting compounds for a three-month period. Test results showed increased urinary flow and decreased prostate size. Many subjects also reported improved sexual function.[16]

Role in Holistic Healing

Because Cordyceps is easy to cultivate and has so many beneficial effects, we see it having a domino effect on society. For example, Cordyceps increases the efficiency of mitochondria, raising ATP levels to improve energy levels.[17] This can allow people to remain more active as they age, continuing to spend quality time with friends and family and living life to the fullest. It is important that we are able to grow fungi that can provide clarity and help sustain energy, even in the face of the toxins in the modern food supply. Many Cordyceps products are now widely available, from chocolate bars to experimental energy drinks.

Preliminary research has found Cordyceps to be an effective treatment for the symptoms of COVID-19 with no significant side effect.[18] So, why not start with this known, ancient medicine, rather than an experimental vaccine?

Overconsumption of sugar and under-exercising are two drivers of chronic disease in modern society. When people recognize these harmful habits and take steps to make changes, Cordyceps can be of support. As noted above, research shows that these fungi can help repair kidney damage that may have been caused by consuming too much sugar. It can also improve lung function, increase energy levels, and reduce muscle repair time, all of which make exercise easier and more enjoyable.

Exposure to environmental toxins can lead to asthma and other adverse effects on lung function. Perhaps you are one of the many people in North America who suffer from asthma. Cordyceps can improve lung function and increase oxygen uptake. I had asthma as a child, even though I was raised in the countryside, away from industrial and urban pollution. Using Cordyceps, along with other healthy lifestyle choices, has increased my lung capacity.

As researchers gain understanding of the life cycles of some species of Cordyceps, more uses are being found for species that parasitize insects that are considered pests. The ability to control pests with biological means is just as important as it was before "Better Living Through Chemistry" came along. For example, a product that targets termites and carpenter ants with a pathogenic fungus and stops them from destroying buildings would be a great benefit. I believe that if humans engage their creativity and intellect to find targeted solutions to pest problems, instead of spraying pesticides and insecticides that kill every insect in their path, these natural secrets would soon be revealed. The old notion that an ounce of prevention is worth a pound of cure rings true here. If people stop spraying harmful chemicals that destroy waterways, beneficial creatures, and human health, then there will be no need to "cure" the problems created by the spraying in the first place.

Cultivation Notes

The purported medicinal activity of Cordyceps has created high demand and driven overharvesting. Even though there is now greater awareness of the scarcity of this mushroom, wealthy people have continued to purchase this rare mushroom, especially in China. It is estimated that the wild population in Tibet in recent decades has dropped by over 90 percent. This has driven prices sky high, reaching upwards of $25,000 per kilo.[19]

C. militaris can be cultivated with relative ease if one can control the environment and create a nutrient broth to provide its mycelium with what it needs to produce a club (fruiting body). No insects need to die in the process. The ability to cultivate copious amounts of this powerful fungus should soon reduce overharvesting of these mushrooms from the wild. Affordable and widely available Cordyceps species is the goal.

C. militaris is cultivated indoors only and requires adherence to strict standards. We may be able to relax these standards as the cultures are developed to be more tolerant of a wider range of growing conditions. Ryan Paul Gates of Terrestrial Fungi is one of the most talented Cordyceps growers in the United States (refer to the Cordyceps cultivation instructions on page 116 for details of his method), so he is a great resource for additional information.

Ethical Wild Harvesting

Cordyceps mushrooms are far too rare to be simply wild harvested for direct sale or even for making dual extractions for sale. The small number of Cordyceps that are found in the wild should be collected only for starting indoor cultures. The number of *C. militaris* fruiting bodies we tend to find in the Southern Appalachians can range from only two or three and up to a dozen or more in really good years. We leave the majority of these where they are and every year we harvest and culture only a few. In Tibet, too, overharvesting of *O. sinensis* is a problem. The market commands high prices on these wild populations, and there has been a sharp decline.

Fomes fomentarius

AMADOU

Amadou, or *Fomes fomentarius*, is a perennial white-rot polypore that grows on various species of trees. Birch (*Betula* spp.) is the most common host here in the Southern Appalachians. Beech trees also play host to *F. fomentarius* in eastern North America. In the western North America, it can be found on alder or aspen trees, and in Europe it is most commonly associated with sycamore. We rarely find it on oak trees (*Quercus* spp.) here in North America, but oak tends to be the most common host in the Mediterranean. *F. fomentarius* occurs in China and Japan and is also found on the African continent. It has been documented in Uzbekistan on walnut, poplar, and apple trees.

Amadou is a saprotrophic fungus, but it is also known to be an enervated parasite, which means it can only parasitize a tree already in a weakened state. Our observation is that many species blur the line between saprotroph and parasite when the hosts are already beginning to weaken for some other reason. The fungi take up a role as natural recyclers of wood into food, housing, nutrients, nurseries, and the next cycle of life as the dying trees are reintegrated into the forest floor.

F. fomentarius goes by many common names: Amadou, Horse's Hoof Fungus, Surgeon's Agaric, Tinder Conk, and Tinder Polypore. And with every mention of *F. fomentarius*, Ötzi the Iceman immediately comes to mind, as well as another of the common names for *F. fomentarius*—Iceman Fungus. *F. fomentarius* is just one of the mushrooms found on the person of this 5,000-year-old

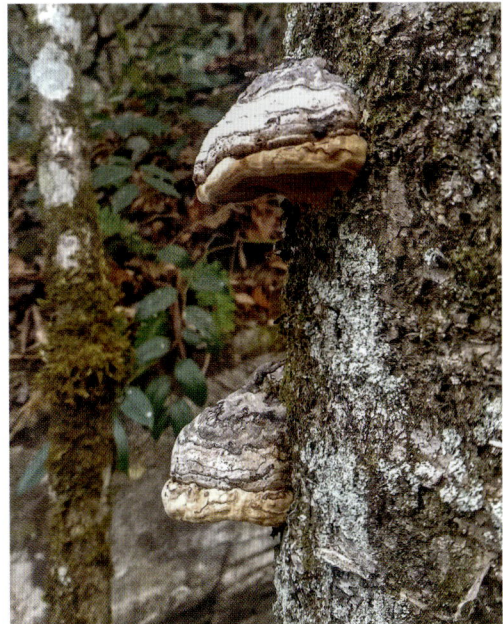

Figure 7.6. Amadou on Yellow Birch (*Betula alleghaniensis*).

155

mummified man from the early Copper Age (around 3250 BCE), which was excavated in the early 1990s in the Italian Alps near the Austrian border. Names for *F. fomentarius* in Norwegian are *Knuskkjuke*, *Knusk* and *Fyrsvamp*; *Duovlečatná*, *Duvle*, and *Tjádná* in Sami; and *Fnöskticka* in Swedish.

Amadou's fruiting bodies persist year to year and occur with a range of colors. Young mushrooms have a light gray or silver cuticle, or the cuticle may be tan or even brown. The fungus appears in tree trunks and has roughly the shape of a horse's hoof (thus the common name of Horse's Hoof Fungus). If *F. fomentarius* parasitizes living trees, the growths will persist even after the death of the host tree. Some years after the tree dies, the fruiting bodies will change color, turning nearly black. In the Southern Appalachians, we find that these fruiting bodies are usually no longer living and are not to be used as medicine, but in other areas of the world, this may not necessarily hold true.

Just as with most of the wood-loving species that we cultivate or wild harvest, *F. fomentarius* enjoys a bit of a nitrogen boost. It has the ability and appetite to break down pollen grains, which are high in nitrogen, to supplement its usual cellulose diet. I wonder if the pollen dispersal times coincide with *F. fomentarius* using this extra boost to produce their massive amounts of spores? This has not been studied yet to our knowledge.

This very hard, woody conk (shelf or bracket polypore) mushroom can live thirty years or longer. The growth layers in the *F. fomentarius* conk provide clues as to the age of the fruiting body—it's similar to counting tree rings. The pattern of layers show that these mushrooms grow very little in the winter. I have observed quite a bit of growth in the springtime and early summer. Our springtime conditions are typically wet, and sometimes there is an early July drought. Rains start back up in August through autumn. In such conditions, is it possible for two distinct growth layers to form in the same year? According to a 2023 report in *Science Advances*, "Typically, between one and three new hymenial layers are produced each year, from which the fungus can release up to 240 million spores/cm^2 per hour."[20] Given that these mushrooms can live to be thirty years old, the number of spores produced in a mushroom's lifetime is frankly astonishing.

Traditional Uses

Regardless of where you live in this world, it is more than likely that your ancestors, only a few generations back, used Amadou in several ways—as a mycotextile to make decorations or hats or for practical medical purposes.

Parts of this fungus have been found in European Mesolithic campsites dating to around 8000 to 7000 BCE. As mentioned earlier, Ötzi the Iceman

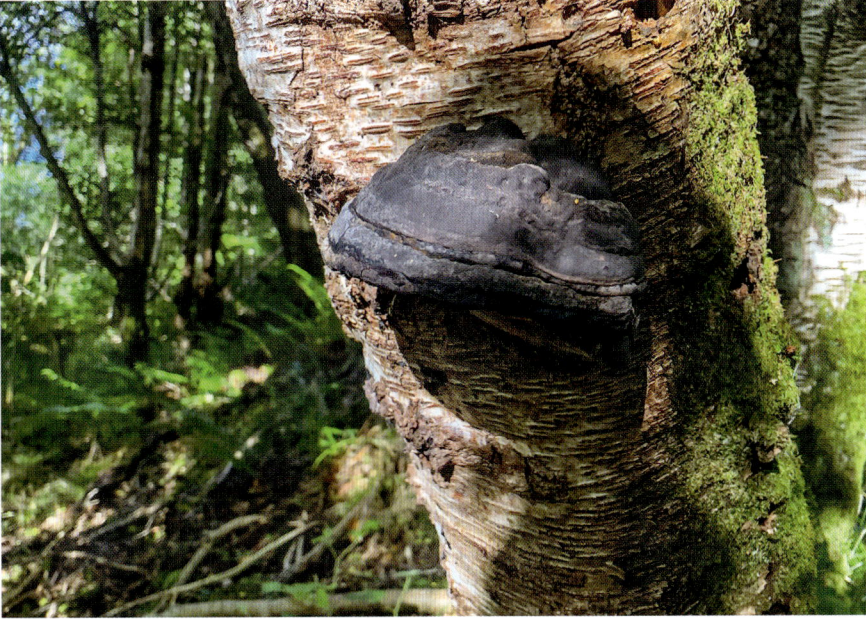

Figure 7.7. Dead *F. fomentarius* still attached to the host tree.

was carrying *F. fomentarius*. It is likely that Ötzi was using the Amadou as a way to carry fire. The conk, when thoroughly dried, can be used to catch a spark or to carry a smoldering ember. The fibers of the conk will keep the ember gently fed. A carefully tended ember can be carried from one site to another, often for many hours, either directly in the conk or in wads of prepared Amadou packed into hollow horns or clay vessels. These smoldering embers could be revitalized into a fire when camp was made. In the driving wind, snow, or rain this could be the difference between life and death. Birch has a terpene-rich bark that burns easily even when moist. This terpene is called *betulin*. When an ember is carefully taken from the *F. fomentarius* container, laid in a nest of fine shavings of birch bark, and awoken from its slumber with the breath, a fire can be quickly kindled.

F. fomentarius is one of the most dominant perennial species in more northern latitudes where the wind, snow, and rain can be deadly for the unprepared. It is the perfect candidate to establish a lifesaving fire in extreme weather conditions, and it also provides an easier method to make fire when the temperature is colder. Amadou will smolder for hours, even days, when occasionally tended. This careful tending and carrying of fire into weather extremes was most likely how humans were able to explore and live in harsh weather regions. It possibly allowed human expansion north after the last ice age.

I have put forth the idea that Ötzi the Iceman was using this mushroom for moxibustion as well as for carrying fire. Moxibustion is the practice of burning an herb (usually Artemisia or Mugwort) to transfer heat close to points on the body to warm a meridian or to drive out cold. Mycologist Peter McCoy has independently come up with this idea too. In fact, Peter has posed the question: Is it possible that what we know as Eastern Medicine may have *not* originated in the East? This is an excellent question, and the traditional uses of *F. fomentarius* may provide an answer.

Ethnobotanist Carl Linnaeus travelled to Sampi, the lands of the Sami people, in the early 1700s. (This area is now parts of Scandinavia and Russia.) Mycologist Ingvar Svanberg reports on Linnaeus' findings:

> *In his itinerary from the summer of 1732 that the Sami in Jokkmokk used* Fomes fomentarius *growing on the south side of birch trees for a kind of moxa-therapy. An amount the size of a pea is placed on the sore place, ignited with a birch twig and allowed to burn away gradually. It is placed where the pain is worst, and the treatment is often repeated two or three times. This causes sores which often remain open for six months, but which must not be treated, being left instead to heal of their own accord. It is used against all pains: headaches, stings, stomach aches, gouty and rheumatic pain, etc. It is a universal remedy among the Lapps.* [21]

The common names of Surgeon's Styptic and Surgeon's Sponge arise from traditional use of *F. fomentarius* by dentists, surgeons, and barbers to absorb fluids and stanch bleeding, and as an antibacterial. This was before the understanding of germ theory, but through observation, people learned that Amadou has the ability to prevent or even treat infected wounds. Armed with this knowledge and the ability to find this mushroom growing in the wild, people in poor, rural areas also made use of Amadou in place of expensive gauzes and manufactured wound dressings.

Surgeons used this fungus to soak up fluids during surgical procedures. Accidental cuts, scrapes, or nicks could be quickly treated with small strips of this fungus to stop bleeding and, more importantly, infection. It would have been difficult for surgeons to count on repeat business if customers ended up with accidental cuts that became infected.

Amadou was also used as a poultice or as bandages to dress wounds; this use was common until the 1800s. The fruiting body was prepared in different ways according to the intended uses. First, the cuticle would be removed along with the hymenium, the spore-producing surface. The remaining center part of the fruiting body is referred to as the *trama*. The trama feels as soft as velvet. It can be wetted and gently pounded to tease the fibers apart until the trama is as thin as needed.

The pounded-thin trama has been used in Eurasia to treat skin conditions and wounds. These bandages can retain their potency for decades. After prepping the fungi for use as bandages, the bandages can immediately be used, or they can be dried and stored in a hemp sack for as long as twenty years.[22] Interestingly, a piece of pounded trama can also be soaked in potassium nitrate (likely sourced from urine) and crushed charcoal to be used as a fire starter.

In many parts of Europe and Asia, trama has been used to make hats, clothing, and decorations. Some of the traditions are still practiced today. Many online vendors offer hats and beautiful vests made from Amadou, as well as finely crafted table centerpieces.

The Khanty People of Siberia burn *F. fomentarius* as an incense in the houses of people who have recently crossed over. Visiting guests would also be ritually purified by smudging with *F. fomentarius* smoke to safeguard themselves and the houses, so they would not fall under any negative influence of the recently deceased.[23]

We have not come across any references to the traditional uses of Amadou in Africa but we did find one tantalizing sentence about an African creation story featuring Tinder Fungus: "The African Pangves originate the creation of Earth and sky from a tinder fungus."[24] This is interesting, and leaves us curious about more of this story.

Research on Human Health Effects

Modern research has validated the ancestral wisdom carried from this mushroom, from its use to cauterize wounds and as a styptic, as well as its anti-inflammatory and antiviral properties and its antitumor effects. The research has not yet made it into human clinical trials but I'm sure that continuing research will reveal new uses and corroborate the ancient uses for this mushroom.

CANCER

The science of using Amadou mushrooms to treat cancer has not yet reached the human clinical trial stage. Laboratory studies have found that extracts of Amadou can cause cancer cell-death and reduce proliferation of human cancer cells including gastric, breast, lung, cervical, hepatocellular, leukemia, bladder, esophageal, and skin cancer cells. A few studies have used Amadou extracts with mice and found them to slow tumor growth and prolong lifespan.[25]

DIABETES

The Amadou fungus excretes compounds that are thought to prevent other organisms from digesting the carbohydrates in the wood that the fungus is consuming. Diabetes researchers reason that these compounds might also inhibit human enzymes responsible for digesting carbohydrates and thus slow the processing of carbohydrates into sugar. Research on this hypothesis is still in the lab phase and not yet being tested with human subjects.[26]

ANTIMICROBIAL

As antibiotic resistance in pathogenic organisms continues to increase, it seems important to keep searching for natural solutions to this human-made problem. Lab work since the 1980s has found Amadou to act against viruses (including HIV), bacteria (gram positive and negative), and fungal infections (such as candida).[27] This work is in the lab phase only. A team from Turkey looked at the impact of Amadou extracts on various microbes that can cause post-surgical infections in hospitals, including some known to be resistant to pharmaceutical antibiotics. Testing the fungal preparation directly against the pharmaceuticals, the researchers found the mushroom performed significantly better.[28]

Role in Holistic Healing

F. fomentarius has been intertwined with human history at least since humans moved into cold climates, and is emerging into modern recognition as a medicinal mushroom that can improve the health of humans, pets, the environment, and the planet overall. The widespread uses of this mushroom by many of our ancestors could do with some rekindling—for incense, fabrics, or simply traditional medicine—as a way to reconnect with those ancestral lineages. Uses of this mushroom are still being uncovered. The deeper understanding of what roles these fungi play in ecosystems offers a better understanding of the world and also helps to unlock the mysteries of nature and develop methodologies to solve potential human-caused problems.

Working with Amadou is a way to reconnect with ancestors. The simple task of using this fungus to carry fire rather than relying on modern matches or lighters is empowering; it gives a deeper appreciation of the many blessings nature makes freely available.

Horse's Hoof Fungus is an important mushroom to carry in an herbal first aid kit. It can be used in conjunction with adhesive bandages to dress deep cuts in situations when immediate medical attention is not available; it could mean the difference between a serious infection and quick healing.

Biosorption of toxic molecules, such as dyes from industrial effluent, is another one of Amadou's superpowers. This ability to clean up waterways is a crucial aspect of healing humanity's relationship with planet Earth. *F. fomentarius* can be cultivated in ways to change the structure of the mycelium to increase the capacity of biosorption. How many other fungi have aspects that can be increased by something as simple as cultivation conditions or methods?

A use could also be found for Amadou as smoke for beekeepers when working their hives. The nature of this fungus to smoke for prolonged periods (as previously mentioned to carry embers) makes a good case for honeybee smokers. The ability of Amadou to hold embers and smoke but not become engulfed in flames also suggests it has some flame-retardant properties (another common name is Tinder Polypore). It is being investigated as a possible insulative material. This may require different growing conditions to produce the desired results of increasing flame-retardant properties and retaining the insulative nature.

Cultivation Notes

The cultivation of *F. fomentarius* on various substrates is similar to the cultivation of other saprotrophic fungi on sawdust or grains. This method of cultivation is typically used to produce mycelium for biomass for biosorption applications. Chapters 4 and 5 covered details of working with sawdust substrate.

Ethical Wild Harvesting

Fall and winter are great times to hunt these mushrooms because they are easier to see without the canopy and understory of leaves blocking the view. This mushroom fruitbody is long lived, so please be mindful to not overharvest the fruitbodies. We typically find trees with ten or more or fruitbodies and then harvest only a few out of each dozen or so conks that I come across.

Fomitopsis betulina
BIRCH POLYPORE

*F*omitopsis betulina (previously known as *Piptoporus betulinus*) goes by many common names including Birch Polypore, Razor Strop Mushroom, Iceman Fungus, Birch Bracket, and Surgeon's Agaric. It grows on dead birch trees (*Betula* spp.) and is occasionally found on beech trees (*Fagus* spp.). Birch Polypores are saprotrophic, and some sources report them as parasitic; however, we have not witnessed this in our Southern Appalachian region. They are common across North America, Europe, and West Asia.

Birch Polypore is a brown rot fungus. Brown rot fungi break down cellulose while altering lignin in their host, which results in a reddish-brown color of the wood. Typically, the wood becomes blocky and brittle or cracks apart into chunks. The fruiting body of Birch Polypore looks like a marshmallow emerging from birch trees. This occurs in early to mid-fall in our region. The young, pure white fruiting bodies eventually transition to a brown or tan cap. *F. betulina* has a springy texture when young and becomes harder and cork-like as it ages. Taking a cross section of this mushroom reveals a pure white interior.

The margin remains white and rolled inward even as the fruitbodies age. Occasionally, the margins may be undulating, giving the mushroom a scalloped bivalve appearance from the top. Fully mature Birch Polypore mushrooms remain on the tree for at least one year and sometimes up to several years. They are annual fungi, meaning they produce growth only in one season. They emerge in the early fall, grow to maturity, release spores and then begin to degrade. Often in the following spring, algae grow on the decaying caps, and mold may develop on the hymenium. It is not recommended to harvest these older fruiting bodies for use in tea or medicine.

Traditional Uses

Birch Polypore has been found on the bodies of ancient people, including spores on the teeth of skeletal remains in archaeological sites. Pieces of Birch Polypore were found, along with *Fomes fomentarius*, in the possession of Ötzi the Iceman, as described in the *F. fomentarius* profile on page 155.

Researchers speculate that Ötzi may have been using Birch Polypore for a spiritual purpose (as a "charm" to ward off spirits that were giving him problems) or for a physical health purpose (as a tea to combat the intestinal parasites, whipworm, he was found to have). Birch Polypore has been traditionally used as an antiparasitic. Some resources claim it has high levels of agaric acid, a fatty acid, but we have not found any research confirming the agaric acid content of Birch Polypore. Some of the compounds in this mushroom are useful in dealing with amoebic parasites.

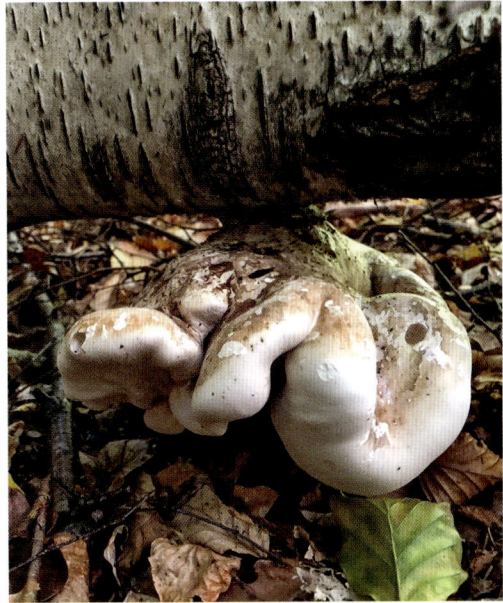

Figure 7.8. Single large Birch Polypore fruiting from under a fallen log in Scotland.

F. betulina accumulates betulin from the bark of birch trees. Betulin is antibacterial, used to help keep wounds clean and speed their healing. The distilled bark of birch trees produces an oil that contains betulin. This oil is highly flammable and it can be applied to the skin as an insect repellent, but it is too toxic to be taken internally or applied to a wound. *F. betulina* accumulates the betulin in doses safe for humans to ingest. The birch trees and the Birch Polypore are inseparable. Indigenous people see and understand such connections. The spirit is the medicine, the tree is the medicine, the mushroom is the medicine, and the medicine is the spirit.

The Birch Polypore was used as a razor strop in Victorian times. A cross section of consistent thickness would be sliced and tacked upon a board so it could be used to put the finishing touches on a straight razor. Possibly, the mushroom's antibacterial, antiseptic, and styptic properties could have been carried over onto the razor being sharpened.

Small slices of this fungi cut out in the shape of corns and blisters have been utilized to provide relief to the affected areas when directly applied. Insect specimens were also mounted on cut fruitbodies of Birch Polypore. The white flesh of this mushroom would provide contrast to obtain a clear, crisp view of the insect being studied.

Birch Polypore has been used in the form of a powder or an ash to stop bleeding. It has been used in the Baltic countries, including Russia, as a wound dressing by being cut into strips and applied to wounds to keep infections at bay and therefore to speed wound healing. This is similar to the

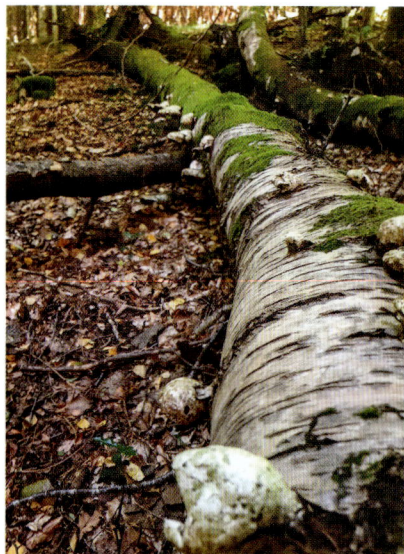

Figure 7.9. Birch polypore fruit bodies in various stages of fruiting and decay (Scotland).

description of such strips in the *F. fomentarius* profile on page 158. A water infusion was used in Baltic countries and Russia as a calming agent, and the dried powder was used as a painkiller.[29]

Research on Human Health Effects

F. betulina is intertwined with human history more deeply than most people realize. From medicine to industrial uses, this mushroom is now receiving attention from researchers and is starting to gain some traction. There is a reason that the uses of these mushrooms have remained with us from lithic technology all the way up through the Information Age. They work. Much work has been done to find new uses for *F. betulina*, and much of this path is still out in front of us.

Most of the research with *F. betulina* is still in the early stages. In the lab it has been confirmed to have antibacterial, antiparasitic, antiviral, anti-inflammatory, anticancer, neuroprotective, and immunomodulating properties.[30] But we have found no reports of human clinical trials and very little in the way of preclinical trials. A handful of studies with mice suggest neuroprotective and anti-inflammatory properties.[31]

CANCER

Birch Polypore ethanol extract has been shown to effectively destroy various types of human cancer cells, while showing low toxicity to healthy surrounding cells. This effect was dose dependent. The more extract applied, the more cancer cells died.[32] Similar results have been achieved with other types of cancers including human lung carcinoma and colon adenocarcinoma, and rat glioma cell cultures.[33]

Some work indicates there may also be a difference in bioactivity between the fruiting bodies and the mycelium. Researchers found that a mycelium extract was significantly active against prostate cancer cells while a fruiting body extract showed moderate activity against both skin and prostate cancer cells.[34]

BACTERIA, VIRUSES, AND PARASITES

F. betulina has been shown to have antibacterial activity against various bacteria, including staphylococcus, and multiple fungal pathogens, including

Aspergillus species, which are known to cause diseases in those with immunodeficiency. The degree of antibacterial activity differs among different strains of Birch Polypore.[35]

Role in Holistic Healing

The historical uses of *F. betulina* are still more well known than the modern science, but science is catching up. This ancient mushroom is being used as an antiparasitic, in the same fashion as Ötzi the Iceman may have used it; this is an example of an unbroken chain of information passed down the generations. There are also new applications for which *F. betulina* shows potential.

Culturing mushroom mycelium in a controlled setting allows for growing and testing different strains for the presence of biocompounds, thus providing standardized medicine. This decreases pressure on the wild populations of Birch Polypore. Mycologists can continue to take samples from the wild, test them for concentrated and stronger values of medicinal compounds, and continue the ancient relationship with this medicinal fungal ally. Birch Polypore naturally fruits only once a year, but in cultivation it can produce year-round and thus be made more widely available.

One of the things that has always excited me about mycology is rediscovering the Indigenous uses. A 2019 article described the traditional uses of Birch Polypore as balls in games by people in Nordic countries. The authors speculate that the "fungi ball" is a forerunner of the rubber ball. At some point these fungi balls fell out of favor because rubber balls took their place.[36] We believe it is very important to carry these skills and crafts such as polypore ball-making into the future. Traditional uses and modern uses of fungi go hand in hand. We have no future without the past. Humanity cannot move forward in the world without the thousands of past generations pushing us forward and supporting us. Making a Birch Polypore ball is an ancestral craft that we may rediscover and pass on to our children, and it is a way of honoring the ancestors.

Most medicinal mushroom research and uses have focused on cancer and immune system modulation, and rightfully so. Piptamine is an antibiotic compound found in Birch Polypore; it is a great candidate for use in the field as an emergency wound dressing. The fresh mushroom is sliced thinly and applied to the wound. Some medicinal compounds found in fungi are only available from the host substrate and the associated fungi accumulate these compounds. Piptamine is different; it will grow in a lab setting and therefore can be utilized in controlled production facilities.

Birch Polypore tissue can also stop bleeding and speed the healing process. I imagine many similar modern uses for fungi. Large sheets of mycelium could be grown out and sliced to the desired thickness and impregnated into adhesive bandage–style dressings. These wound dressings would contain naturally produced compounds that are anti-inflammatory and antimicrobial to speed healing. Studies also show that Birch Polypore can produce certain enzymes that have the potential to prevent dental caries.[37] Yet another example of how we model many things after nature and are continuing to find new ways of copying our natural world and uncovering the secrets that are hidden from view.

Birch Polypore, along with other brown rot fungi, is being investigated for bioleaching heavy metals from woods treated with preservatives.[38] *F. betulina* is also being investigated as an accumulator of arsenic. One study found that Birch Polypores growing close to a contaminated industrial site accumulated ten times as much arsenic as those growing in an uncontaminated woodland.[39] There may be a way to actively use this fungus to clean up polluted soil to return it to agricultural production. These are examples of how this mushroom can work in collaboration with humans to clean up shared ecosystems.

Cultivation Notes

The cultivation of mycelium of Birch Polypore is simple. Outdoor cultivation is possible on birch logs, as described in chapter 2. Indoor cultivation is unknown in my experience; however, other mycologists may be cultivating these indoors.

Ethical Wild Harvesting

Birch Polypore shows up on the same trees year after year in the fall. We harvest only a few of those we find in the forest. The majority of the fruit we see occurs on dead birch trees with a diameter of four to eight inches. Birch Polypore likes colder climates, similar to Chaga, but can also be found in colder microclimates of generally warmer climates, which is why we have them here in the Southern Appalachians. We of course do not recommend harvesting when there are simply a few in an area; wait until you find an abundance, then take only a few, leaving plenty behind. These mushrooms have significant value in human history. Let's not make them scarce.

Ganoderma species

REISHI

Reishi mushrooms in a variety of shapes and sizes are in the genus *Ganoderma*. The Latin root of this genus name means "shiny skin." This quality is apparent to anyone who has seen this mushroom growing in the wild. The caps of these shelf fungi are so shiny they sometimes look artificial, as if a forest nymph had applied a layer of shellac all the way out to the margins. For this reason, they are also called Varnish Shelf.

Reishi mushrooms produce rusty brown spores that are ejected out of the hymenium under forceful hydraulic pressure, which causes the microscopic spores to rise upward, and most end up landing on the mushroom caps. The cap becomes layered in a thick dusting of millions of spores. These spores have a very low germination rate (approximately 50 percent). As a child, I used to watch in fascination as Paper Wasps chewed old wood on the outside of my grandpa's shed. They would use their powerful mandibles to strip the bleached-out cellulose, moving their heads in a side-to-side pattern. Remembering this years later, I realized I was seeing the same exact pattern on Reishi mushroom caps layered with spores. I knew that some types of plant seeds must be *scarified*—their hard shells must be weakened by passing through the digestive system of some animal, before they can germinate. This led me to ask: Is the low germination rate of *Ganoderma* spp. improved by scarification of spores in the digestive system of the insects that create these chewing patterns on top of the fruiting body? I believe that this could be the case. We still know so little about all the nuances of fungi that shape our world.

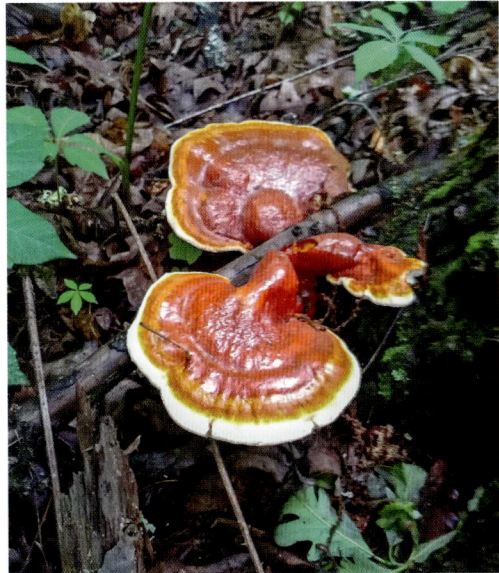

Figure 7.10. *Ganoderma tsugae* (Hemlock Reishi) on dead Hemlock (*Tsuga canadensis*).

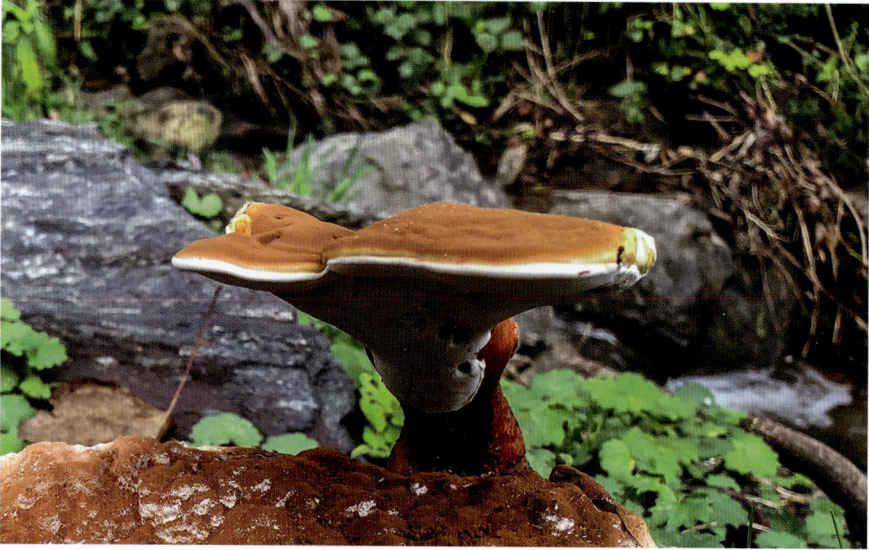

Figure 7.11. *Ganoderma curtisii* (Golden Reishi) growing off substrate block covered in spores.

Reishi are a white rot fungus. This simply means they tend to consume mostly lignin and leave the white fluffy cellulose behind. There are about eighty species in the *Ganoderma* genus. They occupy many forests worldwide and are both saprotrophic and parasitic fungi. Some are considered pathogens and others simply decomposers that recycle woody material back to the forest floor as fertile soils. Just like all mushrooms, Reishi occupy vital niches in ecosystems.

At this point in time, *Ganoderma* species are something of a taxonomic nightmare. As researchers continue genetic sequencing work in the genus, and as more mycologists and mushroom growers study fungi overall, we are sure to sort out more of the species identification and naming. Just like all science, it is a slow and steady process.

Several Reishi species occur in the eastern woodlands of North America. Most of these are saprotrophic. Further south and along southern coastal areas, *Ganoderma zonatum* parasitizes palm trees; once a tree is infected, there is no treatment. The earliest-fruiting Reishi in western North Carolina is *G. tsugae* (Hemlock Reishi), which is endemic to dying Hemlocks (*Conium maculatum*); the occasional outlier is found on White Pine (*Pinus strobus*). *G. curtisii*, also known as the Golden Reishi, seems to have the widest range of host trees. It can be found on oaks (*Quercus* spp.), maples (especially Red Maples, *Acer rubrum*), Honey Locusts (*Gleditsia triacanthos*), Southern Magnolias (*Magnolia grandiflora*) and even Cabbage Palms (*Sabal palmetto*) along coastal salt marshes. *G. sessile* is the last Reishi to fruit in Appalachian forests each year; therefore, we call it Late Reishi. Additional genetic sequencing may reveal that

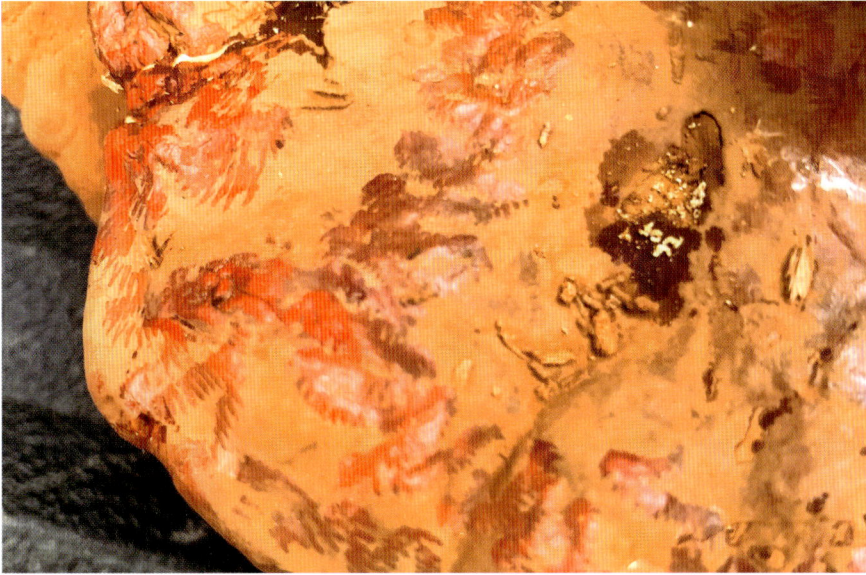

Figure 7.12. Evidence of insects consuming spores off a *G. tsugae* cap.

Ganoderma species that seem morphologically the same are actually different species specific to individual tree hosts. For example, *G. tsugae* has also been identified in China, and the morphology of some *G. curtisii* have been compared to the morphology of *G. lingzhi* (*Lingzhi*) or the *G. lucidum* (*Ling Chih*) from China.

Worldwide, *Ganoderma* species tally up to nearly three hundred. The overwhelming majority of these species have medicinal qualities; some are more widely recognized than others as medicinal. Reishi is one of the most cultivated and popular groups of mushrooms on the planet. Evidence for its powerful medicinal properties is mounting each year as more research is published. Reishi is also a mushroom that can be cultivated and utilized with ease. The Chinese name *Lingzhi* means "The Mushroom of Immortality," or "The Divine Mushroom." The most widely used common name for *G. lingzhi* is Reishi; another common Japanese name is *Mannetake*.

Reishi thrives in hot, humid environments. Most species are found in tropical or subtropical forests. *G. tsugae*, Hemlock Reishi, is an exception. It often occurs in rich coves in the Southern Appalachians where nighttime temperatures will dip into the 40s (°F) during May and June. It is not uncommon for Hemlock Reishi fruiting bodies to grow up to 24 inches in diameter. But in the Appalachian woodlands, Golden Reishi never grow as big as the Hemlock Reishi. This is likely due to the ability of the Hemlock Reishi mycelium to break down its host tree more quickly than the Golden Reishi can consume its preferred host, which tends to be oak. (Hemlock is a much softer wood than oak.)

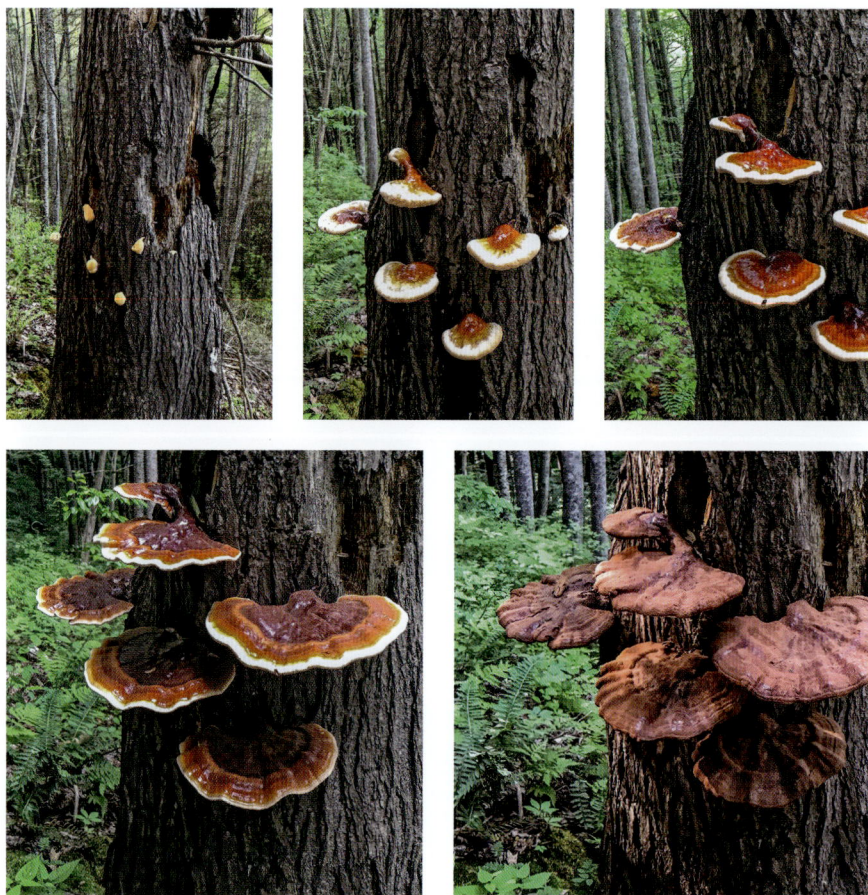

Figure 7.13. *G. tsugae* growing wild over eight weeks. Photos taken (from left to right, top to bottom) on April 21, May 7, May 14, May 22, and June 18.

The Reishi worldwide market was $4.27 billion in 2023. According to the Business Research Company, Reishi mushrooms and supplements will see strong growth within the next several years driven by the awareness of natural products and health and wellness. Functional foods and dietary supplements are expected to boost the growth of the Reishi market. It is estimated that by the year 2028 the Reishi market will be a $6.69 billion industry.[40]

Traditional Uses

In Chinese medicine, and throughout Asia, Reishi mushroom has been utilized for at least two thousand years and possibly much longer. This medicinal powerhouse was mentioned in texts as far back as 100 BCE. Lingzhi has been documented in ancient texts as an effective medicine for a number of ailments, as well as a tonic for strengthening the human body. Sheng-Nong's herbal classic, *The Divine Farmer's Materia Medica*, was composed during the Han Dynasty (25–220 CE), and we can speculate that the knowledge was much older, having been being passed down orally. Information typically stays in a culture to stand the test of time before it is documented, and then the line between information and wisdom begins to blur.

Reishi mushrooms started appearing as a subject in artwork centuries ago. One of my favorite depictions of Reishi is in a soapstone carving of Guanyin from eighteenth-century China, currently held at the Metropolitan Museum of Art in New York City.

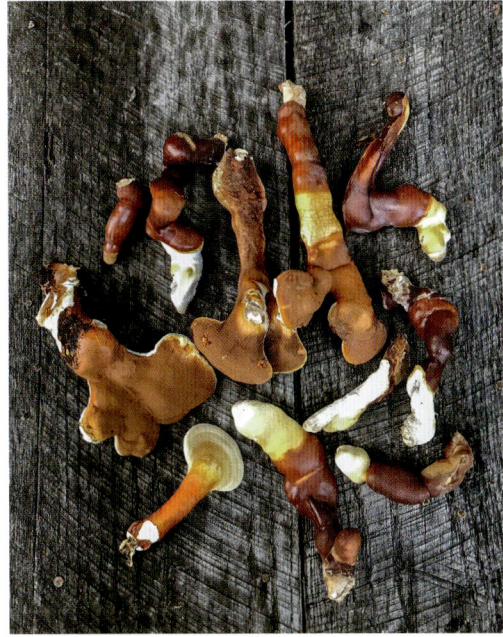

Figure 7.14. Reishi antlers.

We also saw the mushroom wall paintings in the drawing room of Sir Walter Scott's nineteenth-century home in southern Scotland.

The Divine Farmer's Materia Medica shows clearly the importance of various types of Reishi mushroom to Chinese medicine.[41] In these texts, *Ganoderma* species are divided into six categories according to color, and healing properties are assigned to the color of the mushroom dovetailing to the organ or ailment.

Research on Human Health Effects

Reishi continues to be an important mushroom in Chinese medicine and is gaining popularity in the West as more and more scientific research confirms its health-promoting benefits.

Reishi mushrooms influenced the way of life for ancient humans and cultures, and they continue to affect modern humans in the same ways they did our ancestors. New research tools are leading to discoveries that deepen our understanding of species that fall under the umbrella of the *Ganoderma* genus. Laboratory and preclinical studies with Reishi mushroom have found them to have anticancer, antiviral, antibacterial, and anti-inflammatory activity in addition to being of benefit to heart health and in the management of diabetes. Here we summarize a few of the strongest, as well as some more recent, human clinical trials.

CANCER

Western researchers generally agree that Reishi is an effective adjunct therapy for cancer. Use of Reishi can slow tumor growth and improve quality of life, but there is not yet evidence for Reishi to be used as a standalone treatment to cure cancer.[42] We note that all studies published at the time of this writing had worked with people who already had a cancer diagnosis. There are no trials following healthy people over multiple years to gather data on whether use of Reishi prevents, or slows the onset, of cancers.

One international, highly controlled clinical trial with polysaccharides extracted from *G. lucidum* treated advanced lung cancer patients with 600 mg of Reishi three times a day for twelve weeks. The patients who took Reishi showed slower growth of lung cancer, improved quality of life, and increased blood biomarkers indicating a more active and healthy immune system. Use of Reishi was also associated with a reduction in associated issues such as fever, coughing, and insomnia.[43] A hot-water extract of *G. lucidum* has also been found to suppress the growth of precancerous lesions of the large bowel after twelve months of treatment.[44]

G. lucidum spore powder is commonly used in Traditional Chinese Medicine (TCM). In one study, breast cancer patients given 1,000 mg of spore powder extract three times a day for four weeks experienced drastic, and statistically significant, reductions in fatigue, anxiety, and depression and increased physical well-being and quality of life.[45]

INFECTION AND IMMUNE-BOOSTING EFFECTS

In an effort to reduce colds in preschool children in Colombia, a yogurt supplemented with Reishi-derived β-glucans was given daily to 167 children for 12 weeks. Blood samples and physical examinations indicated these children had significantly healthier immune systems and suffered fewer colds than children who did not receive the Reishi yogurt. This method is being investigated as a possible way to reduce the spread of infections in young children.[46] Similar work looked at the effect of Reishi-derived β-glucans (200 mg daily) on healthy adults over a twelve-week period. Researchers found increased biomarkers for a healthy immune system.[47]

CARDIOVASCULAR EFFECTS

Reishi's cardioprotective effects seem to be due primarily to its beneficial effects on levels of blood glucose and blood fat, blood pressure, and the liver. Reishi has been shown to reduce inflammation in the heart and blood vessels, which has a protective effect against heart disease.[48] A daily dose of 540 mg Reishi-derived β-glucan for people diagnosed with atrial fibrillation (irregular heartbeat) over ninety days resulted in significant improvements in systolic blood pressure, heart rate, anti-inflammatory markers, compounds that reduce tumors, energy, and quality of life, as well as reduced fatigue, pain, and physical limitations.[49] In patients with coronary heart disease, a twelve-week treatment of daily Reishi extracts reduced various heart-related symptoms and resulted in a higher likelihood of a normal ECG reading, all while reducing blood pressure and serum cholesterol levels.[50]

One study looked at Reishi as a possible preventative medicine for heart disease by studying people who had mildly elevated blood pressure and cholesterol levels. The participants took 1.44 g Reishi for twelve weeks. Researchers saw improvements in levels of beneficial cholesterol but no significant change in blood pressure. They did, however, find improvements in blood plasma insulin levels, suggesting a possible antidiabetic effect.[51] These results are promising, but more research needs to be done.

DIABETES

Two tightly controlled studies have looked at the effects of Reishi in people with type 2 diabetes. The first study found a significant beneficial effect, but the second study found no effect. Two possible factors might explain this disparity of results: the studies may have used different extraction methods, and patients were given different dosage levels. The study that found a significant result used Ganopoly, which is a patented commercial Reishi-extraction product. The study results don't state exactly what is in Ganopoly nor how it is produced.[52] The study that found no effect used "*Ganoderma lucidum* extract and spores." This is also not a precise description, but it is clearly different from the content of Ganopoly.[53] The study that showed significant results used a much higher dose (5,400 mg per day) than the study that didn't find an effect (3,000 mg). The studies were conducted in different countries, and thus different dietary habits or other cultural differences could have impacted results as well. More research is needed.

ANTI-INFLAMMATORY EFFECTS

Chronic inflammation may underlie many diseases, including cancer. Reishi has been shown in lab studies to reduce inflammation. A handful of human clinical trials have tested Reishi's effects on inflammation in a few disease states. Results are mixed, but one promising example is fibromyalgia, which is characterized by chronic and widespread pain throughout the body without a clear cause. Understandably, secondary impacts include depression, anxiety, and reduced quality of life. A study of female patients who received 6,000 mg of micro-milled Reishi antler daily for six weeks showed a distinct trend toward greater happiness and life satisfaction and reduced body pain and depression compared to baseline.[54]

Role in Holistic Healing

This mushroom is on my top-three list of mushrooms to never be without. When my oldest daughter was two years old, she was bitten by a Brown Recluse spider on her pinky toe. Anyone who has had the pleasure of getting to know these bites understands they can be very difficult to treat. Brown Recluse venom causes necrosis, essentially cell death, of the tissue. My daughter's toe had swollen to almost double normal size. The whole toe extremity was bright red, and the skin had started to crack. Her toe was so tender that she cried when it was touched. After she went to sleep, I was able to gently open up the wound. I applied ground-up Reishi (dried wild *G. curtisii*) to her tiny toe and bandaged it.

Ground-up fresh Reishi takes on a puffed-up appearance similar to ground bark. It is fibrous and hard to pack, but the fibers act as a sponge to draw out poison from a wound, or to draw out excess liquids. Within two hours the swelling was reducing, and the skin color had returned to nearly normal. At about five hours the swelling and redness had started to return. I gently removed the Reishi from the wound and applied new Reishi powder. I did this two or three times a day for about ten days until her body was clearly up to the task of finishing healing the wound on its own.

For several days, every time I changed out the Reishi, the wound seemed to get deeper as the Reishi absorbed the poison. The Reishi was not only acting as an anti-inflammatory and antinecrotic, but it was also absorbing the spider venom so that her body could heal.

With good reason, more people are looking to this medicinal heavy hitter for holistic support in their modern day lives. As both an immune system and blood pressure modulator, Reishi seems a natural candidate to be a cornerstone medicinal mushroom for helping

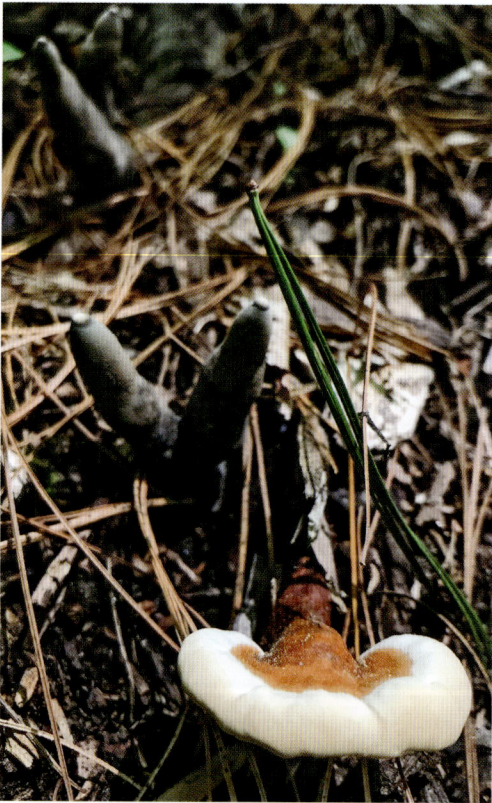

Figure 7.15. Outdoor-cultivated Reishi. The black protuberances near the Reishi are Dead Man's Fingers (*Xylaria polymorpha*).

people cope with stress-filled lives. Using Reishi can help restore balance by counteracting stress hormones that increase inflammation in the body.

We need the medicine of such powerful mushrooms to help regulate heightened states of stress and anxiety. Although some humans can thrive in fast-paced modern environments, it appears that most of us cannot. Humans need physical connection to the Earth to remain healthy. Although this notion was thought to be crazy or woo-woo as recently as about fifteen years ago, research studies now support the benefits of *grounding*, simply having our skin in direct contact with the earth, to increase blood viscosity. One study showed that just two hours of grounding had dramatic effects on red blood cell aggregation.[55] As described in "Cardiovascular Effects" on page 172, Reishi provides some of the same benefits to cardiovascular health as grounding does.

Reishi has a deep untapped potential to change the lives of people in communities lacking medical infrastructure close at hand. Underserved populations in the United States, and worldwide, can start to improve the quality of their lives by growing their own medicine and creating supportive, mycelial-like connections with neighbors and those in need. Will you be a node in the web to connect your community?

Cultivation Notes

The patience required to grow Reishi has lessons for us mushroom cultivators. If you haven't started cultivating this mushroom yet, I encourage you to try it! The joy it brings, the grounding that comes from being in contact with your medicine, the empowerment that arises from knowing you can take charge of your health—these are feelings that no amount of money can buy.

Reishi is easily cultivated on sawdust substrate in controlled environments. This can allow the grower to manipulate carbon dioxide levels, which can facilitate the formation of antlers. Outdoor cultivation is possible by partially burying small-diameter logs horizontally. Larger- diameter logs should be buried vertically. See the Reishi profile on page 167.

Ethical Wild Harvesting

Wild Reishi can be a rare find, seeming to show up on only one dead tree out of hundreds. Yet at times, we find a hillside where almost every dead oak tree has Reishi fruitbodies.

Some species of Reishi are plentiful only because of the demise of their host trees. *G. tsugae* is the best example in Appalachia. This species is endemic on Hemlock trees that are dying due to infestation by the Hemlock Woolly Adelgid (*Adelges tsugae*). This will often result in huge flushes of Reishi in parts of forests that had groves of hemlocks. It is easy to imagine these hundreds of pounds of mushrooms as a never-ending supply. But in order to continue flourishing, this species will need to make a leap onto other tree species as a host once all the hemlocks have died out. (We and other mushroom hunters have occasionally found it on White Pine.) A lot of bad advice is circulating about harvesting Hemlock Reishi—to harvest too early, or to harvest all you can get, predicated on greed. We must find a balance between harvesting the current bounty and conserving enough to allow the fungus to adapt and change over time.

Other *Ganoderma* species are much less plentiful. For example, we may find only a few Golden Reishi (*G. curtisii*) while on a five- to ten-mile trek through the forest. If they are this scarce in your region, the recommendation is to pick a small percentage of what you find and leave the rest intact. Along the coastal regions in the southeast, we find Golden Reishi to be pretty common among live oaks and even Cabbage Palms. The fact is that if harvesting is not done correctly, then the population dwindles and the medicine is no longer available. Culturing and growing naturally on logs on your own property is the best and most consistent way to obtain Reishi.

Grifola frondosa

WISHI, MAITAKE

In the Cherokee language, *Grifola frondosa* is called *Wishi*. It is hands-down my favorite mushroom on the planet. Wishi is an important cultural part of the Cherokee fall diet. Of course, some people do not like them, but in my experience, those people are very few. My Auntie Gail told me that my cousin thinks they taste like dirt. He probably needed to be checked for a fever! We find them to be amazingly meaty and crunchy, with a mild but remarkably full flavor.

G. *frondosa* belongs to the family Meripilaceae, which is in the phylum Basidiomycota. Most mycologists consider *G. frondosa* a saprotrophic fungus; some say it is slightly parasitic. It is a polypore mushroom with a long shelf life; it stays fresh in the fridge for several weeks when picked at its peak. In North America, it is a fall-fruiting mushroom, found almost exclusively on oak trees (*Quercus* spp.). I

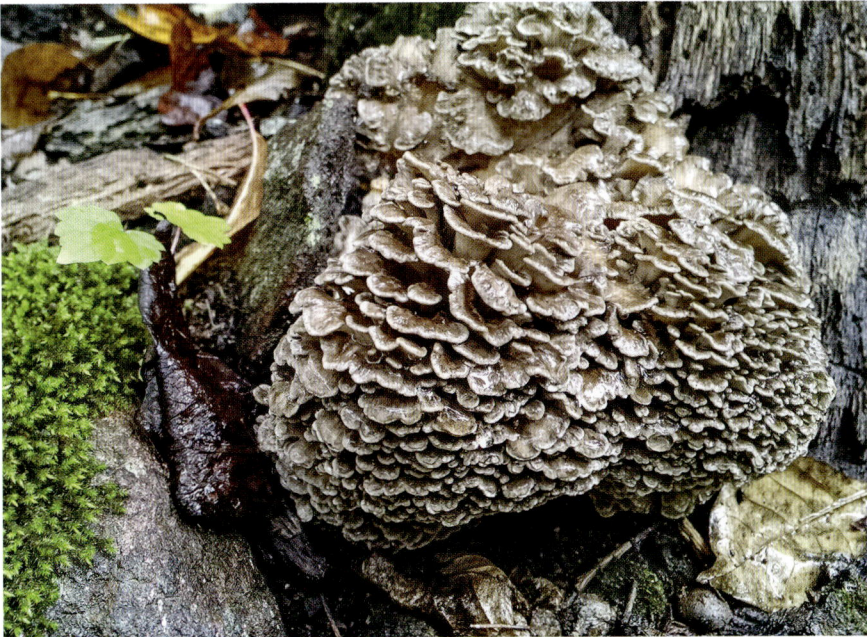

Figure 7.16. This wild maitake is thriving at the base of a dead oak tree.

have found it growing on birch (*Betula* spp.) only once, and once on a maple tree (*Acer* spp.). I have heard reports of it growing with other old hardwood trees, but this seems to be a rarity. *Grifola frondosa* translates to something comparable to "fish net" or "basket" because *Grifola* means "intricate or braided" and *frond* means "leaflike" or "leaf" (and the *-osa* suffix means "abundant"). The Japanese name for this mushroom is *Maitake*, which translates to "dancing mushroom." The name in Chinese is *Hui Shu Hua*, which translates to "Grey Tree Flower."

In North America, people use different names for *G. frondosa* in different regions. I have heard people from Pennsylvania call it Sheep's Head mushroom. In the Northeast, it can be called Ram's Head. And the name Hen-of-the-Woods seems to be common in all parts of the United States.

Superficially, *G. frondosa* looks the same wherever it is found in the wild, from China to Eastern North America. But although the morphology is the same worldwide, I am sure that Wishi, just like other mushrooms, develops different flavors according to the host tree species. I have found this to be true with Shiitakes, for example. Those cultivated on Wild Cherry (*Prunus avium*) have a less umami flavor than those grown on oak.

And interestingly, a 2002 study revealed that eastern North American and Asian *G. frondosa* are genetically different. The study included only one European isolate, which also proved to be different from both the others.[56]

This polypore mushroom has leaflet-like layers of varying sizes often arising from one strong central stem. It is a fungus that fruits on the cusp of change, at the interface of two different environments, where the wood meets the soil. Occasionally they can be found growing on the trunk of a tree, but most often you will find them at the base of a tree or stump. They are overwhelmingly associated with old trees. If a Wishi has ever been found at the base of a young tree, I have not heard about it. Wishi can also be found a short distance away from trees, fruiting off the large leader roots. It is not unreasonable to estimate that some of these mycelial colonies consuming the dying wood in old trees may be hundreds of years old. This leads me to realize that my ancestors likely harvested Wishi from some of

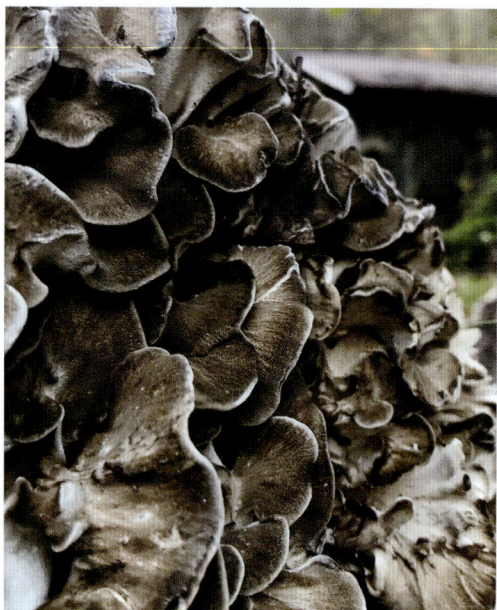

Figure 7.17. Close-up of wild-harvested Maitake.

the same trees I do. If people do not kill these big trees, but leave them to die naturally, it is reasonable to assume that the Wishi from those trees can feed multiple generations of people. These are the long memories of Indigenous peoples: not only thinking of ourselves, but setting up food systems that will support people for thousands of years.

Traditional Uses

Indigenous cultures of North America tend to have oral traditions, and as such, information about Wishi and some other species of mushrooms is limited. I know these mushrooms for being delicious and for making me feel great

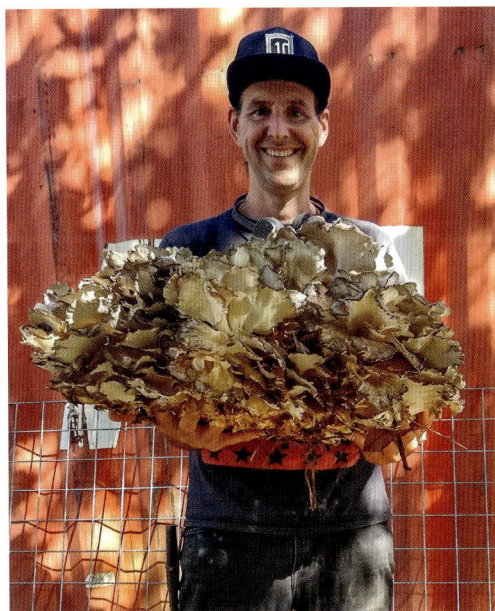

Figure 7.18. Author Chris with large Maitake from an old oak tree. Photo courtesy of Adawehi Parker

after I eat them. The Western Cherokees have held onto this mushroom as part of their traditional foods even after they were brutally removed from our ancestral land. Wars, famines, and forced relocations have all played a part in people who are from the land losing their cultural inheritance in many ways, including traditional medicines and foodways. I am happy that Wishi grows in Oklahoma so the Cherokee people can continue to enjoy this traditional fall delicacy.

In Traditional Chinese Medicine (TCM), *G. frondosa*, or Hui Shu Hua, is used to calm the mind. It cleanses or clarifies heat and replenishes the *qi* of the spleen. It has also been used in TCM to tone the liver and kidneys. It is associated with the heart, large intestines, and stomach channels as well as regulating the intestines. Hui Shu Hua has also been used to protect the body from external aggressions.

During "The Age of the Warrior" (1185–1603 CE) in Japan, the *shoguns* (warriors) had more power than the emperor, and the Maitake was worth its weight in silver. That would be enough to make any mushroom hunter dance! (And that's the origin of the common name *Maitake*, meaning "Dancing Mushroom.") Can you imagine paying approximately $300 per pound for *Hen-of-the-Woods*? The 30-pound fruit we once found would be worth $9,000!

In Japan *G. frondosa* is used to support well-being and the immune system while being considered a broad health tonic. Herbalists in Japan traditionally used dried *G. frondosa* by slicing it and steeping it in hot water for a few minutes to make a nourishing tea, often in combination with other fungi. Maitake continues to play a major culinary role in Japanese culture.

Research on Human Health Effects

Wishi is a mushroom that has many applications beyond a food source. We are continuing to develop new and creative ways to grow, use, and display this fungus. This mushroom has a long history with humans and our cultures in the northern hemisphere. Some of our threads of cultural knowledge have been continuous and some have been broken. We are mending some of these broken links, while adding to the fabric of knowledge. The research on the many applications of *G. frondosa* supports the traditional understanding of the medicine that it holds for human and planetary health. Not only does it help our bodies, but it can clean up environmental toxins, from petroleum products to bisphenol A (BPA). The research is helping us understand the larger role this mushroom can play in our lives. A strong body of scientific evidence for the medicinal value of Maitake mushrooms has been gathered over the past thirty years. The majority of this work, done in mice and rats, shows strong effects: Maitake is immunomodulatory, antitumor, antiviral, antidiabetic, antioxidant, antibacterial. Studies also show effects on the regulation of lipid levels and hypertension. There are some publicly available reviews of this science, but here we focus on the smaller body of research with human subjects.[57]

CANCER

Human clinical trials have shown that Maitake seems to stimulate the immune system to fend off cancers. Maitake's action on the immune system is complex and not yet understood. In a sample of women who had undergone surgery for breast cancer, researchers found that Maitake extract resulted in a highly significant dose response on 24 of the 146 immune parameters measured. Maitake extract enhanced some immune parameters and suppressed others. Optimal dose differed depending on the immune parameter targeted. An intermediate dose of 5 to 7 mg per kg of body weight per day was associated with the most benefits.[58]

In cancer patients not being treated with any other anticancer drugs, Maitake was found to both reduce metastatic expansion of cancer and decrease the expression of cancer biomarkers. Simultaneously, the activity of natural killer cells, the white blood cells that destroy infected cells, increased.[59]

VIRUSES

Maitake's ability to stimulate the innate immune system has also been shown to help us fight flu infections. In one study, people took 7 g powdered Maitake extract daily for twelve weeks; at week four they also received an influenza vaccine. Researchers found that Maitake extract increased levels of antibodies and reduced cold symptoms as compared to placebo. Interestingly, the positive benefits of Maitake extract were even stronger in participants over sixty years of age.[60]

DIABETES

In one small, uncontrolled study with seven type 2 diabetes patients, the subjects took Maitake extract three times a day for four weeks. All seven patients showed a significant decline (between 30 and 63 percent) in fasting blood glucose levels over the trial period. Significant improvements were seen with just two weeks of treatment, and blood glucose levels continued to gradually decrease over the next two weeks.[61] These results could be attributed to the placebo effect, but they warrant further research.

Insulin resistance is a feature of diabetes, and also of polycystic ovary syndrome (PCOS). A small study of women with PCOS showed the positive benefit of increased ovulation from supplementing with Maitake.[62]

PROTECTION AGAINST TOXINS

Bisphenol A (BPA) is a known endocrine disrupter that can be absorbed through skin contact. It can cause skin damage and produce proinflammatory proteins connected with skin diseases. A water extract of Maitake has been shown to stop the cell death and inflammation caused by BPA in human connective tissue cells cultured on petri plates.[63] Whether this result will translate to human use remains unknown. We hope that future research will pursue this question.

Role in Holistic Healing

Something deep within me stirs every time I pick these mushrooms and hold them in my hands. The feeling transcends me as an individual human, more powerful than my single experience. Perhaps it is a deep ancient connection to this medicinal food, this mushroom that is so celebrated by my people.

Research in Japan has investigated some possible uses of *G. frondosa* in cleaning up toxic waste from various industrial processes. One study from 2011 found the enzyme laccase produced by *G. frondosa* effective in degrading BPA and decolorizing synthetic dyes.[64] Mushroom farming operations in Japan that produce loads of spent substrate are a source of mycelium from which to source laccase. Laccase is stable even at high temperatures and a wide range of pH, making it a candidate for potential industrial and biotechnical applications.

The ability of Maitake to degrade polychlorinated biphenyls (PCBs) was established as early as 1999.[65] Researchers experimented with growing the mushroom in various substrates. They used low-, moderate- and high-nitrogen mediums; some were supplemented with lignin, and others not. Adding lignin significantly increased the ability of the culture to increase degradation of PCBs. It is thought that the presence of lignin may have allowed for the increase of the enzyme peroxidase, which is associated with the breakdown of lignin and PCBs alike. *G. frondosa* degraded forty components in the major forty-one PCBs within sixty days.

G. frondosa has traditionally been used as a food and medicine. That is still true today. As we harvest, cultivate, and use this mushroom, we become an important part of perpetuating it. Indoor production of this mushroom as an important food for people across the globe has increased, and it is expected to increase beyond 2030. These fungi are grown on substrates that are or were seen as waste products: for example, sawdust and waste logs from the logging industry. Finding ways to transform these substances into food and medicine is beneficial to all of us.

When we cultivate these fungi indoors, we also end up with a waste product in the form of the spent substrate blocks, and yet these blocks have many functions. They can be collected from farms to extract extracellular metabolites. One significant enzyme, mentioned earlier, is laccase. Laccases can be extracted from these blocks and used for other commercial, industrial and environmental applications. Some of these laccases can be used in the treatment of water to break down phenolic compounds. So a waste product (sawdust) is used to grow a nutrient-dense food loaded with medicinal properties. When that is finished, another waste product, the sawdust substrate, is then processed and enzymes and metabolites are extracted to be used in biological or industrial applications, including environmental remediation to remove pollutants. *G. frondosa* is another tool in our fungal toolbox that we can use to break toxins down, to help clear out our ecosystems, and to improve our bodily health.

Cultivation Notes

The first artificial cultivation of *G. frondosa* was in Japan in the 1980s. Methods for bottle, bag and sawdust, and sterilized log-in-bag cultures were developed.

Wishi can be cultivated indoors on sawdust substrate or outdoors on logs in a natural setting. Log cultivation lends itself well to the sterilized-log method. Once incubation is over, logs are placed partially buried in the forest to simulate natural production. Wishi only produces in the wild and outdoors one time per year. See "Maitake" on page 43.

When growing indoors these delightful beings can be grown year-round under consistent temperature control. *G. frondosa* takes a bit longer to produce than most indoor mushrooms, and a few nuances need to be followed.

Ethical Wild Harvesting

The wild harvesting of Wishi arrives at my favorite time of the year. The leaves are all showing their true beautiful colors, acorns are dropping, chestnuts have just finished up, and black walnuts are still falling. This seasonal change really drives us to get out and pick our favorite mushroom. We keep track of dozens of trees producing Wishi and have been doing this for more than twenty-five years. These trees do not produce fruit every year, but some are more consistent. We typically harvest about 50 percent of what is on the tree. Because these mushrooms come off oaks that are sometimes hundreds of years old, there is lots of energy in the tree that the mushrooms feed on. We harvest from one set of trees one year and another set of trees the next. We rotate our harvesting to allow diverse spore dispersal.

These mushrooms have an affinity for cleared, park-like settings. Even in the forest, we find them on ridges or open hollers where there is not a lot of underbrush. Most people that are members of the Eastern Band of Cherokee Indians (EBCI) have a close relationship with this mushroom. I think back to when the forests were more carefully managed with fire and recall de Soto's observations of the eastern woodlands being open. I marvel at how much more plentiful Wishi and other foods would have been when our ancestors were shaping the forests to support so much more life.

Wishi is native to many parts of eastern North America. It can also be found across Europe and Asia. The fruiting bodies can be substantial when the right conditions occur. We have found specimens that weigh as much as 30 pounds. Often when hunting Wishi, we look up into the treetops for a helpful clue. In October the trees are starting to change to their brilliant reds, yellows, and oranges. Look past all this beauty to spot large limbs, and especially tops, that are completely dead. The dead limbs are a sign of a higher probability of heart rot, and they will oftentimes lead you to *G. frondosa* fruitings.

In years when autumn is dry, we often find Wishi only on completely dead trees and stumps because the dead wood acts like a big sponge, creating the moist conditions the fungus needs. When ample rain falls in October, the bigger the tree, the bigger the Wishi. Our biggest haul was nearly 75 pounds from one stump that had several clusters. (And we did not take all of them.)

Hericium erinaceus

LION'S MANE

*H*ericium erinaceus, or Lion's Mane mushroom, is a widespread wood-decaying species prominent in cool climates across North America, Europe, and Asia. It is a distinctive mushroom that appears as a white mane on dying wood. It can seem as though Gandalf's white beard has suddenly grown out of a standing tree's trunk. *Hericium* species typically produce striking fruiting bodies in the fall and winter months, but occasionally fruit in the spring.

The Japanese name for *H. erinaceus* is *Yambushitake*. "Lion's Mane" and "Monkey Head Mushroom" are translations of the Chinese common names. The German name, *Igel-Stachelbart*, translates to "Hedgehog Quill." In the Cherokee language, we call this mushroom *Uguku*, which is the same word for the Barred Owl (*Strix varia*).

The first time I found Lion's Mane while mushroom hunting, they were on a dead log lying on the forest floor. I got the impression that these mushrooms

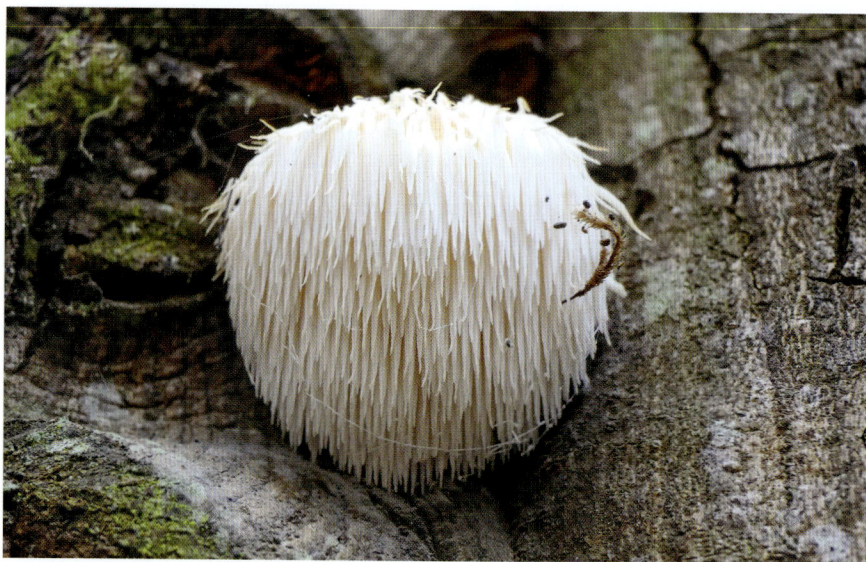

Figure 7.19. The white color of a Lion's Mane fruiting body stands out against a forested background, like a beacon calling to us from a distance. Photo by PlazacCameraman / iStock

always grow on dead logs. It took me several years to figure out that these mushrooms are usually found in old but still living trees, up in spots where you might see an owl. This is another good example of why slowing down and paying attention is important when we are in the forest seeking mushrooms.

I have come to understand that if something comes from an old tree, then it likely carries more wisdom, more power. It has been here for longer, so it has a greater stored intelligence. It has seen more winters, more changes. The tree it came from likely has heart rot or dying limbs, so it has been through some hard times. Lion's Mane will often slowly feed on and decompose the deadwood sloughed off by the tree, sometimes over a period of decades. As a saprotroph, Lion's Mane will not harm the tree's living wood—it consumes only the dead wood. We can learn from this. Carrying burdens that we should no longer hold onto, can keep us from growth. Dragging around the "deadwood" of life's struggles is exhausting. That deadwood could be transmuted into something fertile, where seeds can germinate, or that others can use as fertilizer. We can use this "deadwood" ourselves as fertile ground for growth. But it serves no one if we do not let it go.

Like the human brain, a Lion's Mane fruiting body branches out from one central

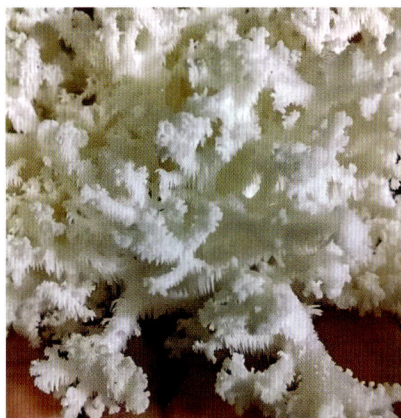

Figure 7.20. *H. coralloides*, aka Coral Tooth Fungus.

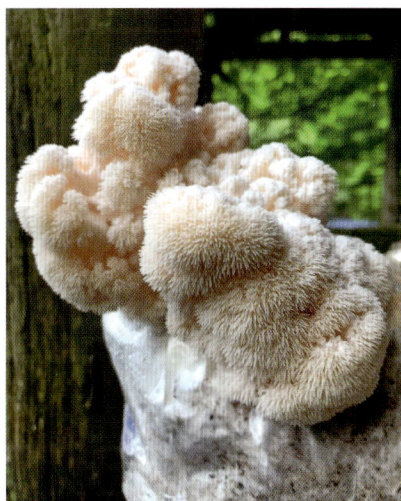

Figure 7.21. Young Lion's Mane on substrate block.

base into many intricate parts. A mushroom's stem is called a *stipe*, but Lion's Mane appears to squat and sit directly on a branch, just like an owl. It does not have a proper stem. Some species of *Hericium,* such as *H. americanum* (Bear's Head Tooth), are particularly branched (see figure 7.20). The Doctrine of Signatures—an ancient understanding that the physical appearance of a plant or fungi may give clues to its potential medicinal use in treating a similar looking body part—suggests Lion's Mane could be beneficial to the brain. Turns out this is beyond true: the research suggests these mushrooms are really amazing for our brains.

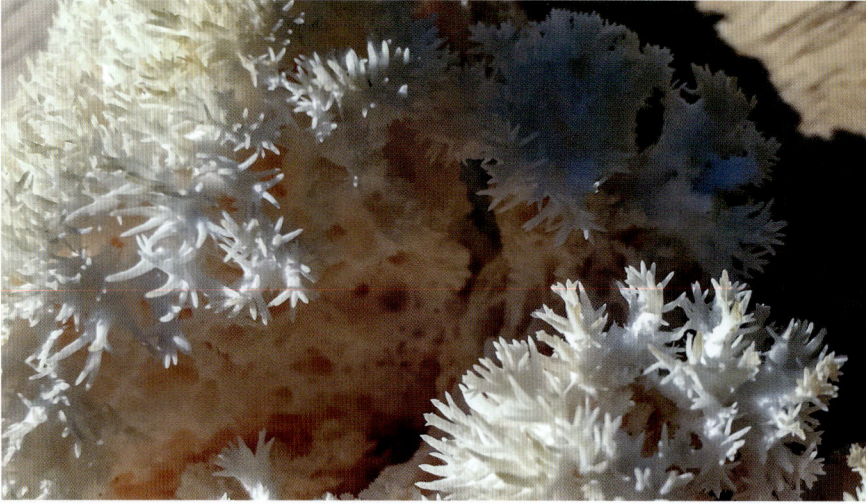

Figure 7.22. Lion's Mane branching pattern.

Traditional Uses

H. erinaceus has a long history of use in Asian cultures. In Traditional Chinese Medicine (TCM), Lion's Mane is used for the five internal organs: liver, spleen, kidney, heart, and lungs. It has also been recommended in TCM for gastric ulcers and chronic gastritis. This mushroom also affects some characteristics of qi deficiency such as insomnia and hypodynamia (the loss of power or strength). It is also known for its effects on the nervous system, which we explore below in "Research on Human Health Effects."

Some Indigenous American nations used Lion's Mane to prevent bleeding, and the first scientific description of this fungus occurred in North America.

In Europe, it has been used as a food source for a long time, but its wild habitat has become fragmented and Lion's Mane is listed as an endangered species in thirteen European countries. This fragmentation has likely led to the loss of knowledge about traditional roles that this mushroom played. It is now so rare in the United Kingdom that it is protected by law; sale and picking of wild Lion's Mane have been illegal since 1998.

Research on Human Health Effects

I first read a study about the beneficial effects of Lion's Mane in 2007. I remember feeling excited and delighted about the potential of this humble mushroom to do so much. It took persistent education to convince people to try eating this strange looking, from-under-the-sea-like fungi, much less use it as a medicinal mushroom. Now in our classes and in conversation, we meet many people who are taking

Lion's Mane supplements because their doctors have exhausted all other avenues without desired results. The knowledge spores have landed in fertile areas and germinated, and now the mycelium is running through our society.

Hundreds of research papers have been published covering the health benefits of using Lion's Mane. *H. erinaceus* has been shown to have numerous health benefits, such as antioxidative, antidiabetic, anticancer, anti-inflammatory, antimicrobial, and possibly antidepressant and antianxiety effects. There are many reports on laboratory and animal studies. In the following we focus on human trials centered on mood and cognitive performance. Human trials also show some possible effects on diabetes and general gut health.

DEPRESSION AND ANXIETY

Pharmaceutical antidepressants can have serious, unwanted side effects for many people. *H. erinaceus* may be a superior alternative. In one study, thirty-six menopausal women ate four cookies enriched with 0.5 g powdered Lion's Mane daily for four weeks. The results suggest a positive effect of Lion's Mane extract by significantly reducing subjects' anxiety and depression over four weeks. Participants did not report any impact on sleep quality.[66]

A later study with more patients and a longer duration showed an increase in sleep quality as well as reduced anxiety and depression. This study was conducted with people affected by obesity. The *H. erinaceus* supplement consisted of 20 percent fruiting bodies and 80 percent mycelium, extracted in both water and ethanol. Patients took three 500 mg capsules a day for eight weeks.[67]

COGNITIVE PERFORMANCE

The effects of Lion's Mane on diseases of the aging nervous system, including Parkinson's, Alzheimer's, and stroke, are the field of widest research. At the time of this writing, there is no cure for these diseases, and pharmaceutical treatments will likely come with unwanted side effects and costs. Medicinal mushrooms may offer a safe, and widely available, alternative.

Preclinical research has found that neuroprotective compounds called *hericenones* and *erinacines* are present in Lion's Mane. These compounds can easily pass through the blood–brain barrier and stimulate production of various neurotropic factors, proteins that are crucial to the growth and maintenance of neurons, including brain-derived neurotropic factor (abrineurin or BDNF) and nerve growth factor (NGF), helping to maintain brain health. BDNF is a key molecule that promotes brain plasticity and neuron growth. Animal research has shown that Lion's Mane increases neuronal growth in brain areas key for cognitive functioning.

Research in humans has focused on treatment for those already experiencing cognitive decline and at effects on cognitive performance in healthy adults.

In a study of adults aged fifty to eighty years with mild cognitive decline, those who took 250 mg Lion's Mane powder tablets (four tablets three times a day for sixteen weeks) saw a significant increase in cognitive performance. After an additional four weeks of not taking the Lion's Mane, their cognitive performance scores had significantly declined, underscoring the importance of continued supplementation. No one reported any side effects.[68]

In a later study, people of a similar age group who had hearing loss took Lion's Mane (2,000 mg per day) for eight months. For people over sixty-five years of age, but not for the younger patients, there was a significant improvement in hearing and a simultaneous increase of NGF in the blood. Levels of BDNF increased but did not reach statistical significance. This suggests that use of Lion's Mane stimulates the brain's production of compounds that aid the nervous system in repairing itself.[69]

In a forty-nine-week trial with people fifty years and older diagnosed with mild Alzheimer's disease, patients were given 5 mg of erinacine A daily, and various cognitive tests and other evaluations were performed frequently. The participants showed improvement in cognitive abilities and performance of tasks of daily living. Testing of a control group who were not receiving Lion's Mane showed that they continued to decline. Brain imaging found that some key brain areas in patients treated with erinacine A showed less decrease in brain matter, and visual tests showed an increased ability in those patients to perceive contrast. The researchers suggest Lion's Mane may be important in preventing, or slowing, the progression of Alzheimer's disease.[70]

Could Lion's Mane benefit younger people, or those without any sign of cognitive decline? A 2023 study with forty healthy volunteers, aged eighteen to forty-five, looked at both the immediate (after sixty minutes) and longer-term (after twenty-eight days) impacts of ingesting 1.8 g of Lion's Mane daily. The results showed that volunteers who took Lion's Mane performed significantly faster on one cognitive test 60 minutes after the initial dose but not on a different test. After twenty-eight days, the group taking Lion's Mane reported a strong trend toward feeling less stressed.[71]

An eight-week trial, during which participants over age fifty-five ingested a total of 3.44 mg erinacine daily, found a significant improvement in cognitive function, assessed by two non-verbal speed tests. Simultaneously, levels of the brain booster BDNF significantly increased. The control group showed a decrease in BDNF over the eight weeks. Participants taking Lion's Mane also showed an increase in the diversity of their gut microbiota that positively correlated with neuropeptide Y (NPY), a molecule known to regulate the production of BDNF. This research uncovered for the first time a complex system that involves gut bacteria aiding in the breakdown of chitin in fungal cell walls and in the body's ability to produce BDNF. These friendly gut bacteria seem to make the hericenones and erinacines from Lion's Mane more available for use.[72]

GUT MICROBIOTA

One pilot study looked specifically at the impact of 3 g daily of Lion's Mane mushroom powder taken for just seven days on the gut microbiota of thirteen healthy volunteers with an average age of thirty. Researchers found significantly increased gut flora diversity, an increase in the relative abundance of some short-chain fatty acids and beneficial bacteria, and a reduction in some harmful bacteria. These gut flora changes were correlated with positive, health-promoting changes in various blood chemicals.[73] It seems that Lion's Mane may have general health benefits mediated through interactions with gut microbiota.

DIABETES SUPPORT

Research on Lion's Mane's effects on diabetes is still in the laboratory phase at the time of this writing. Studies show that compounds isolated from the mushroom can inhibit human enzymes that break down glucose, thus slowing the transformation of carbohydrates to sugar.[74] Studies with mice and rats have found Lion's Mane to help reduce blood sugar levels and suggest it may be helpful in preventing diabetes. More research with Lion's Mane in this area seems important, given the clear evidence that sugar intake is associated with a greater incidence of dementia.[75]

IRRITABLE BOWEL SYNDROME (IBS)

Lion's Mane has been found to be anti-inflammatory, but this action has not yet been studied in humans with IBS. A 2023 study used intestinal tissue samples from people with IBS to investigate the effects of a nutraceutical (fortified food) containing Lion's Mane and other compounds. Researchers found a positive effect on the tissue cells in that the supplement helped reduce inflammation.[76] This, along with research showing that Lion's Mane can help to increase beneficial gut flora, is a promising start to its potential use for those with IBS.

Role in Holistic Healing

As we move around on this planet, we accumulate experiences. In traditional cultures this is honored; life experience is valued and sought out. We are encouraged to listen to our elders, human and beyond-human, and to listen to the wisdom of the planet. Slowing down enough to actually pay attention is vital, just as it was for me to be able to find Lion's Mane in the wild. Those that have these gifts of experience and wisdom to pass on to the next generations are vital to our cultures, our individual balance, and our very survival on this planet.

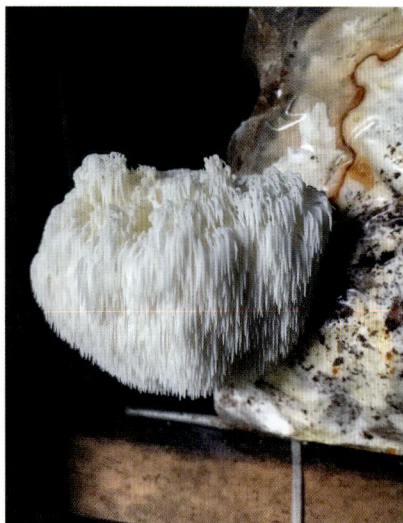

Figure 7.23. Lion's Mane fruiting from substrate block.

Careful observations and experiences of the elders are shared with the younger generations, because they have learned from past mistakes or past successes: this is how cultures are developed over many millennia.

It is unfortunate that a lifetime of experience and wisdom can be lost when a person develops Alzheimer's or dementia, and that no significant scientific advances have been made in the treatment of Alzheimer's for the last twenty years. Lion's Mane research over the past twenty-five years has shown its potential as a tool for preventing or slowing cognitive decline in our aging population due to its compounds that can regenerate damaged neural pathways.

The "silver tsunami" is already here, an aging demographic that is larger than ever before. This brings challenges through the rise in conventional healthcare costs. Many people have found that the Western medical model does not serve them well. Providing the medicine that Lion's Mane mushrooms offer can be an affordable way of helping people continue to have a good quality of life as they age.

Lion's Mane mushroom can be incorporated into the diet to help sufferers of inflammatory bowel diseases (IBD) by regulating gut microbiota and inflammation. *Helicobacter pylori* is a bacterium that replicates in the lining of the stomach and leads to inflammation. It is known to cause peptic ulcers and, in some people, has been linked to stomach cancers. Lion's Mane has been shown to inhibit the growth of this potentially harmful bacteria. People that suffer from stomach lining issues from the abuse of alcohol may see some benefits from *Hericium erinaceus* without the side effects of the pharmaceuticals typically prescribed.[77]

The quality of our lives as modern humans has been improved in many ways, and yet we are still living with a lot of stress and anxiety. Another promising aspect of Lion's Mane as medicine is its unrealized ability to help relieve some of the stresses of life in congested cities and fast-paced environments. Results from clinical trials are promising. For example, obesity is stigmatized in many societies, and it is difficult to overcome. Emotional state plays a role in our ability to lead a healthy, active lifestyle. Finding the inspiration or energy to make a change is arguably a major hurdle.

Another example may be sleep disorders, which can affect a person's energy level. After a sleepless night, I need to consume more calories to function in my day-to-day life. The studies cited in the previous section suggest that Lion's Mane is a game changer when it comes to better sleep quality, which helps us find motivation and enjoy all that life has to offer.

Many supplements containing Lion's Mane have arrived in the marketplace. Exercise caution when purchasing these products. Quality varies, and some supplement companies, driven by investor demands, put a premium on profit rather than product results. For most types of mushrooms, the fruiting body is the part that contains the highest number of medicinal compounds. But some mushroom coffee products are made from myceliated rice rather than the fruiting bodies of mushrooms. If the mycelium is grown on organic brown rice, then often the supplement is 40 to 60 percent carbohydrates. How are these products being processed? Are they just being dehydrated and ground up? Are they using a long hot-water extraction method? Processing is undoubtedly important to free up the mycocompounds. When you are paying a premium for a mushroom-based coffee substitute, you want to get a premium product. Refer to chapter 6 for a discussion on how to process mushrooms for maximum benefits.

Cultivation Notes

It is now easier than ever before to access these enchanting mushrooms as more and more people are learning how to grow them. If you live in an area where you do not have access to Lion's Mane, perhaps it is an enterprise you could participate in.

Lion's Mane mushrooms can be grown indoors with ease and don't require purchasing a lot of equipment. This is a way to grow food and medicine that gives a deeper sense of satisfaction. We are improving our own health and also improving the lives of everyone around us.

Lion's Mane mushrooms are very productive in a controlled environment. Lion's Mane and other *Hericium* species can be grown on sawdust substrate for consistent indoor production. A wide variety of types of wood can support the growth of Lion's Mane outdoors on logs. The hardwoods will support production longest, and softer woods produce earlier but will be shorter lived. Chapters 4 and 5 cover details of sawdust substrate methods. See the Lion's Mane profile on page 42 for log cultivation tips.

Ethical Wild Harvesting

Lion's Mane can be safely harvested from the wild, sometimes for decades from the same trees. Figure 7.24 shows a Lion's Mane that my dad found. We ate it for over a year once processed.

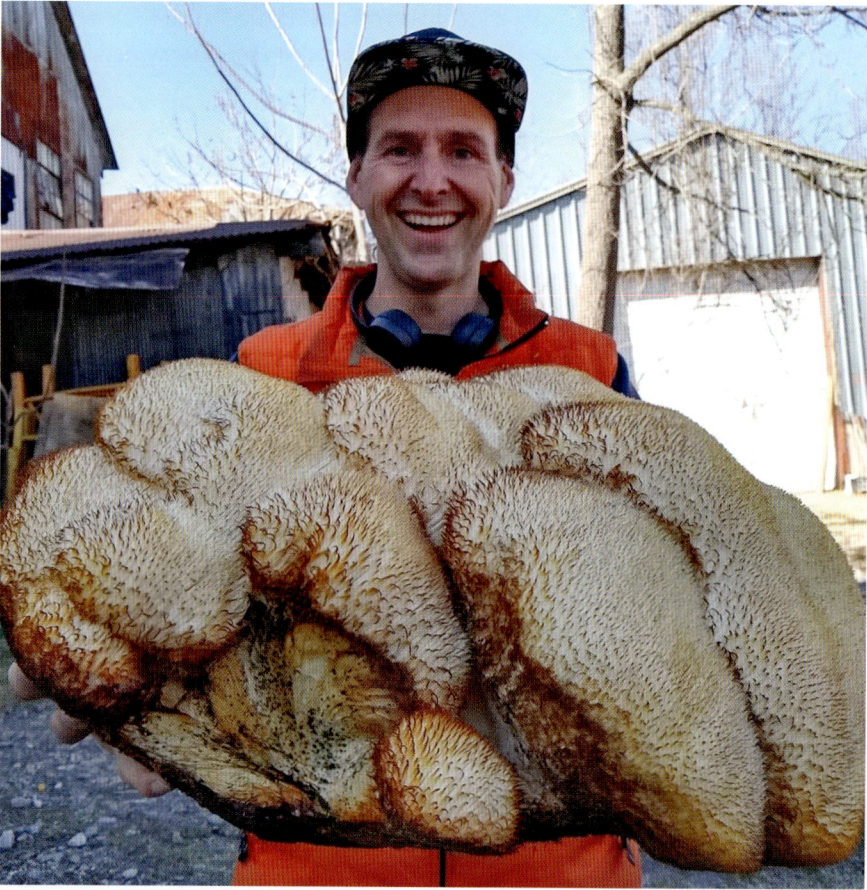

Figure 7.24. Author Chris with large wild Lion's Mane. Photo courtesy of Adawehi Parker

Of course, it is not advisable to take all of the wild fruitbodies you find every year. The smaller trees or dead wood that support Lion's Mane growth will usually last only a few years. Large trees that can be hundreds of years old such as oak (*Quercus* spp.) or black walnut (*Juglans nigra*) can provide opportunities to harvest year after year, occasionally for decades. But taking all of the mushrooms will interrupt spore dispersal for new generations in new locations. This is important to remember, because interrupting spore dispersal too often can reduce Lion's Mane populations in the wild.

Cityscapes are great locations to find Lion's Mane, especially on maples (*Acer* spp.), which are commonly planted because of their attractive growth patterns and quick-growing nature. These trees are subject to frequent trimming because of power line rights-of-way or proximity to buildings. The cut limbs that die back are commonly hosts to Lion's Mane. It is often the case that more Lion's Mane can be found growing in cities than in forests.

Inonotus obliquus
CHAGA

Chaga mushroom (*Inonotus obliquus*) is a parasitic fungus that lives mostly on birch trees (*Betula* spp.) in cool conditions—either in more northerly latitudes or at high elevations. In the Southern Appalachians, it typically occurs at about 3,500 feet (1,100 m) or higher in elevation. Further north, it also grows at lower elevation. Occasionally it grows on trees other than birch. In the twenty years that I have been harvesting and using Chaga, I have seen it growing on White Oak (*Quercus alba*) only once.

Chaga is packed full of antioxidants, proteins, fiber, vitamins, and minerals and has been widely used to treat cancers, reduce inflammation and oxidative stress, boost the immune system, and improve insulin resistance. Chaga produces medicinal compounds called *betulin* and *betulinic acid*, but only when it is grown on birch. The name for this mushroom in Chinese, *Bai Hua Rong*, translates to "Diamond of the Forest." The Japanese name, *Kabanoanatake*, translates to "Mushroom of Immortality" (which, not to confuse things, is also the translation of the Chinese name for Reishi mushrooms).

Chaga is slow growing, and it can take five to ten years to accumulate enough growth for sustainable harvesting. The part harvested is not the fruiting body but rather a sclerotium, which the mushroom produces as an energy reserve (as described in "Fungi Shape Their Environments" on page 18).

Chaga plays the long game, parasitizing living birch trees and slowly moving toward its goal of killing its host. At some point the tree will either succumb to the fungus or it will fend off the

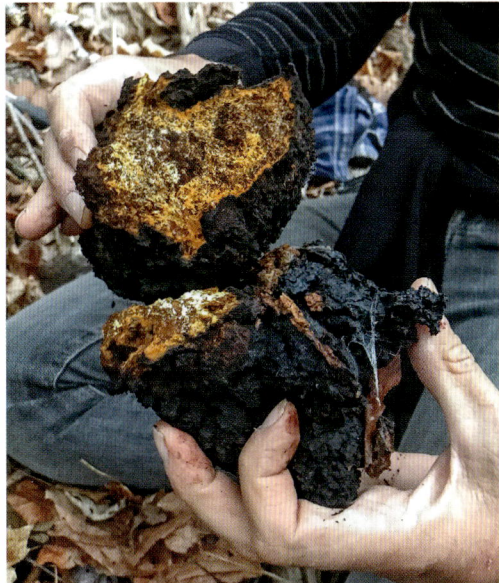

Figure 7.25. Harvesting Chaga from a dying birch tree.

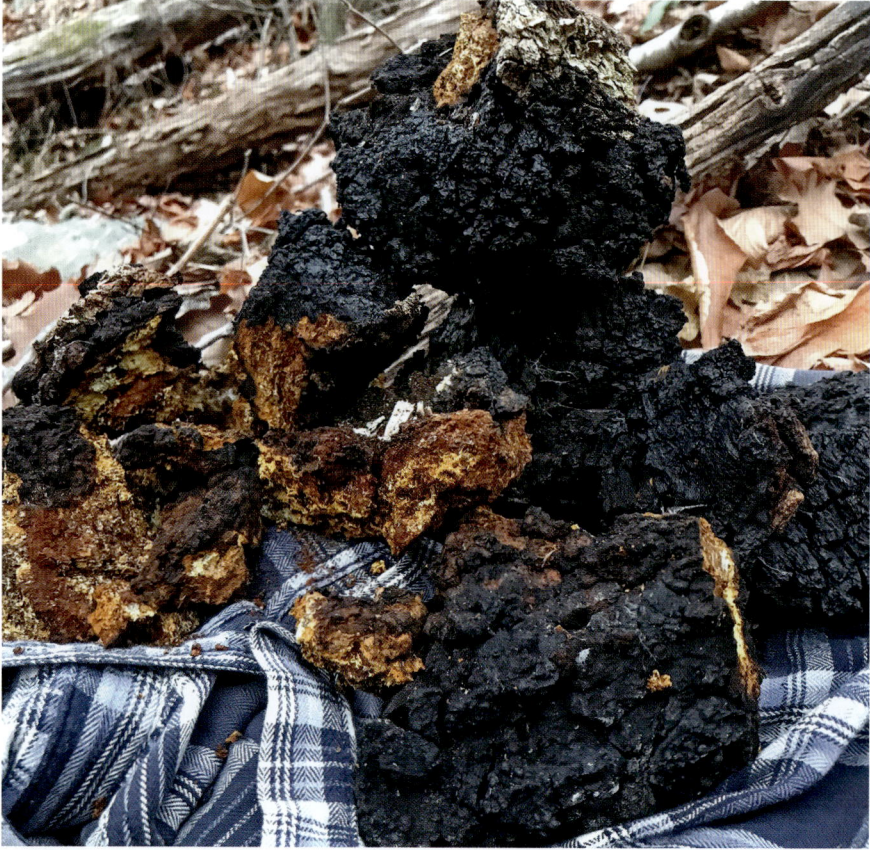

Figure 7.26. An abundance of chaga from one tree.

"infection" by this parasite and return to a healthy state. This battle has been going on between Chaga and birch trees for somewhere between 66 and 145 million years.

Chaga produces a fruitbody only after the host tree dies. Once the tree is dead, and the environmental conditions are right, the mushroom withdraws energy from the sclerotia and directs that energy toward production of a thin, silvery looking skin, which is a type of fruitbody called a *crust fungus*. I have seen this type of crust in the wild only once. It is difficult to spot because it grows under the bark of the dead tree and is readily consumed by insects.

Traditional Uses

The use of Chaga spans continents and cultures in higher latitudes. The birch forests of the world are full of healing stories and Indigenous uses, from Siberia to Alaska. Chaga has proven itself over the centuries to be a strong and needed medicine.

People have been using Chaga mushrooms as folk remedies for an extraordinarily long time. Indigenous people in the Baltic region, including Russia, still use this mushroom as they did centuries ago. People in rural Siberia grind up the mushroom and add it to everyday soups, beverages, and stews. Through long use, they discovered that eating Chaga protects them from the onset of degenerative diseases and supports vitality and longevity. They also use this mushroom to make a coffee-like drink to ward off parasites, to treat tuberculosis, to cure gastritis and other digestive disorders, and even to prevent cardiac or hepatic illnesses.

The Khanty people from Siberia have been documented to use Chaga in numerous ways, including "by infusion, inhalation, or maceration in water of the charcoal obtained after burning to make body soap, which was used as an antiseptic."[78] The soap water was used for ceremonial cleansings, especially after menstruation and childbirth. There are apparently written records of Chaga being used in Eastern Europe as far back as the twelfth century, although it is not clear how accurate these reports are. Likely, of course, it has been used for much longer than these written records allow us to see. Modern-day Russian hunters and foragers use Chaga to increase their endurance.

Russian scientists have noted that cancer is absent among people who traditionally harvest Chaga. Aleksandr Solzhenitsyn's novel *The Cancer Ward* mentions the use of Chaga mushrooms in gulags, Soviet-era prison camps. Chaga is now being investigated for cancer fighting properties. We have seen a small pile of Chaga lying close to the base of a birch tree, and then looked up to see a healed-over knot. The tree won that battle. According to the Doctrine of Signatures—an ancient understanding that the physical appearance of a plant (or fungi) may give clues to its potential medicinal use in treating a similar looking body part—this is a textbook example of what it takes to cure cancer.

In *Braiding Sweetgrass,* botanist Robin Wall Kimmerer of the Potawatomi nation describes how the black Chaga conk appears burned, but when cracked open, it reveals bands of bronze and gold. Using the native Potawatomi name for Chaga, she writes, "Shkitagen is a tinder fungus, a firekeeper, and a good friend to the People of the Fire. Once an ember meets shkitagen it will not go out but smolders slowly in the fungal matrix, holding its heat. Even the smallest spark, so fleeting and easily lost, will be held and nurtured if it lands on a cube of shkitagen."[79] Her reverence for this mushroom draws from a long history of the Potawatomi people tending the birch forests of the land now called the Great Lakes region. Keeping an ember smoldering can be crucial to life, as discussed in Amadou and Birch Polypore profiles (pages 155 and 162).

Canadian Indigenous populations used *I. obliquus* for the treatment of many diseases. Various preparations were created specific to an affliction. Preparations included soap water, smoke, tea, infusions, syrup, burning, moxibustion, and lotions. Chaga has been used to treat heart disease, infections, liver disease, stomach disease, tuberculosis, arterial disease, wounds, joint diseases, arthritis, and toothache. It can be used as a wash after childbirth or during menstruation.[80] Indigenous people have a deep history and relationship with Chaga. In the form of incense, it is used to carry prayers. Research has shown that some ergosterol derivatives in Chaga, after being consumed, turn into vitamin D when skin is exposed to sunlight.[81]

Research on Human Health Effects

Indigenous uses tell us that this mushroom helps with treating cancer, prevents oxidative stress, modulates the immune system, and reduces inflammation and infections from viruses, bacteria, and parasites. Despite the widespread, long-term use of Chaga among many northern Indigenous people, scientific research lags. This may be because Chaga is found only in extreme climates and has not been very accessible to the Eurocentric scientific community. Clearly, we need

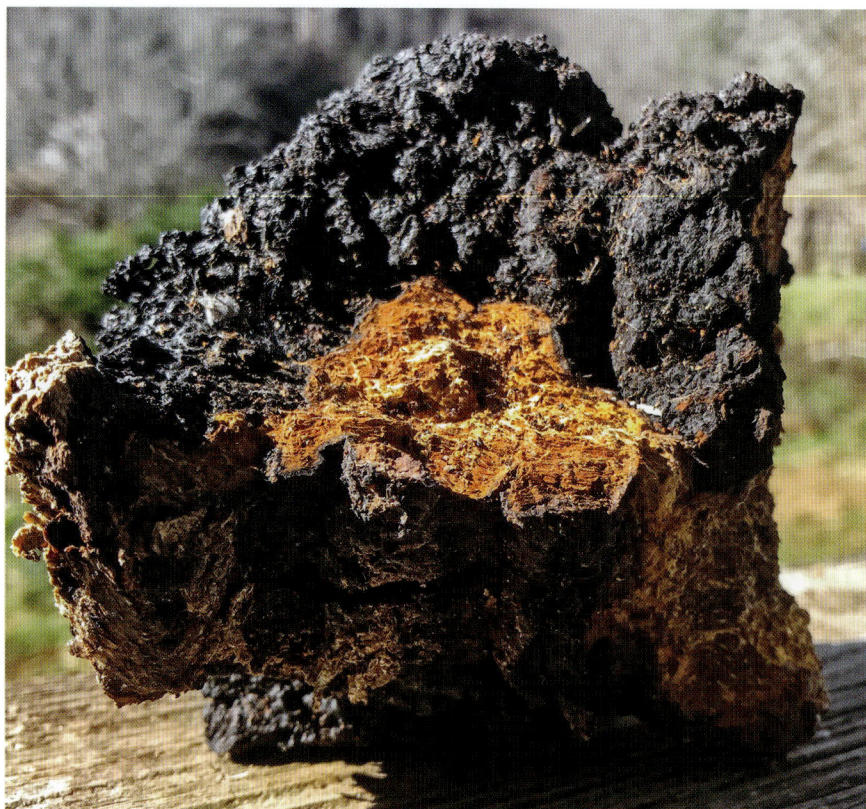

Figure 7.27. Close up of internal structure of Chaga.

more research to uncover the properties in *I. obliquus* and to effectively utilize it as medicine.

ANTIOXIDANT EFFECTS

Studies with Chaga in the lab and with mice have demonstrated antioxidant effects through encouraging cellular expression of antioxidant genes and through reducing free radicals. In mice bred to have neurodegenerative diseases such as Alzheimer's and Parkinson's, these antioxidant effects are seen to be neuroprotective.[82]

CANCER

Most of the scientific research on Chaga has focused on fighting cancer. Scientists are studying effects of Chaga extracts on human cancer cells in laboratory settings. Chaga extracts have been found to be effective against human breast, cervix, lung, colon, gastric, liver, mouth, brain, and pancreatic cancer cells.[83] These studies have found that the active compounds in Chaga extracts include various triterpenoids (including betulinic acid and betulin) and ergosterol. These compounds act in a variety of ways, including killing cancer cells, preventing cancer cells from growing, and suppressing the metabolism of cancer cells. Research has now progressed to using mice in whom cancer has been induced, and this research is finding Chaga extracts to reduce tumor size.[84]

IMMUNE SUPPORT AND ANTI-INFLAMMATORY

Studies with mice uphold the Indigenous understanding that Chaga may support the immune system and act to reduce inflammation in the body. A preparation named Episalvan containing 80 percent betulin was available in 2022 and approved as a prescription medication by the European Medicines Agency for superficial skin wounds and second-degree burns.[85] It has been shown to be far superior to conventional treatments.[86]

ANTIVIRAL, ANTIBACTERIAL, ANTIPARASITIC

A few reports show Chaga to be effective against human and feline herpes viruses, HIV, and SARS-CoV2 (COVID-19) in laboratory studies.[87] Chaga has also been shown to help regulate gut flora, act as a probiotic in mice, and reduce infections of the parasite *Toxoplasma gondii* in mice.[88]

Role in Holistic Healing

The role that *I. obliquus* could play in holistic healing is multifaceted. Chaga can teach us about sustainable harvesting and the long-term effects of our actions on the forests. Clear-cutting reduces the soil and insect diversity that keeps forests resilient and flourishing. As we weaken forest soils, we weaken the whole system. The trees that eventually grow back do not have the full range of community partners they need to thrive. Chaga seems to have the ability to choose the trees that have a weakness we humans may not see. Culling out weak trees and leaving healthy ones standing is intelligent forest management. Slow, methodical observations over generations are the only way that we sustain our medicine and our culture. Chaga shows us that the forest left intact is more valuable in the long term.

Chaga shows up as a "cancer" on birch trees, and therefore, through the lens of some traditional medicinal practices, it is a likely candidate to be used in treatments for cancers, and most of the modern research supports this traditional use. Science is slowly progressing toward recognizing other wide-ranging benefits of this mushroom, including as an antioxidant, an immune modulator, and an anti-inflammatory agent, as well as an agent that reduces infections from various pathogens.

Because Chaga has specific temperature requirements, it is not a widespread mushroom globally. Now that worldwide shipping of products has become commonplace, we are concerned that Chaga populations will be depleted. The modern marketing machine has already taken hold of Chaga, promoting it as a superfood.

Manufacturers of Chaga products make grand claims about its health benefits, but because of the lack of human clinical trials, marketers draw on its Indigenous history to back up these claims. Jonathan Robbins, a historian of commodities and colonization, points out that this tends to ignore the Native American relationship with Chaga to focus on Eurasian uses. This, he believes, is designed to make the use of the mushroom more comfortable for Anglo-American and European consumers. He says, "The selective use and misuse of history presents chaga as heritage recovered, rather than appropriated."[89]

Cultivation Notes

Chaga mycelium can be cultivated on petri plates, and in grain and sawdust. We have inoculated living birch trees with myceliated plugs, but these limited trials have produced no results. It is important to note that cultivating the mycelium of Chaga on substrates will not result in the important compounds that the fungus accumulates from the living birch trees. More experiments are needed. As described above, birch trees must be living to produce Chaga sclerotia, which is the part we wish to harvest. When the birch tree succumbs to the fungus, all energy is removed from the Chaga sclerotia and transferred to the fruiting body. If the tree is dead, the Chaga sclerotia are dead.

Ethical Wild Harvesting

Chaga is one of the only fungi harvested during the dormant stage. Chaga overharvesting, by those that have not visited the fungus or do not have a relationship with the fungus, is definitely a problem. Chaga is essentially a protector. Humans, when using the medicine as protection, should return the favor and protect this fungus.

The wild harvesting of Chaga has been a subject of tension because it has been overharvested and used in everything from shampoo to teas. Education around *I. obliquus* and its life cycle is desperately needed to prevent overharvesting. How often it can be harvested, how fast it grows, and how much is *over*harvesting are all legitimate questions when our goal is preserving and encouraging the proliferation of a fungus that we use medicinally, as well as the trees that support it. Occasionally the birch tree is able to fight off the fungus. It seems more often the fungus wins and kills the tree. How do we participate in this balance?

One midsummer, we harvested Chaga from a Black Birch (*Betula lenta*) tree approximately 12 inches in diameter that was bursting with Chaga on all sides. It looked as though the tree would not survive much longer: Most of the leaves in the sparse canopy were yellow instead of bright green. We harvested 4 to 5 pounds, a heavy harvest, because we assumed the tree was going to die. Three years later, we came back and saw that the tree had new growth and some Chaga had grown back. We did not harvest any that time. Three years later, we returned yet again and harvested 1 to 2 pounds, leaving approximately 4 pounds intact on the tree. The following winter we checked on the tree and found it was dead. We concluded that removing some of the Chaga can be beneficial and help extend the life of a tree, especially a tree that appears close to dying. Striking the balance to properly harvest Chaga requires careful observation and thought.

If all the Chaga growing on a tree is harvested, does the mycelium double down on extracting sustenance from the tree? Does leaving a part of the Chaga weaken the mycelium because there are still energy reserves in the form of sclerotia? Does harvesting at a certain time of the year increase the tree's ability to resist the fungus? The jury is still out, but we do know that harvesting incessantly is *never* sustainable.

Lactarius and *Lactifluus* species

MILKY CAP MUSHROOMS

People in many cultures around the world have consumed Milky mushrooms as a nutritious food. Milky mushrooms are a group of fungi that span several genera, and over 150 species occur in North America alone. *Lactarius*, *Multifurca*, and *Lactifluus* are three genera of these mushrooms that exude a "milk" when bruised or cut. *Lact-* means "milk" and *flu-* is "flow," so *Lactifluus* translates to "flowing milk" or "milk flows." A range of reactions can occur when these fruiting bodies are bruised or cut. Sometimes a small amount of "milk" oozes out, and other times there is an amazing overflow, as if the mushrooms are bleeding; the amount of liquid seems to depend on that individual mushroom in that moment. The milk can stain everything it touches a brown color. Sometimes the liquid immediately shows up as white, but later it changes color; this varies by species.

Milky mushrooms are ectomycorrhizal and show up as fruiting bodies in the forest floor at varying times of the season. They typically have sturdy stems centered under the cap with flesh and gills that can be brittle.

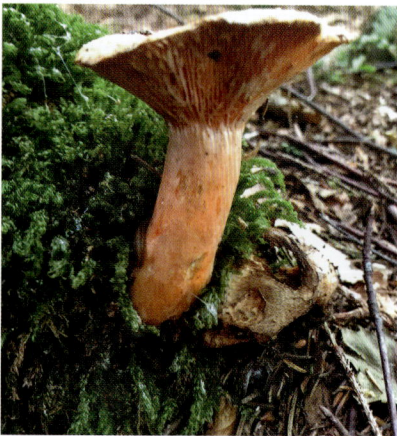

Figure 7.28. *Lactarius deliciosus* (Saffron Milk Cap) in Scotland.

Mycologists have reclassified many *Lactarius* species, placing them in the genus *Lactifluus*. Over 200 species of *Lactifluus* are reported worldwide. Some are generalists that can pair up with a range of tree species. Others are exclusive to individual species of trees or shrubs. For example, *Lactarius paradoxus* (Silver-Blue Milk Cap) associates with White Pines (*Pinus strobus*) in forests in the eastern United States. Identification of some species of Milky mushrooms can be easy, but others can be difficult. The results of DNA investigations seem to point toward more diversity within the genera than previously assumed, and

200

some species may be specialized to be in relationship with only one, or a very few, plant species.

One day as I was sitting down to watch Ground Squirrels (*Tamias striatus*) shredding *Lactifluus corrugis* (Corrugated Milky Cap), it occurred to me that they were not only eating these mushrooms but also probably helping to distribute the spores. Adawehi, my oldest daughter, calls this behavior *squirrelifying* mushrooms. The squirrels rip the mushroom apart, digging into the fruiting body as if hoping to find a prize buried within the cap. (They also do this with Maitake/Wishi and other fungi.) The squirrels seem to do this only during the first seven to ten days of the Milky mushroom season, though. After that they seem to become disenchanted with them. On the day I was watching the Ground Squirrels, I noticed them taking parts of the

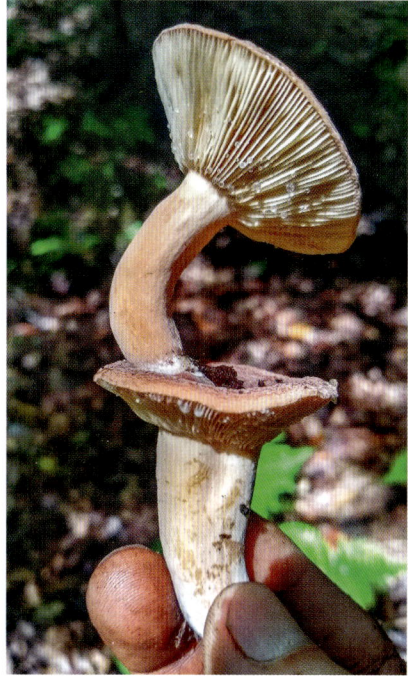

Figure 7.29. Milky Cap with unusual morphology.

cap back into their dens in the ground. I thought about how the squirrels would later eat the shredded mushrooms, and the spores would end up in scat in their burrows. (I've also observed lots of squirrel scat just outside the burrow entrance.) The squirrels would also end up with spores all over their upper bodies, paws, legs, and face. The realization then struck me that these little fast-moving beings scurrying around industriously from place to place are a major spore dispersal partner to the fungi. *Tamias striatus* translates to "striped steward." What a fitting name! This also led me to wonder how the spores might be affected by passing through the digestive tract of animals (like my musings about *Ganoderma* spores eaten by insects). Would it help increase germination rates, or decrease them? I don't think anyone has studied this.

A taste test of Milkies here in the Appalachian region can yield some intriguing results. (Note: Taste testing in this way is not recommended for other types of mushrooms!) With a Milky Cap mushroom, it is safe to touch your tongue to the fresh milk to taste it. Milk from the edible species will have a slightly sweet flavor. Let the flavor develop for a moment. Some Milky Cap species are sweet at first but sneak up on you after you have let the milk reach the back of your throat, producing an acrid burning sensation that slowly moves across your soft palate to the top of your throat. This often will leave your mouth with a dry, cottony feel and a lack of saliva. These experiences of tasting Milky

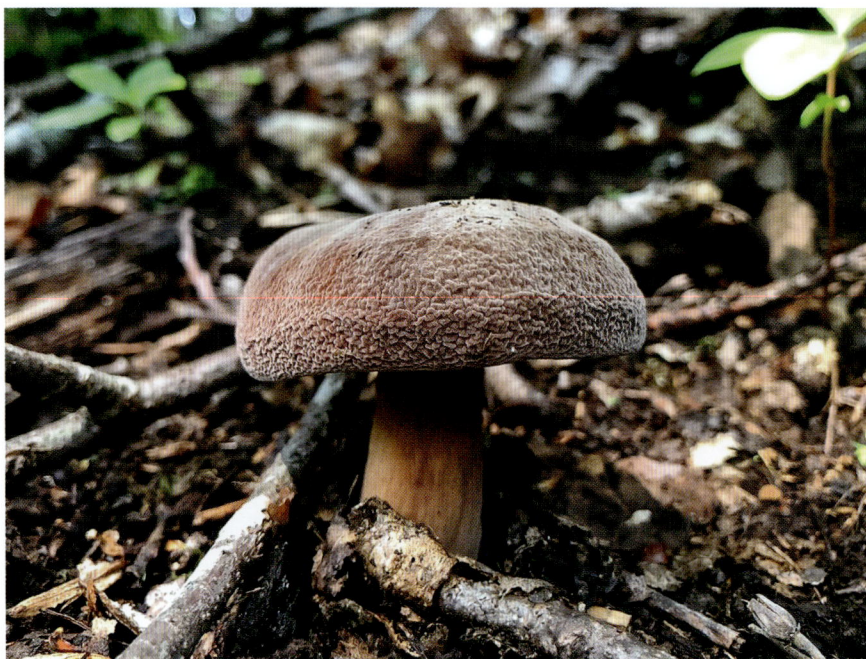

Figure 7.30. Milky Cap button after a forest fire.

mushrooms have led me to wonder whether this "milk" could possibly be used to deter insect pests of food crops in home gardens.

Traditional Uses

Milky mushrooms have played a large part in the diets of native peoples on every continent. Just a few examples: People in the Himalayas and China eat various species, differing according to the region where they live. Milkies are also eaten in Mexico, and many members of the Eastern Band of Cherokee Indians (EBCI) still consume them.

Chocolate Milky Cap (*Lactifluus corrugis*) is my second-favorite mushroom to eat (after Wishi). This mushroom grows in abundance in the Southern Appalachians, often within rhododendron thickets. In season, it is not uncommon to be able to pick 10 pounds in as little as 15 minutes. This mushroom has a meaty texture that I find similar to ground beef when chopped finely and cooked with appropriate spices.

The ethnomycological reports about Milky mushrooms are comparatively few in number compared to other mushrooms, but Milky mushrooms have likely been used as medicine as well as a food source in past times. In 2008, mycologist Gastón Guzmán wrote a paper studying the diversity in the traditional fungal medicines of Mexico. In Mexico, there are approximately ten

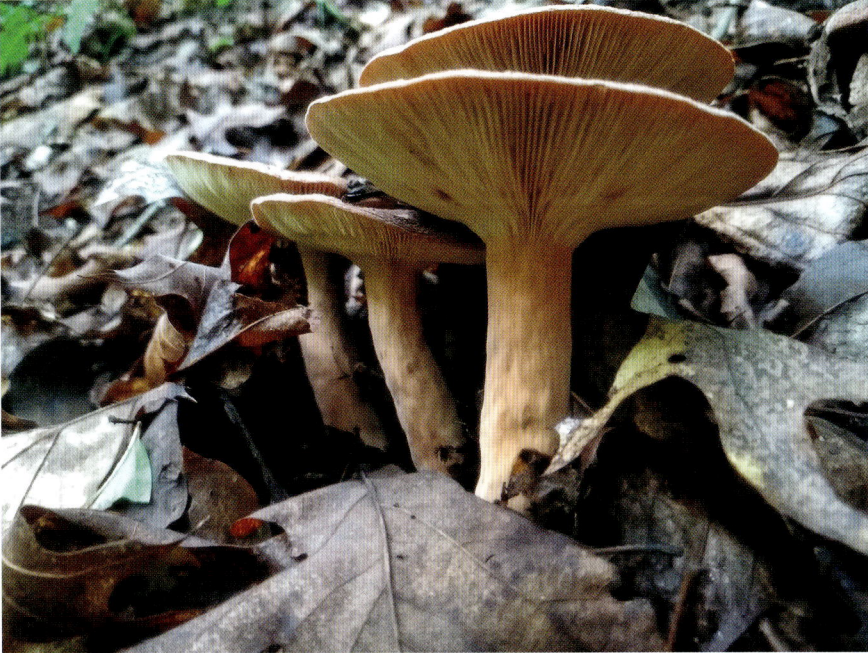

Figure 7.31. Milky mushroom cluster.

ethnic groups and over sixty different Indian cultures. These cultures have a vast knowledge of edible and medicinal mushrooms. It is estimated that there are over 200,000 species of fungi in Mexico, and only about 5 percent of those have been studied.

Guzmán reported that traditionally in Mexico, *Lactarius indigo* (Indigo Milk Cap) was used as a purgative and a laxative. *Lactarius deliciosus* (Saffron Milk Cap) and *Lactarius salmonicolor* (Salmon Milk Cap) were both used to reduce fever, and to treat headaches, indigestion, and intestinal pains.[90] Researchers are still discovering new compounds in *Lactarius* and *Lactifluus* species that have profound medicinal qualities.

In traditional medicine, Milky Caps are used in the treatment of urinary tract diseases and are considered to have a positive effect on the regulation of urine formation. *Lactifluus piperatus* (Peppery Milk Cap) is also considered to have beneficial effects on joint and muscle relaxation.

Research on Human Health Effects

We could not find reports of human clinical trials within the Milky mushroom complex. As the science of medicinal mushrooms moves forward, and these mushrooms become more popular, we hope that clinical trials in humans will be carried out for the benefit of those consuming or using these fungi as medicine. Here we summarize some interesting preclinical studies that show the potential of these mushrooms.

MINERAL CONTENT AND SAFETY

Initial work has looked at the mineral content and safety of *Lactarius* mushrooms. *Lactarius* species are good sources of potassium, magnesium, and iron, and specific composition differs among species.[91]

ANTIMICROBIAL

Mature fruiting bodies of *Lactifluus piperatus* and *Lactarius deliciosus* with mature spores have been found to have lower microbial activity against bacteria and fungi compared to the immature mushrooms.[92] Both ethanol and methanol extracts of *Lactifluus piperatus*, *Lactarius quietus* (Oakbug Milk Cap), and *Lactifluus vellereus* (Fleecy Milk Cap) show promising antibacterial, antioxidant, and antibiofilm properties.[93]

CANCER

Lactarius deliciosus has shown strong microbial activity in addition to cytotoxic activity against human skin, lung, and colon cancer cells.[94] Extracts of wild-harvested *Lactarius zonarius* (Ringer Milk Cap) have shown high antioxidant properties, cytotoxic effects, and strong antiproliferative activity against human lung, liver, and colon cancer cells. This species has low toxicity to other healthy human cells.[95]

One study offers promise for future research on the effects of Milky mushrooms on brain cancer. In this study on glioblastoma (the most commonly occurring brain cancer in adults), *Lactarius deliciosus* ethanol extracts were found to decrease metabolic activity in human glioblastoma cells at varying levels.[96]

Role in Holistic Healing

Many species of *Lactarius* and *Lactifluus* mushrooms are eaten and used for medicine, and there is potential for their use by underserved communities in rural areas. More educational efforts are needed. We feel that there is much still awaiting discovery about the healing powers of *Lactarius* and *Lactifluus* species.

Milky mushrooms also serve the bigger purpose of multispecies connection within an ecosystem. They support the trees and they support us as a long-term food source. We hope that people will reject the notion that Milkies are simply a source of new bioactive compounds to be exploited by pharmaceutical giants to make soaring profits.

The complex relationship that Milky mushrooms have in our forest ecosystems is still poorly understood. They play an important role in forest ecosystem resiliency, as food sources for mammals, insects, amphibians, and reptiles (especially turtles), and as hunting grounds for Red-Spotted Newts (*Notophthalmus viridescens*). As mentioned earlier, Milky mushrooms also have potential for use in our gardens as biological pest control, increasing disease resistance of the plants with which they have mycorrhizal relationships.

Cultivation Notes

Propagating Milky Caps is a simple method that is done right while harvesting them in the forest. This technique works for many mycorrhizal species. While picking the perfect Milky mushrooms to eat, also pick a few mushrooms that are past their prime. Take note of the species of trees and plants in the area too. As you continue mushroom hunting, watch for other spots where those same trees and plants are growing. That's where you'll "plant" the past-prime mushrooms you've collected. Use your foot to move the leaf litter aside and drop parts of the caps or whole mushrooms on the ground surface, then cover them up with leaves. This drop-and-cover technique takes only a few seconds. This is best done right before a rain, if possible, which will help ensure good spore germination and lead to mycelium leaping from the tissue into a relationship with the plants or trees.

Milky mushrooms are mycorrhizal and depend on their partnerships to survive. They cannot be cultivated in an artificial environment. The demand for these mushrooms is not high enough to stimulate interest in exploring techniques for cultivating them at scale. Their power lies in being a part of that forest ecosystem that supports trees, insects, and other animals, including us. Milky mushrooms are there to help remind us of the deep connections we are part of on this planet. Cooperation is their lesson, not isolation.

Ethical Wild Harvesting

Occasionally, Milky mushrooms can be the dominant species on the forest floor during their fruiting season. When they are, harvest them and help them to spread using the technique described previously in "Cultivation Notes." In areas where Milky mushrooms are not prolific, we do not recommend harvesting. Give them an opportunity to expand a fruiting colony for future enjoyment.

Lentinula edodes

SHIITAKE

Shiitake mushrooms are the type of cultivated mushrooms that are most widely grown outdoors. They are very popular among beginner growers because of the ease of cultivation and their abundant production. Shiitakes produce several flushes in the spring and several in the fall. Even after more than thirty years of my journey with mycology, I still experience childlike excitement when I see Shiitakes emerging from the logs in the forest.

Lentinula edodes is native to East Asian countries, including Taiwan, China, and Japan, where it can be found growing wild in mountainous regions. In Japanese, *shii* is the word for Chinquapin Oak (*Quercus muehlenbergii*) and *take* (pronounced "tah-kay") is the word for mushrooms. Thus, Shiitake is "Oak Mushroom" or "Chinquapin Mushroom." Other common names for *L. edodes* include "Oakwood Mushroom" or "Black Forest Mushroom." Oak is the best type of wood on which to grow this culinary delight.

The Chinese name for this mushroom, *Xiangu*, translates to "Fragrant Mushroom." It is also known as the "Queen of Plants." Of course, modern taxonomy no longer classifies fungi as plants, but this does not change how highly these fungi were and are still regarded in their native range. The Latin root *Lent-* means flexible or pliable, and *-inus* means "resembling." *Edode* means "edible." So, it seems *Lentinula edodes* is "Resembling Flexible, and Edible."

Shiitake mushrooms are deep brown to nearly black in the button stages, becoming mostly lighter tan with age. The button stage displays a cottony, scale-like growth on the caps that fades after the caps open and enlarge. The edge of the cap (margin) flattens out and then often becomes undulating or wavy. The stem can be long or very short, according to the variety. The spores are white and often stand out well against the contrast of the brown logs on which they are cultivated. Cap size ranges from a diameter of 2 inches (5 cm) to 10 inches (25 cm). The flesh is firm and has an umami flavor that we find earthy and woodsy. It is one of the favorites in our kitchen.

Up until 1972, it was illegal to import Shiitake mushroom cultures into the United States. Bureaucratic powers thought that Shiitakes would colonize and damage railroad sleepers. (Similar to *Neolentinus lepidus*, a mushroom called TrainWrecker, which can consume treated wood and railroad ties.) Although

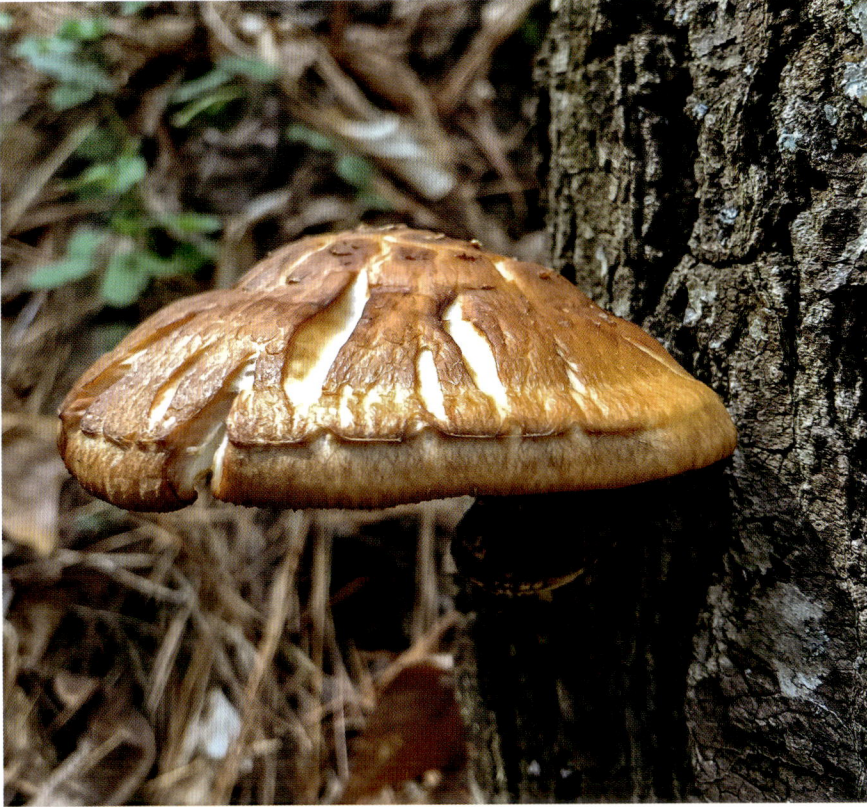

Figure 7.32. Donko Shiitake on oak log.

the bureaucrats were wrong about Shiitake, we agree it is wise to be cautious in introducing new species to an area, because they could end up displacing native and important species.

By the 1980s, people in the United States had started cultivating Shiitakes, and now *L. edodes* is escaping from cultivation across the world. In the Appalachian Mountains, environments similar to the mushroom's native habitats are proving to be hospitable to Shiitakes. While out mushroom hunting over the years, I have found four different locations of Shiitakes that have escaped cultivation, growing on logs or trees in the woods. And over the years, many people have brought me wild Shiitakes for culturing. Out of nearly a dozen different samples from the wild, only two have been proven to be highly productive strains.

Traditional Uses

The traditional uses of *L. edodes* are limited to the region of Asia where it is native, which represents a smaller geographic area and range of cultures than most of the other mushrooms we discuss in this book. The following description of Shiitake cultivation is from the first verified written record, which roughly translates as the *Records of Longquan County* by He Dan, written in 1209 CE. This information, documented over eight hundred years ago, describes the full process of selecting trees, cutting the logs, and harvesting and drying the mushrooms. He Dan also describes the properties of the mushrooms at each stage of processing. This writing reflects a deep observation of the process, which likely had been followed for a long time before anyone wrote it down.

He Dan writes, "Fragrant mushrooms (*xùn*) are only found in the deep and shady places of the mountains. The method is: use dry heartwood olive wood, called mushroom wood, first cut it down to the ground at the foot of the mountains, use an axe to cut the mottled bark, wait for it to be soaked, and it will start to emerge after two years, and in the third year, the mushrooms will emerge on the side. After the beginning of spring, the earth's qi will be released, and thunder and rain will shake, and the mushrooms will emerge on the wood."[97]

He Dan also describes how the mushrooms can be hung on bamboo strips to dry and notes that spring flushes tend to be heavier than autumn flushes. He describes the cultivation technique of striking the logs to force mushrooms to fruit, one that is still used today.

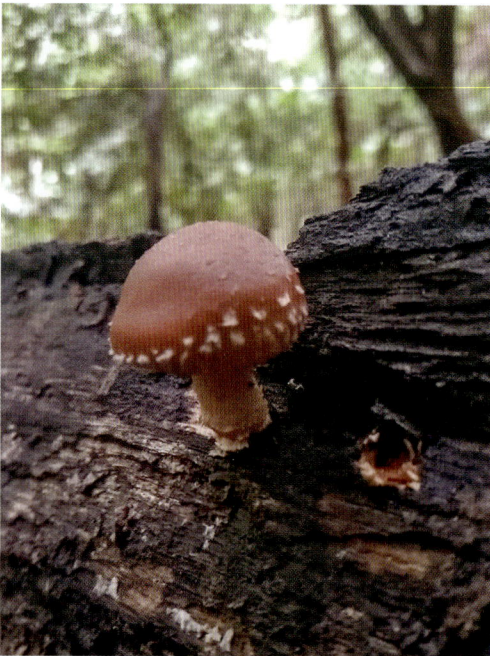

Figure 7.33. Wild Shiitake that escaped cultivation.

Local legend says that the first cultivation of Shiitakes dates back close to one thousand years ago, and was begun by a wood cutter and charcoal maker, Wu Sangong (whose name might have been Wu Yuyu) from Longyan Village in Longquan County. Wu Sangong noticed that where his axe had cut dead logs, mushrooms later appeared. He decided to mix fresh logs in with the fruiting logs, and thus Shiitake cultivation was born.

While the Chinese were beginning to cultivate Shiitakes, the Japanese were still wild harvesting only. By the mid-1500s there were many mushroom farmers in China.

Nearly six hundred years after the publication of He Dan's Chinese text, in 1796, Sato Narihiro wrote *The Shocking Mushroom Record*. The author was a Japanese forest scientist, and the work references He Dan. Sato Narihiro compiled, improved, and summarized He Dan's *Records of Longquan County* and other subsequent writings for *The Shocking Mushroom Record*. Sato Narihiro's work catapulted the innovation of Shiitake farming and production in Japan. The significance of Sato Narihiro's historic work cannot be overemphasized. Cultivation of Shiitakes has accelerated since, and in 1906 the Japanese began artificial cultivation, birthing the techniques still used today. This technology also spread to Korea and then to Taiwan.[98]

Shiitake is renowned in these East Asian countries as a highly nutritious food. It is high in protein (20 to 30 percent), carbohydrates, fiber, and various nutrients, including selenium, an antioxidant that may prevent cancer and promote cognitive function. Shiitake also has a long history of medicinal use. A Chinese text from 1620 refers to two-hundred-year-old knowledge stating that *L. edodes* "accelerates vital energy, wards off hunger, cures colds and defeats body fluid energy."[99]

Research on Human Health Effects

Some research suggests that Shiitakes have a positive effect on treating cancer indirectly or may be used as an adjunct therapy for cancer treatment. Shiitakes contain lentinan, a polysaccharide and β-glucan, that is effective and safe for the treatment of cancers. Lentinan was discovered in the 1970s, and it was largely ignored until recently. In 2022 researchers found that lentinan protects the body from oxidative damage and that a diet with lentinan can modify the intestinal microbiota.[100] This has the potential to support the gut lining and enhance intestinal immunity.

Lentinan is likely also responsible for Shiitake's ability to support many facets of our immune systems. This support often leads to cancer cells being uncloaked so that the cancer can be dealt with by our immune function.

In Japan, Shiitake is used in treating diseases that suppress the immune system, including AIDS, cancer, allergies, candida infections, and recurrent colds and flu.[101] Shiitake extract is used in Japan to treat various cancers, including stomach cancer.[102]

CANCER

Extracts from Shiitake mycelium have been studied extensively for effects on cancer. In mice, Shiitake has been found to act against carcinogens, modulate the immune system to improve outcomes, stop tumor growth, and reduce blood sugar levels.[103] There are well-controlled trials with humans undergoing standard cancer treatments. A three-year trial in which liver cancer patients received 1 g of Shiitake mycelium extract daily for the first year found a significantly lower rate of cancer recurrence and reduced tumor size.[104] In another trial, patients who had head and neck cancers received 3 g of Shiitake extract daily for two weeks before radiation and chemotherapy and also for two months afterward. Researchers found significantly higher levels of various healthy blood markers and less weight loss in patients using Shiitake extract than in the placebo group. Additionally, there was less treatment-related toxicity in those taking Shiitake. The Shiitake patients reported significantly higher quality of life, and the study's authors noted that receiving Shiitake led to better clinical outcomes.[105]

People undergoing radiation and chemotherapy can experience chronic fatigue syndrome (CFS), which may be related to having a low, or acidic, overall pH level in the body. Over six months of Shiitake extract treatment, combined with heat therapy, cancer patients suffering with CFS reported significantly reduced (that is, improved) CFS scores while their body pH values had returned to neutral (that is, normal).[106]

VIRUSES

Shiitake extracts appear to boost the immune system and reduce rates of infection due to various viruses. Shiitake has been shown to reduce occurrences of the common cold and speed recovery time in the elderly.[107] It has also been shown to significantly reduce viral load in those with hepatitis C, without side effects.[108] One exploratory study analyzed blood from healthy volunteers who had already been taking a Shiitake extract for a year. Researchers injected COVID-19 into the blood. Results suggest that consuming Shiitake primed the volunteers' blood to launch an immune response to the virus. More antiviral agents were found in the blood of the Shiitake eaters compared to control.[109]

LIVER DISEASE

In patients with nonalcoholic fatty liver disease (NAFLD) who took 2 g of Shiitake daily for ninety days, a biomarker of liver disease (alkaline phosphatase) was found to significantly decrease. Other biomarkers suggested that the Shiitake had an immunomodulating effect. No participants reported any adverse reactions or problems with the treatment.[110]

IRRITABLE BOWEL SYNDROME (IBS)

In a human trial with those suffering from IBS, patients took 2 g of Shiitake extract daily for four weeks. Results showed that 63 percent of the treatment group, compared to 30 percent of the placebo group, felt their symptoms were improving. Various markers of immune system functioning and anti-inflammatory activity were significantly improved in the treatment group.[111]

Role in Holistic Healing

L. edodes is the second-most widely consumed mushroom and the oldest known saprotrophic cultivated mushroom on Earth. With all that this gastronomic delight has to offer in the way of high-protein and high-nutrient content, as well as medicinal qualities, it is no wonder it has been sought after by urban-dwelling mushroom growers, forest farmers, and mycologists alike. The desire for Shiitakes is largely responsible for advancement in the production and cultivation of mushrooms.

Though Shiitake may not be the medicinal powerhouse that some other mushrooms are, it still holds its own in the realm of medicinal mushrooms. Reishi, for example, is arguably more medicinal, but due to its bitter medicinal compounds, it is not pleasant to partake of. Shiitake, on the other hand, has one of the best umami flavors. It's easy to incorporate into nearly any diet. For us, the importance of this mushroom outweighs many other medicinal fungi because of its cultural significance, history, medicinal qualities, ease of cultivation, high-quality nutrition, and adaptability. We hope it will soon replace the ubiquitous White Button mushrooms (*Agaricus bisporus*), which lack much medicinal benefit and are potentially harmful due to their tendency to hyper-accumulate heavy metals.

L. edodes is a perfect example of a mushroom with an ancient history that has been fully incorporated into modern times. As the years go by, researchers are uncovering more facets of Shiitake's medicinal qualities. With these findings, more people are beginning to use the Shiitake as medicinal instead of as just a culinary mushroom.

Shiitakes are now grown in high-tech, climate-controlled environments with all the bells and whistles one can dream of. There are also forest farmers like us who are growing these mushrooms with essentially the same methods as they were grown hundreds of years ago. Across the United States you can find Shiitakes served in restaurants and sold at grocery stores and farmer's markets, and we encounter many people who tend Shiitake logs in their backyard.

A research paper published in 2016 explored the potential of Shiitake as a treatment for dental

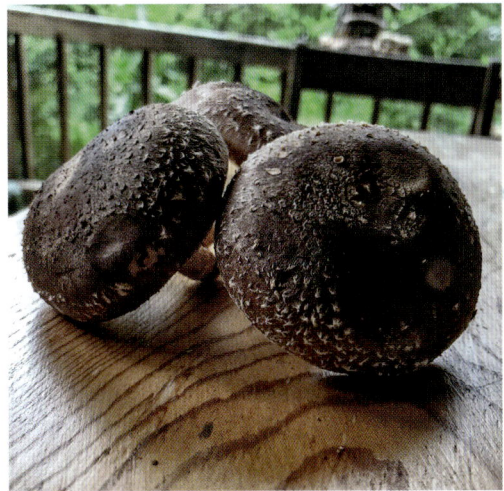

Figure 7.34. Log-grown shiitakes.

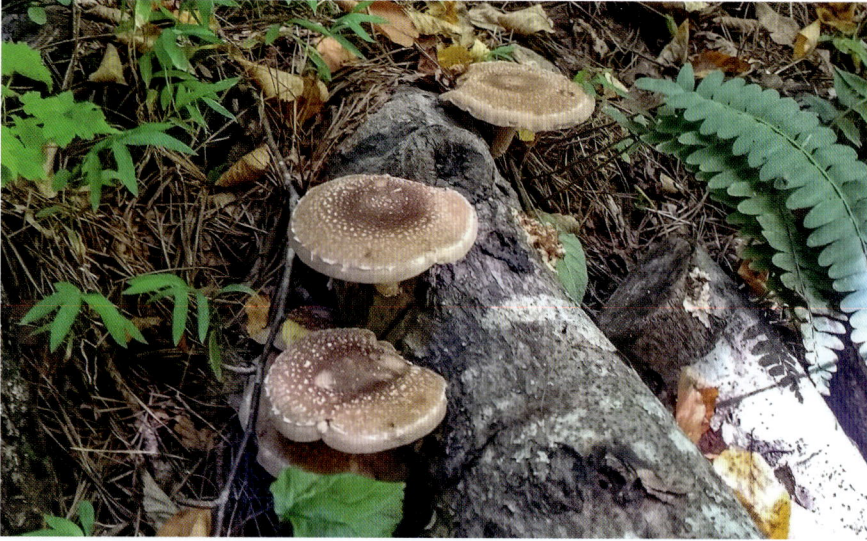

Figure 7.35. Shiitakes growing on oak logs.

cavities, with extracts shown to have powerful antifungal and antibacterial activities related to tooth decay.[112] Perhaps Shiitake will someday be incorporated into oral care products as a healthier alternative to chemical-laden fluoride toothpastes.

L. edodes can also help clean up environmental toxins. Dichloropropenes (DCPs) are volatile organic compounds (VOCs) used in pesticides. And 2,4-DCP is one of the most toxic and can cause lung problems and kidney and liver damage in humans. A paper from 2013 studying the remediation effects of Shiitake mycelium found that adding vanillin (from the vanilla bean) to *L. edodes* mycelium increased the efficacy of the mycelium in breaking down 2,4-DCP from 15 percent to 92 percent.[113] Exciting findings like these continue to show that new things in the world of mycology are waiting to be uncovered and implemented.

Cultivation Notes

Log cultivation is the easiest and most hands-off method for growing Shiitakes, and Shiitakes produced outdoors are far superior to those produced indoors. Indoor production is a viable option for Shiitake cultivation, but it requires more involved methods than other easier-to-grow species. See Shiitake log cultivation on page 41 for more details.

Because Shiitakes have been cultivated for so long, growers have had ample time to select for desirable traits. For example, we have strains of Shiitake that will produce mushrooms at over 80°F (27°C), and others that will thrive on substrates that mushrooms would not typically grow on, including waste products such as wheat straw. Other strains are cold-weather specific, and still others straddle both heat and cold, growing in a wide variety of temperatures. Compared to other types of fungi, Shiitake cultivation techniques are literally thousands of years ahead, thanks to having our ancestors' hands and the fungi themselves as our guide.

Ethical Wild Harvesting

As mentioned above, Shiitakes are not native in North America, and the species has escaped cultivation in some areas. We know the location of five trees with wild shiitakes. Some believe that wild Shiitakes could become invasive or push native species out of a niche. This is possible, so we harvest them just like we would any other useful invasive species in our region. We harvest as much as we need without concern for their survival, knowing they are more successful than many native species.

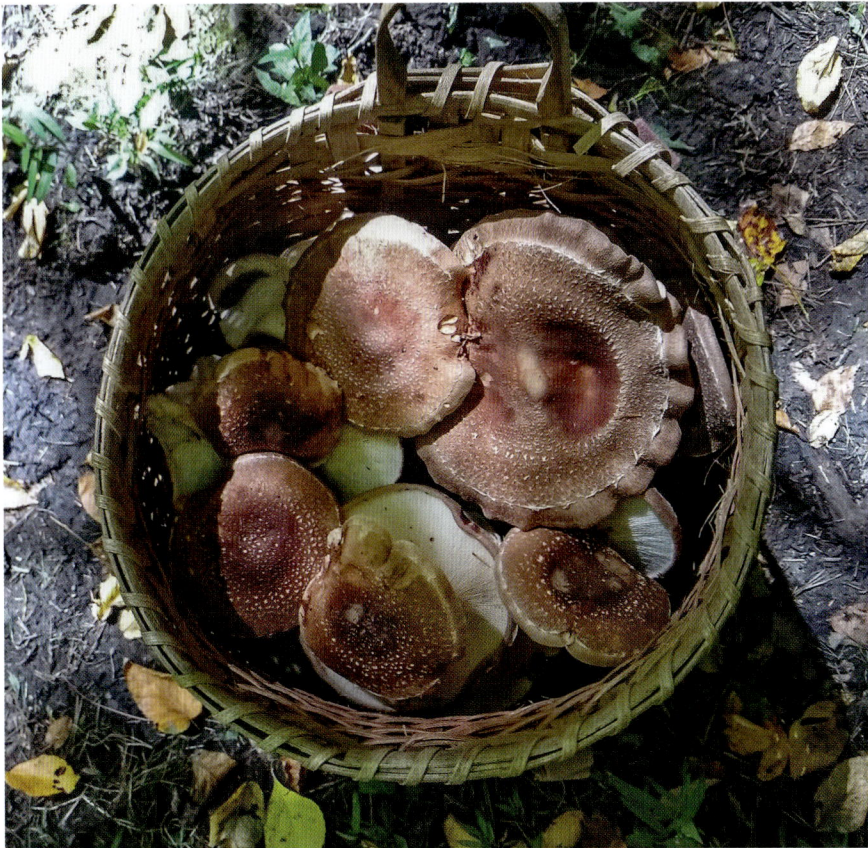

Figure 7.36. Shiitakes collected from our logs.

❖ ❖ ❖

Penicillium species

MEDICINAL MOLDS

*P*enicillium is a genus of "imperfect fungi," meaning they engage only in asexual reproduction, or that may have sexual reproduction methods as yet not detected. The name *Penicillium* derives from Latin meaning "painter's brush," in reference to their conidiophores, which are spore-producing structures that look like upright paintbrushes, bristles pointing skyward. These fungi do not produce a complex, fleshy fruiting body with an obvious hymenium.

One common form of *Penicillium* fungi is the powdery green mold that grows on the skin of citrus fruits left on the countertop too long. These are not mushrooms, but they are fungi. They are part of the same phylum, Ascomycota, as cup fungi, the highly sought after truffle (*Tuber* spp.), and the often-elusive morel (*Morchella* spp.) mushrooms. The developmental similarities of *Penicillium* spp. and *Morchella* spp. place them in the same category. It is the sac-type structure of the conidiophore, containing four to eight spores, that places *Penicillium* in this common branch of ancestors. The mycelium is highly forked or branched, with the spores (conidia) produced on the conidiophores, which are oriented erect.

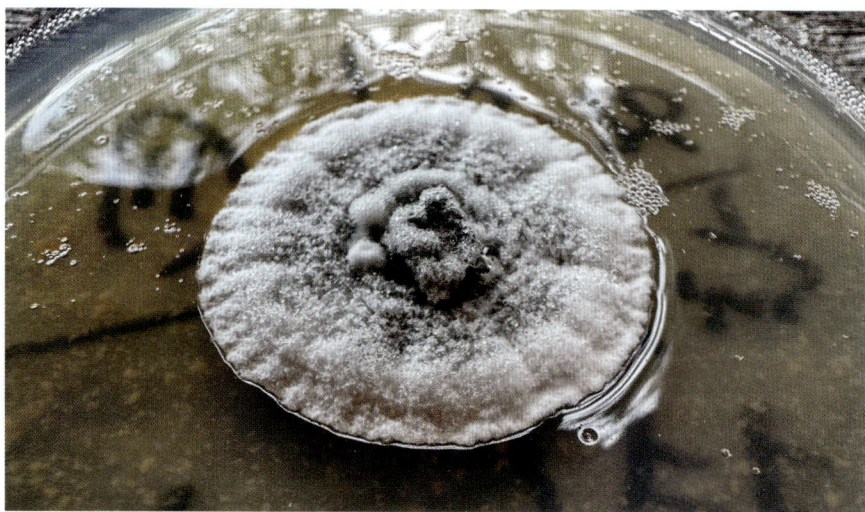

Figure 7.37. *Penicillium* on petri plate.

Because these fungi produce asexually, a single cell of these spores contains all the genetic information needed. When a spore lands in a suitable environment it will germinate, colonize the substrate, and continue to propagate the species. Spores are lightweight and can be carried by the wind. Asexual spores have a distinct advantage because, in theory, a single spore could be picked up on the wind and carried across continents, then land and start a colony thousands of miles away from where it originated.

Penicillium has spread worldwide. I find it surprising that there are only about 350 species in this genus. (By comparison, there are more than one thousand species in the genus *Ganoderma*.) I wonder whether this is because *Penicillium* species are general decomposers, not specialized to a specific plant or tree, allowing each species a potentially large range. Or the lack of recorded species may be due to a deficiency in the study of soil microbial communities. As more soil microbiologists are trained and turn their attention to the life-filled layers below the surface, more species of *Pencillium* may be identified. Similarly, scientists have barely scratched the surface in the exploration of undersea fungi, and initial findings are tantalizing.

When an anatomical structure in fungi has remained unchanged for millions of years, it speaks to the success of that organism. *Penicillium* have the same basic structure of fungi that have been foundational to all life on Earth, from the first vascular plants to ancient megafauna and the creatures that walk with us now. They have become part of a wide variety of ecosystems, and they will be here long after us humans.

Penicillium can cause problems for humans. For example, it can cause allergic reactions in individuals. At larger scale, it can cause losses in the food industry. *Penicillium* molds produce mycotoxins.

The genus *Penicillium* has been reconceptualized to include species from other genera such as *Thysanophora*, *Chromocleista*, *Eladia*, *Torulomyces*, and *Eupenicillium*. This is a rare occurrence in the world of mycology. According to a 2022 review of the genus, published in *Studies in Mycology*, "The genus currently contains 354 accepted species, including new combinations for *Aspergillus crystallinus*, *A. malodoratus* and *A. paradoxus*, which belong to *Penicillium* section *Paradoxa*."[114] Some of these species are known to be plant pathogens; some are known to solubilize phosphates. Some are known to have symbiotic actions with other organisms that survive in harsh environments. Often it is these fungi, or similar fungi, that will survive the onslaught of tilling machinery and chemical weed suppressants or insecticides. They exist in these agricultural battlefields where they can adapt to consume chemical compounds and utilize them as a source of energy. Then they become a pathogen on the very plants farmers were attempting to protect. In conventional systems, farmers then pour on more chemicals, rather than understanding the problem as an ecosystem out of balance. In order to regain balance, we must integrate these fungi into our crop systems and allow them to help us in new ways.

Traditional Uses

Molds were not understood in ancient times to the degree we understand them now, but there is evidence they may have been used for medicinal purposes. The biological mechanisms of the healing actions of molds were not fully understood for hundreds or even thousands of years. But it is well known that many of our ancestors used moldy bread to directly treat skin wounds.[115]

South of Egypt lies the ancient Nubian kingdom. Human bones in the ancient Nubian kingdom dating to 350 to 550 CE were discovered to contain traces of the antibiotic tetracycline. Modern tetracyclines were only "discovered" in 1948. Researchers wondered how the bones of these ancient people came to contain a modern antibiotic. They hypothesized that the fermentation process of making beer could have pulled in the bacteria streptomyces from soil. Turns out, tetracycline is a metabolite of streptomyces. It could have been transferred from batch to batch of beer through the starter used for each new batch. The research team found that the skull of a four-year-old was full of tetracycline and speculated that this child had an illness his people were trying desperately to cure.[116] The researchers were not clear whether the Nubian people were deliberately making antibiotic-rich beers or if they simply noticed the effects that certain brews were having and did their best to repeat these processes.

Many traditional peoples relied on invisible organisms in brewing beer and making bread. Saccharomyces, or yeasts, were used for food and to purify water by making beer. Even low levels of alcohol produced by these fungi can effectively kill some water-borne pathogens, including parasites and bacteria. Traditional peoples were wielding the power of these tiny beings without a scientific understanding of their potential power.

The ancient Egyptians harnessed this power of moldy bread, as did the Chinese, approximately 2,500 years ago, creating their first antibiotic. At that time, soybean curd or tofu was used to treat boils. This tofu had been colonized by an unidentified mold, and it began to be administered as a standard treatment. Scientists hypothesize that this mold could have been producing penicillin. In parts of Europe, moldy cheese has been used to fight off infections in wounds for at least one thousand years.[117]

Research on Human Health Effects

In 1928 Alexander Fleming, a Scottish physician, discovered that *P. rubens* inhibited bacterial growth. A petri plate he had inoculated with the bacteria

Staphylococcus aureus became contaminated with *Penicillium*. In the area surrounding the fungus, the bacterial colony died out. Fleming cultured the fungus and found that it produced a substance, penicillin, that acted as a powerful antibiotic against bacteria and other pathogens.

Nearly a decade after this initial discovery, penicillin became famous in Britain during the Second World War. Research on mice had already shown that the fungal extract showed promise as an antibacterial agent. The research was given a rapid boost by the need for a remedy for allied soldiers dying of sepsis and gas gangrene during the last two years of the war. The Rockefeller Foundation gave a $25,000 grant to two Oxford-based researchers, Ernst Chain and Howard Florey, who had come across Fleming's original research. They developed a team to start the Penicillin Project at Oxford in England. Building on previous research on penicillin in animals, their team gave the first intravenous injections of penicillin to people suffering with severe sepsis in 1941.[118]

Penicillin became one of the most widely used antibiotics across the world. Resistance to penicillin is a new outcome resulting from overprescribing. This is part of the challenge with commercial production. But the use of penicillin as an antibiotic is so widespread that we do not cover it here. Instead we discuss some novel uses of *Penicillium* species.

COGNITIVE PERFORMANCE AND SLEEP

Surprisingly, one *Penicillium* species, *P. camemberti*, has been found to positively impact cognitive performance and sleep. Camembert cheese is made through a process of fermenting milk with this white mold. Oleamide, a compound produced during the fermentation process, has been found in animal studies to enhance sleep and learning. In a trial in humans, people fifty to seventy-five years of age with mild cognitive decline took oleamide (60 μg) daily for twelve weeks. The results suggest that both oleamide and oleamide-containing foods (that is, the cultured milk and Camembert cheese) are safe and help improve cognitive functions (particularly short-term and working memory) while enhancing sleep.[119] Good news for cheese lovers! *P. camemberti* is the only excuse we need in our household to eat more cheese.

PRECLINICAL WORK IN CANCER

Penicillium species are often endophytic: they live inside plants, feeding on plant cells. In the process they produce secondary metabolites, including indole alkaloids. A group of researchers extracted an indole alkaloid from a *Penicillium* mold living on the leaves of olive trees in Egypt (*P. chrysogenum*), then tested its effects on various human breast cancer cells. One indole alkaloid, meleagrin, inhibited the growth of human breast cancer cells, blocked receptors shown to play a role in the development of breast cancer, and reduced the movement of breast cancer cells into other cell lines.[120]

P. citrinum lives in the ocean. One of its secondary metabolites, penicitrinine A, has shown antitumor effects against human melanoma (skin) cancer cells. It reduced their proliferation rate, increased cell death, and reduced the degree of metastasis.[121] This type of work is progressing and may yield some novel cancer treatments.

According to one lab-based study, *P. vulpinum* may be able to prevent the recurrence of lung cancer. It was also found to stop certain types of lung cancer cells from replicating and migrating, in addition to causing them to die.[122]

DIABETES

In the search for novel antidiabetic drugs with fewer side effects than conventional pharmaceutical treatments, a team of Asia-based scientists screened various fungal metabolites to find chemical structures with the potential to serve as nontoxic drugs. The compound that showed the most promise was pinazaphilone B, a secondary metabolite of a *Peniciullium* fungus.[123]

Role in Holistic Healing

Penicillium fungi have played a historic role in human history. This group is found on every continent of this shiny blue planet. It is present in many strata of soil, and in the human gut (although it is not a resident there). And it's safe to assume that many species remain to be discovered and documented.

It is not rosy with all molds though. Many millions of pounds of food are lost each year because of mold growth. Some of these molds can make people or pets deathly ill, and they can make houses sick too. In moist conditions, *Stachybotrys chartarum,* known as Black Mold, can flourish and produce mycotoxins that cause a whole range of symptoms. *Aspergillus niger* is another toxic black mold. If you live in a humid and warm summer climate like the Southern Appalachians, then black mold is a serious health concern.

The other side of that coin is that some species of *Aspergillus* have the amazing ability to transform humble soybeans into soy sauce or tamari (aged soy sauce). And inoculating partially cooked soybeans (sometimes mixed with grains) with aspergillus results in delicious tempeh. The action of this mold can increase nutrients in a food or make something less than desirable into a food with wonderful umami flavor. Groups in many parts of the world have used mold organisms to change their culture and to shape their foods. Just as Asian peoples fermented soybeans, European peoples used various species of fungi to cure and store milk from sheep, cows, and goats—an otherwise quickly perishable commodity—so it could become a staple food that kept people from starving. Modern research studies have given us more insight into the possible benefits of these tiny imperfect fungi. The possibilities are not limited to what we currently understand about fungi in general but include soil health, human health, industrial applications, animal (wild and domesticated) health, ecosystem balance, nutrient upcycling, and more.

Combined knowledge of ancient techniques and modern observations of the secondary compounds that *Penicillium* produce is leading to deeper understanding of what these fungi are capable of. Some species of *Penicillium* are endophytes, meaning that they live symbiotically inside the tissues of plants aboveground. These fungi use sugars produced by the plants as a food source, and in return they produce metabolites that are beneficial to the plants. They promote plant growth, provide drought tolerance, and more. Note that although plants have the capacity to produce secondary metabolites, when fungi collaborate with plants, it is often the fungi that produce the compounds protective to the plants.

Given the impactful results humanity has seen from just one *Penicillium* metabolite, penicillin, the potential benefits of other such compounds is very exciting. Researchers are describing hundreds of new metabolites produced by plant endophytes. A 2023 article in *Microbial Biotechnology* reported that among 302 endophytes isolated from 30 wild plants, 70 compounds (23 percent) exhibited activity against pathogens.[124]

P. pinophilum is a root-associated fungus that has the ability to increase plant growth and output by secondary metabolite production. A 2020 study found that co-inoculation of three arbuscular mycorrhizal fungi (AMF) and *P. pinophilum* was more successful in comparison to using only one inoculant in both tomatoes and lettuce.[125] It is clear from this study that there are applications for *Penicillium* species in modern agriculture to improve soil conditions, plant growth, and production.

Penicillium as an endophyte is able to fill many ecological niches and respond to environmental stressors by producing metabolites that protect and strengthen the organisms around them. In this way they may actually be mutualists—that is, these organisms benefit from having each other around but do not necessarily need each other. They may have something to teach us about healthy relationships.

Research on *Penicillium* has moved beyond looking for antibiotic compounds. The medicinal benefits are pretty obvious with *Penicillium* species and their counterparts. Many species of *Penicillium*, *Trichoderma*, *Verticillium*, and the like, are known to be antagonistic to nematodes, the miniscule worms that cause gardeners and farmers all sorts of problems. Work is being done to develop products to help combat nematode infestations. We advocate being careful of introducing fungi from thousands of miles away to treat our local crops, because of the possibility of displacing our native fungi and getting our-selves into a situation we didn't predict. It is important to get people out into the field as much as possible to find local solutions to local problems.

Cultivation Notes

We do not cultivate *Penicillium* fungi in our lab because we lack the equipment to extract medicinal compounds, and because *Penicillium* is typically consid-ered contamination in the kinds of fungi we do cultivate. If you feel inspired to cultivate *Penicillium,* we suggest using a facility separate from your other mushroom growing operation. *Penicillium* species can be easily cultivated on any grain.

Wild Harvesting . . . Ethically?

The sheer abundance of *Penicillium* fungi on planet Earth makes it seem impossible to overharvest them. One method to demonstrate this is to place a container of partially cooked rice in strategic areas, such as a forest or field or near buildings, and see what you have captured in a few days. A mix of various wild imperfect fungi will grow. *Penicillium* typically shows up in the mix, but it takes skill to identify it.

Pleurotus species

OYSTER MUSHROOMS

Oyster mushrooms are the second-most widely cultivated, wild-harvested, and popular edible mushrooms worldwide. *Agaricus bisporus*, the White Button mushroom, is the first. We would like to see this preference flip, because Oysters have the potential to be grown in a variety of environments and provide many more medicinal benefits.

Oyster mushrooms are a readily available, inexpensive, non-harmful source of macro- and micronutrients. They have been part of human diets for longer than we know and may hold a key to providing healthy food in countries that struggle with food shortages. In addition, these mushrooms are highly efficient at restoring forest ecosystems, breaking down pollutants, and turning waste into delicious, nutritious food.

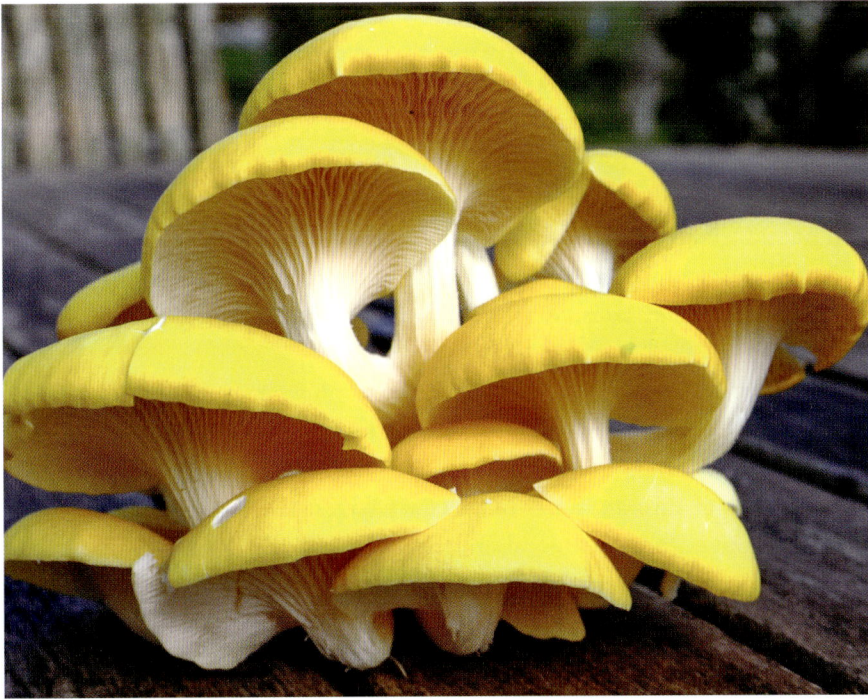

Figure 7.38. Summer-fruiting Golden Oysters (*P. citrinopileatus*).

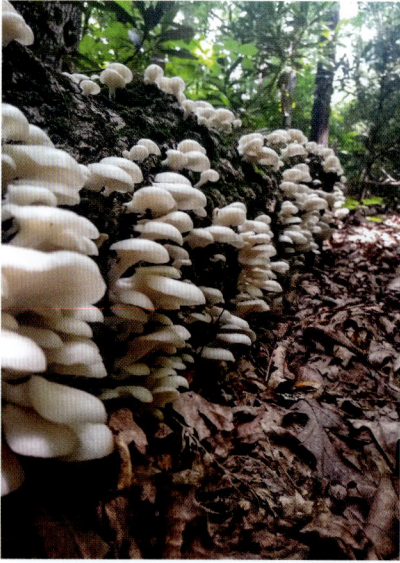

Figure 7.39. Wild Pearl Oysters (*P. ostreatus*).

Many people are unaware of the medicinal properties of Oyster mushrooms. Oysters show exciting promise to help with major diseases of the Western lifestyle, including diabetes and cardiovascular disease. Scientific research on the medicinal benefits of this mushroom is in its infancy, but the wealth of evidence from thousands of years of traditional use points to Oysters as a significant medicinal mushroom. And they seem to have no nasty side effects, so why not add them to our diets?

The Latin and Greek root of *Pleurotus* translates to "side ear," a reference to the way in which an Oyster mushroom's cap grows away from the stem or stipe (see figure 7.38). Stipe size varies across different species and varieties. Some Oysters grow in immense clusters covering dead trees and others grow as a single specimen. Colors range from deep blues, hot pinks, and striking golden hues to whites, blending-into-the-forest browns, and steel grays. Thus, some Oyster clusters stand out boldly against their environment and others camouflage themselves perfectly into the natural landscape.

More than two hundred species have been identified in the genus *Pleurotus*. Some of these species coexist in the same forests, while others seem to have exclusivity in certain forests. They can be found in every temperate, tropical, and subtropical forest in the world, surviving in frigid climates as well as hot and humid tropical rainforests. Oysters have a voracious appetite for cellulose and an ability to adapt and change in response to their environment. There is no doubt that *Pleurotus* is one of the most useful and adaptive genera of fungi in the world.

The morphology of the many species in this genus is puzzling to the untrained eye because of their wide range of shapes and colors. There are basic structural similarities, though. The caps are offset and off center from the stem and enlarge out into an oyster-like shape. At first the fruiting bodies have a beautiful convex form; within about forty-eight hours, the cap evolves into a concave, upturned margin. This concave older stage of growth is what we prefer to eat. The spores are the same color across species with only slight variations, from off-white to a grey-lilac or pale salmon.

The King Oyster Mushroom (*P. eryngii*) develops large and heavy stems and nearly no cap. Some King Oysters can grow upwards of a pound apiece!

They have a hearty meaty texture. On the other side of the spectrum, Golden Oysters (*P. citrinopileatus*) have a slight citric-acid flavor and are so delicate that I jokingly tell people that they prep themselves in the bag on the way home from the market!

Oysters are part of a community of pioneer species that reforest a swath of forest after a disturbance, whether due to a forest fire, clear-cutting, flooding, or, in extreme case, a meteor air burst. Oysters consume many pioneer species such as Tulip Poplar (*Liriodendron tulipifera*). In boreal forests the pioneer species are White Birch (*Betula papyrifera*), which reestablishes first, followed by spruce and fir trees (*Picea* and *Abies* spp.). Oysters are one of many fungi that break down the dead or dying softwoods and softer hardwoods, quickly and efficiently, to rebuild the topsoil. When some of these pioneer fungal partners show back up in the landscape, at first glance, they may seem to be singular islands of life among the devastation that has recently occurred. But these fungi serve as pioneers to incorporate other life forms back into the landscape.

Traditional Uses

It is safe to assume that Oyster mushrooms have been used as a food source for more than ten thousand years. This includes by Indigenous Americans in North America, and by pre-Hispanic cultures in Central America and Mexico that have used *Pleurotus* as a staple food source within their traditional diet.[126] Oysters were also an important food source for the ancient Greeks and the Romans. Asian peoples too have been implementing these mushrooms into their diet and medicine for several thousand years.

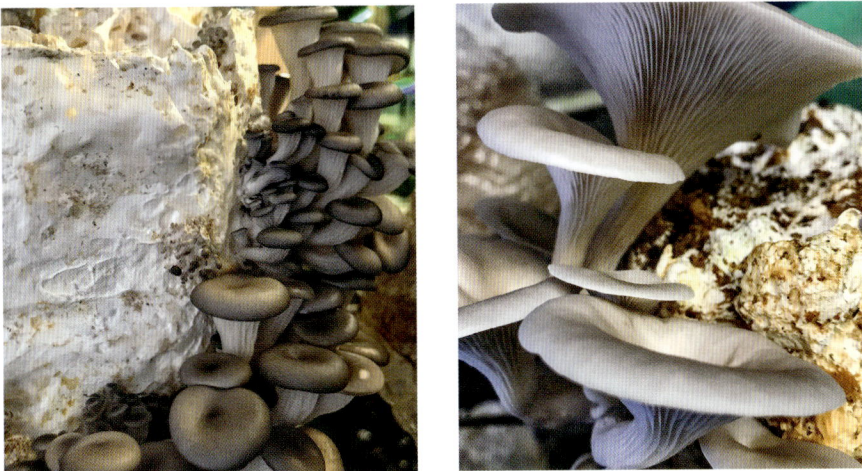

Figure 7.40. Mature Blue Oysters (*Pleurotus ostreatus* var. *columbinus*) growing indoors.

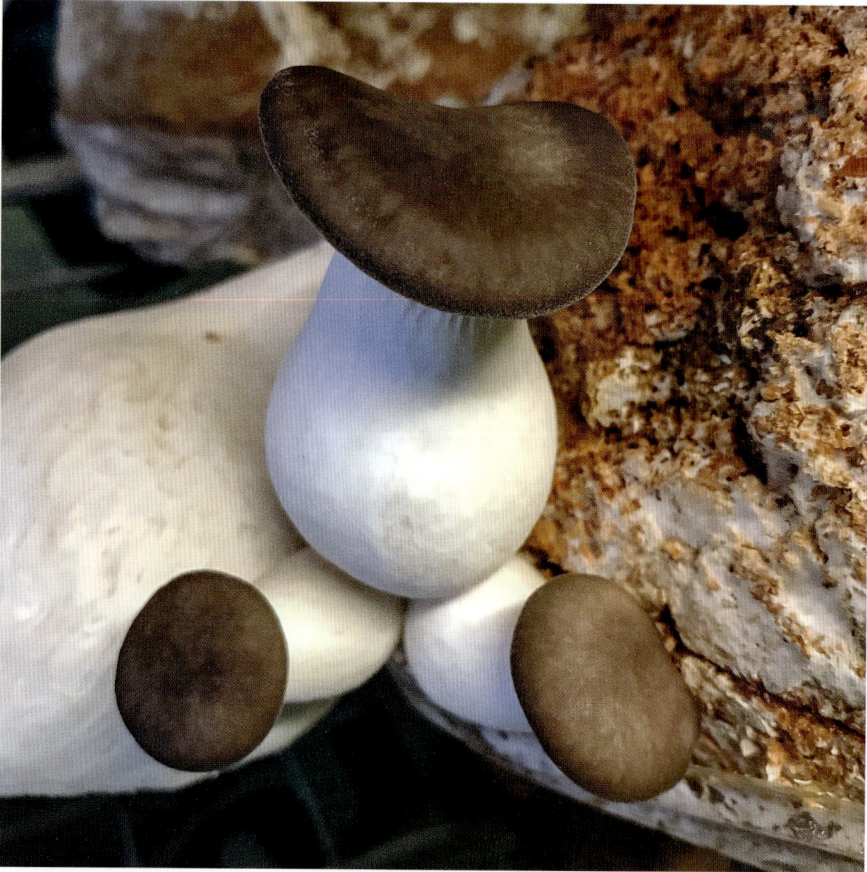

Figure 7.41. *Shimofuri Hiratake*, a popular culinary type of Oyster mushroom.

Research on Human Health Effects

Clinical trials for *Pleurotus* species are limited. Some human clinical trials have investigated the use of Oysters against viral infections, to promote heart health, and to diminish problems with metabolic disorders, including weight gain and diabetes.

ANTIVIRAL EFFECT

Two well-controlled human clinical trials underline the potent antiviral effects of Oyster mushrooms known, either explicitly or implicitly, by cultures around for world for thousands of years. These trials focused on the polysaccharide pleuran-β-glucan, extracted from *P. ostreatus* (Pearl Oyster), used against viral infections. In one twelve-month trial, pleuran-β-glucan was given daily in a syrup to children five to eight years of age who experienced recurrent respiratory tract infections. Researchers found considerably lowered occurrence of infections in these children.[127]

Another trial looked at pleuran-β-glucan for the treatment of herpes simplex virus 1 (HSV-1), one of the most prevalent viruses in humans. Asymptomatic participants ingested pleuran-β-glucan daily during a 120-day preventative period. These participants were more likely to show no HSV-1 symptoms, and a considerably diminished course of symptoms, compared to the placebo group.[128]

METABOLIC DISORDERS, INCLUDING DIABETES

Four clinical trials with people with diabetes or metabolic disorders show that Oyster mushrooms can be effective at reducing cholesterol, triglycerides, blood sugar, and blood pressure levels. All of these are markers for diabetes and the assumption is that their reduction will lead to better outcomes for patients. The studies varied in how people ingested the mushrooms. In one trial, people with diabetes ate 150 g of cooked Oysters each day for seven days.[129] In another trial, intake was 200 g of Oysters a day for 360 days.[130] The daily dose in a third study was 3 g of powdered Oysters.[131] Another trial provided a daily snack of dried, seasoned mushroom slices.[132] One trial followed people for almost a year, and saw positive benefits continue to the end of the study.[133]

CARDIOVASCULAR HEALTH

A systematic review from 2020 from a research group in Germany found eight published human trials that addressed Oysters in relation to the known leading causes of cardiovascular disease: high blood glucose, high blood pressure, and high levels of blood lipids.[134] Some of these studies were done with people with diabetes or hypertension, and others were done with either healthy people or those with hyperlipidemia (that is, high levels of cholesterol and triglycerides).

All the studies found beneficial results of consuming Oyster mushrooms, as evidenced by reductions in the parameters measured. The reviewers point out that it is hard to draw conclusions from these studies because of the different methodologies, different parts of the mushroom used, and the different ways of preparing and serving the mushrooms. The studies are few in number and the sample sizes were small. The reviewers conclude, however, that the evidence so far warrants more studies on the effects of Oysters on major contributors to heart disease.

Role in Holistic Healing

The phrase "Greater than the sum of its parts" is credited to Aristotle. In holistic healing, Aristotle's concept is an ever-moving thread. Many herbalists, mycologists, wild foragers, and cultivators have known or recently discovered the positive health benefits of various *Pleurotus* species. Oysters are used as a deeply nourishing and healthy food source to help combat viral loads, reduce bad cholesterol levels, support diabetics, and potentially speed wound healing. Oyster mushrooms grown on straw substrate indoors are a substantial food source composed of 63 percent carbohydrates, 12 percent crude fiber, 29 percent protein, 7 percent ash, and 1 percent fat.[135] When we make bone broths and soup stocks, we like to add Oyster mushrooms for a nutritional boost. (In chapter 6, we describe other ways that we use Oysters and other mushrooms.)

Several years ago, a holistic healer from San Francisco contacted me and asked to purchase every *Pleurotus* culture in my library. This was an unusual request. I learned that they were helping people in their area counteract symptoms of ulcers, irritable bowel syndrome (IBS), and leaky gut by making and distributing vegan broths with Oysters as the star of the concoctions.

Ergothioneine (EGT) is a modified amino acid found in Oyster mushrooms. Its name is based on the ergot fungus that parasitizes grain or cereal crops such as rye. This compound is widely distributed in plants and animals. EGT has been studied as a protective agent in kidney disease, cardiovascular disease, cancer, neuron damage, eye disorders, and cellular aging.[136] The presence of EGT in Oyster mushrooms may explain why some naturally occurring statins in *Pleurotus* species do not have the same detrimental effects on the kidney and liver as pharmaceuticals.

Plants receive EGT through association with mycorrhizal fungi, but animals are able to absorb ergothioneine only through diet. Consuming mushrooms is the easiest way to ingest EGT. This compound seems to have a preference to end up in tissues that have been exposed to stress, oxidation, or injuries. Many researchers are looking to EGT as a potential therapeutic treatment for serious conditions of oxidative stress and inflammation. At the time of this writing, there are no clinical trials of EGT's potential to prevent or treat chronic diseases.[137]

Studies are underway in various countries to assess the efficacy of the powerful Oyster mushroom for turning agricultural waste into high-quality food. One study in India found a yield of 300 g of fresh mushrooms for each kilogram of dried cotton stalks used as substrate.[138]

It is only in relatively recent times that growers have been able to cultivate Oyster mushrooms on a large scale. And it is only within the last seventy-five years that research has focused on learning about medicinal compounds in this humble and wide genus.

Approximately 92 million Americans take some type of statin drug to help control high cholesterol.[139] Statins work by blocking the enzyme that signals the liver to produce cholesterol. Unfortunately, some of these drugs can cause kidney failure, liver disease, and significant muscle soreness.[140] There is also growing data on the risk of dementia with statin use.[141] A natural statin called lovastatin is found in low concentrations in Oysters. Lovastatin may help reduce cholesterol levels. It has no contraindications when it comes to pregnancy, liver disease, or kidney disease.

When we cook Oysters, we start the process of breaking down the mushrooms' cell walls. Some of the best medicinal compounds—such as the polysaccharide chitin—are in the cell walls. Think of a crab shell, which is mineralized chitin, sitting on a sand dune for years. Eventually, exposure to wind, rain, and sun will break down the shell, but it takes a long time.

When I first started making medicinal mushroom extracts over twenty years ago, chitin was not well known as a medicinal compound; it was simply a block to getting to other medicinal polysaccharides. But Oyster mushrooms have been found to possess prebiotic properties in the form of indigestible compounds such as chitin and glucans.[142] Supporting the growth of healthy and beneficial gut bacteria is essential to maintaining a balance of microbiota, improving health and reducing the need to take antibiotics. If we all used fewer antibiotics, we would reduce the risk of developing antibiotic-resistant strains of pathogenic microbes. Consuming Oysters is a good way to help prevent the growth and proliferation of harmful gut bacteria by maintaining healthy balance. Although further research is needed to understand how we can best utilize these fungal partners, it is safe to assume that including Oyster mushrooms in our diet is a way to start supporting a healthy gut and reducing the need for antibiotics.[143]

In holistic healing it is important to emphasize the "whole" in holistic. We need to heal not only our bodies but also our "house"—our house being our planet. One of the many amazing things that Oysters can do is to break down petroleum hydrocarbons. The hydrogen–carbon bond found in ligneous (woody) plants and in trees is similar to that found in petroleum products. Oyster mushroom mycelium produces lignocellulosic enzymes that break down lignin, cellulose, and hemicellulose into simpler forms such as glucose. This means that Oyster mushrooms can be used to clean up petroleum spills in waterways or on land. The standard approach to cleaning up oil spills is to remove contaminated soil to a landfill. But this doesn't solve the problem; it simply relocates the pollution. It turns one toxic problem into someone else's toxic problem. We need to implement alternative, cost-effective ways of combating spillages, and Oyster mushrooms can be part of a true solution.

The special enzymes that Oysters produce are why we often grow them on straw produced by non-organic farms. The Oysters break down the hydrocarbons from any pesticides or artificial fertilizers present in the straw. The fruiting bodies are contaminant free and provide us with nutritious, medicinal food. The potentially toxic straw has been removed from the ecosystem, and we can use the spent straw in our organic garden.

Oyster mushrooms are also an example of science becoming more outlandish than fiction. Oyster mushrooms consume tiny creatures known as nematodes, which are one of the most prevalent organisms on the planet. They are found on every continent and in the oceans. Some types are beneficial, but others are parasites on animals (including humans), and still other species can attack plants or spread plant viruses. Exactly how Oyster mushrooms feed on nematodes was unknown until recently. The mushrooms produce 3-octanone, a biochemical that seems to be key to their ability to entrap nematodes by causing paralysis and cell death. It is estimated that nematodes cause approximately $157 billion worth of damage to crops worldwide annually.[144] Oyster mushrooms have the potential to be used as a natural and efficient biological control of these crop pests.

Cultivation Notes

Oysters are one of the easiest mushrooms to acquire, whether you purchase them from a local grocer or know someone who grows them locally. It is one of the mushrooms we focus on in our classes. We teach people simple ways to grow these humble and powerful beings. Various companies online sell grow kits that can sometimes "break even" for what you would pay retail for the mushrooms, and you cannot buy the joy it provides of growing your own. We tell people that the biggest advantage of a grow kit is that it can be expanded onto other substrate, such as logs, straw, and so on, which can then provide ten to fifteen times the yield of fresh mushrooms you would get from the kit alone.

The *Pleurotus* genus is perhaps the easiest mushroom for beginners to grow. The most experienced cultivators often use this one as a staple of their production, for the simple fact that it is one of the most versatile mushrooms for cooking and it can be grown on a wide range of substrates. Oysters have a forgiving nature when it comes to types of substrates and a voracious appetite for anything that produces enough cellulose. This mushroom is a perfect candidate for both indoor and outdoor cultivation.

One of the only drawbacks to indoor cultivation is that a small percentage of people can develop an allergy to the spores. Be mindful of this. If you have allergies to many different plants, particulates, or animal dander, this could be an indicator for you.

Oysters, when cultivated on a large or small commercial scale, can trigger allergic reactions for those who are working with them closely. Day after day of exposure to heavy spore dumping can lead to the development of allergies. Symptoms range from itchy eyes and throat to constricted breathing and severe headaches. A friend of mine became allergic to Oysters so badly that he could not even be in the same car with them. Once cooked, however, he could eat them with no ill effects.

By growing a range of *Pleurotus* species, you can achieve nearly year-round production. Choose hot weather strains such as Golden Oyster in the summer, cold weather strains for winter production, and types that tolerate a wide temperature range for spring and fall. Cellulose-rich agricultural wastes are a viable source of substrates for indoor or controlled outdoor cultivation. Log production outdoors is the same as for other mushrooms. See "Oysters" on page 43 for details on how we grow Oysters using the totem method.

Ethical Wild Harvesting

Even if you try to harvest all the Oyster mushrooms you find, they have ways of stopping you. Insect damage is one obstacle. Plus, Oysters do not produce all their mushrooms at a perfect size at one time. A portion of the flush will be perfect, but the others will only be pins. Once, we harvested Oyster mushrooms from a dead American Ash (*Fraxinus americana*). About 2 pounds were the perfect size with no insect larvae. But most were still clusters of pins approximately 1 inch tall. Of course, we left the pins to mature, knowing we would not be back that way again soon. When you find Oysters in the wild, about one-third of them will be perfect—be grateful for the ones ready to harvest and don't take the ones that aren't ready. This mushroom's staggering of fruiting is a natural way of ensuring plenty of the fruitbodies make it to maturity to disperse spores and perpetuate the species.

Psilocybe cubensis
PSYCHOACTIVE MUSHROOMS

*P*silocybe cubensis is one of many species of mushroom that produce the psychoactive compounds that are much sought after and that have received so much attention. Not all species in the *Psilocybe* genus produce these compounds, and many other genera of fungi do produce them, yet *P. cubensis* has become the focus because it easy to grow and to extract compounds from. Psychoactive fungi have a wide geographical distribution and have been used in countless cultures for their mental, emotional, and spiritual healing capacity.

The twenty-first century has brought a shift in attitudes about *P. cubensis*, and this psychoactive mushroom is now being given a chance to address some of the most pressing concerns of modern society, from depression to fear of death in the terminally ill. It is a powerful ally that is relatively easy to grow. The natural distribution worldwide, from the tropics to temperate areas, makes this mushroom widely accessible. *Psilocybe* species have likely served as catalysts for change throughout history.

At the time of this writing, the use of *P. cubensis* is legal for therapeutic use and decriminalized for personal use in some states of the United States. Possession has been decriminalized in specific states, while remaining a felony in most states. At the federal level, it is considered a Schedule I drug, which is defined as addictive with zero medicinal benefits. In light of the research that has been done on the beneficial effects of *Psilocybe* (we summarize some of that research later in this profile), we believe that the classification should be changed.

Psychoactive mushrooms offer a way to reconnect with a sense of hope and wonder. In modern society, dysfunction has been normalized. People feel isolated, and many believe they live in a soulless, mechanical universe with no purpose. But as human beings, we are most happy when we have community interaction, when we are in contact with nature, when we move our bodies freely, when we eat nutrient-dense food, and when we are in touch with Spirit, something beyond the human. Psilocybin fungi can play an important role in supporting a shift to a more fulfilling life.

It is time to let go of the "Reefer Madness"-type panic about *P. cubensis* and other hallucinogenic fungi and allow these fungi to take their role as healers in global human society. Powerful little beings lie at our fingertips, able to bring us back to living in balance if only we get out of our own way.

P. cubensis is one of the few mushrooms described in this book that are not saprotrophic. Instead, it is a secondary decomposer, working alongside bacteria in the soil to continue breaking down organic residues after primary decomposers do their work. This secondary decomposer, alongside *Amanita muscaria* (Fly Agaric), is one of the most significant mushrooms that have changed the course of the human story. As we noted in the introduction to this book, some people believe that exposure to psycho-

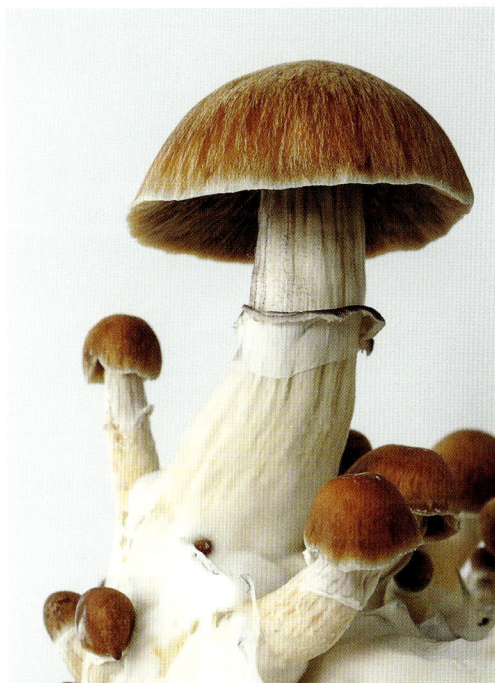

Figure 7.42. Indoor-cultivated *P. cubensis*. Photo by Cannabis_Pic / Adobe Stock

active mushroom compounds over a prolonged period of time influenced human evolution. Some people use these fungi as a powerful tool for developing their insight, coping strategies, and adaptive responses, as well as to alter perceptions and challenge preconceived notions. I notice that it increases my intuition.

If humans had not developed mental filters to block out distractions in their environment, humankind would have gone extinct a long time ago, likely while staring at leaves moving in the wind while a ravenous bear moved in for a juicy meal. But ingesting fungi that contain psilocybin expands our view of the world by helping us temporarily drop these perceptual filters—rigid ways of perceiving—that we have gathered over the years in order to function in ordinary reality. Ingesting these fungi can also dissolve the sense of self, of who we think we are. This can allow for the emergence of new ways of thinking, feeling, and acting. Neuroimaging studies of people who have used psilocybin suggest that changes in corresponding brain networks can last up to four months or longer.[145] These mushrooms have the power to bring into one's awareness the connectedness of all being, including the non-psychoactive mushrooms we discuss in this book.

Numerous psychologists, philosophers, and other theorists have proposed that psilocybin played a role in human cognitive evolution. Terence

McKenna, an American ethnobotanist and philosopher, in his 1992 book *Food of the Gods*, proposed a hypothesis known as the "stoned ape theory." However, not much evidence has been gathered to support his thinking, and thus it remains a hypothesis. I find the "stoned ape" language unhelpful because there are so many mushrooms that provide a wide variety of medicinal benefits. We do not need to perpetuate the idea that these powerful beings exist only to help people get high. I am in full support of recognizing *Psilocybe* as a sacred mushroom and using it as a powerful ally just as our ancestors did.

As megafauna grazed prehistoric savannahs, they would have ingested spores from *Psilocybe* fruitings. Whenever they left piles of manure under shady trees, thermophilic bacteria and other organisms would break it down. When the manure cooled enough, the *Psilocybe* mycelium would run from the spores, and when it reached the edge of the nitrogen-rich pile, and there was enough rain, it would have produced fruitbodies. Our human ancestors, who were tracking these animals as game, would of course see these mushrooms growing in the manure. At some point they tried eating them and the knowledge of their effects would have spread across the human groups. We can speculate that the humans revered the animals as a sacred source of food, just as Indigenous Americans revered the American Buffalo, and Indigenous Europeans revered the Reindeer and the Deer. So it makes sense that mushrooms found in the sacred animal's dung would be received as an offering from the gods. Spores that traveled through this animal held information that, when ingested, gave insights to the humans.

Some psychologists and anthropologists suggest that consuming these mushrooms at microdose level (that is, not enough to be psychoactive) would have increased visual acuity and color perception, giving our ancestors an advantage in finding food, detecting hidden predators, and navigating the terrain. At higher doses, psilocybin predictably creates what are known as boundary-dissolving experiences, which facilitate optimal group coordination, crucial for small bands of humans trying to survive in a dangerous world. At even higher doses, ancestral humans would have had transcendental visionary experiences and likely constructed rituals to make sense of them. Some theorists believe that these psychedelic experiences may have led to the creation of myths as a way to explain the experiences, which then formed the basis of religions. In *The Psilocybin Connection,* medicine guide Jahan Khamsehzadeh writes that academics widely accept the assertion that the first form of religion among humans worldwide was shamanism, an animist worldview that sees the world as alive and interconnected. Khamsehzadeh contends it is likely that these fungi, and other natural psychedelics, played a large role in this development.[146]

Traditional Uses

Some of the oldest records of humans using *P. cubensis* come from Mesoamerica. The "mushroom stones" from ancient Guatemala are one example. These stones are estimated to be up to three thousand years old and are assumed to be associated with mushroom-focused religious, spiritual, or healing practices. The stones are carved with various effigies including Jaguars, human figures, or phalli.

The late archaeologist Dr. Stephan F. de Borhegyi, who studied Mayan culture,

> *was convinced that hallucinogenic mushroom rituals were a central aspect of Maya religion. He based this theory on his identification of a mushroom stone cult that came into existence in the Guatemala Highlands and Pacific coastal area around 1000 BCE along with a trophy head cult associated with the Mesoamerican ballgame. In most cases, the mushroom imagery was associated with ritual sacrifice in the Underworld, with jaguar transformation and calendar period endings, and with the decapitation and resurrection of the underworld Sun God by a pair of deities associated with the planet Venus. Mushrooms were also closely associated with Tlaloc and the ritual warfare carried out in his name that is known as Tlaloc warfare.*[147]

Unknown numbers of codices were destroyed by the invading Spaniards in a systematic, aggressive pursuit to destroy the Indians' ancient belief systems. Catholic missionaries made a crusade of destroying as many of the "mushroom stones" as possible. Over two hundred, however, escaped the feverish destructive obsession of religious zealots. It is probable that more of these historically significant stones are lying under the soils of Mexico and Central American countries.

In 1957 Gordon Wasson, an American banker and ethnomycologist, blew open the generations-old healing traditions of Southern Mexico. He documented the Curanderos' traditional use of psychoactive fungi for ritual purposes and, with an article in *Life Magazine*, kicked off the cultural revolution of the 1960s.

Mushrooms that, to my eye, look like *P. cubensis*, or a comparable species, growing from a jar are clearly depicted in ancient Egyptian images. This is an interesting parallel with modern-day cultivation methods, which still cultivate psilocybin-containing fungi in jars. Most Egyptian archaeologists deny any association between the ancients and these powerful medicines. However, the ancient Egyptians participated in a number of ritualistic drinks or concoctions

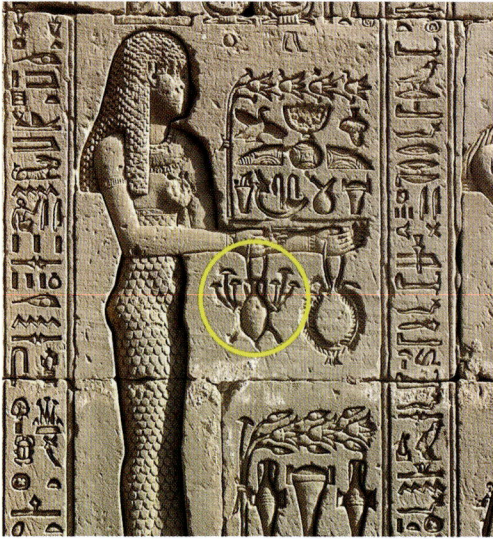

Figure 7.43. Possible depiction of psychoactive mushrooms fruiting from container. Photo by Chaetomiopsis / Wikimedia Commons

made from alcohol, opium, cannabis, Blue Lotus flowers (*Nymphaea caerulea*), and other plant medicines.[148] Why not mushrooms? It is not out of the realm of possibility that they would have used a fungus that commonly grew on piles of manure. Figure 7.43, which shows one of these ancient images, is clearly a fungus growing on soil.

The ancient Egyptians associated these mushrooms with immortality and believed them to be a gift from the god Osiris. Common people were not allowed to eat, or even touch, these special mushrooms, which were guarded for the elites. Psychedelic mushrooms are depicted in various temples throughout the regions and in hieroglyphic texts. Some archeologists hypothesize that some temples were actually designed to resemble giant mushrooms and that the shape of crowns worn by rulers of ancient Egypt were inspired from the primordia of *P. cubensis*.[149]

Recent study of the Egyptian pyramids suggest they are much older than the four thousand years generally cited by archaeologists. This includes investigations by author and researcher Dr. Robert Schoch, who has contended that certain damage to the Sphinx could have only resulted from amounts of water that have not been seen in the Nile valley for at least ten thousand years.[150] This view could push the depictions of fungi in Egyptian temples back much further in the historical record as well.

Research on Human Health Effects

The United States has led the colonial suppression of psilocybin through its "war on drugs." The federal Controlled Substances Act (CSA) of 1971 put the brakes on research and official use of this Indigenous medicine. Psilocybin mushrooms were placed under Schedule I, which states that they have no medical use or medicinal value, despite thousands of years of worldwide use and a large bank of scientific evidence (over one thousand published papers) concerning their unique medicinal value. The CSA has put our knowledge base about psilocybin mushrooms fifty years behind. It was driven by ignorance and fear among politicians who perceived a moral panic, and by the careless use of these medicines by young people at that time.

Now people are rediscovering what these ancient beings are offering. In 2018, the FDA declared psilocybin had "breakthrough therapy" status for major depressive disorder and treatment-resistant depression, which has opened the doors to a frenzy of clinical research. This rapid growth of scientific interest in psilocybin is likely due to the combination of the profound states it creates in people, the size of the unsolved depression epidemic, the mystique created by the outright banning of this mushroom, and positive popular media reports known as the "Pollan Effect." Many other countries are also part of the resurgence of psychoactive mushroom medicine research. This research, by no means yet conclusive, is paving the way for more and more decriminalized and legalized supervised use in the United States and Europe. Alongside these developments is a burgeoning industry, focused on profit, ready to take full advantage of this sacred medicine. How this will play out remains to be seen.

MICRODOSING

Microdosing refers to taking amounts of psilocybin small enough to allow you to go about your day without any psychoactive effects. There is no consensus as to what amount constitutes a safe microdose. It is likely that the safe dosage level varies among individuals. People usually start by taking between 0.1 g and 0.5 g and then proceed by trial and error. Microdosing started gaining traction around 2015, possibly in Silicon Valley to improve job performance. Microdosing has become popular because of purported mental health, cognitive, and general well-being benefits.

A recent review identified nineteen published placebo-controlled trials of microdosing. The reviewers concluded that these studies showed that microdosing with psilocybin or LSD (another fungal-derived psychoactive) leads to changes in "neurobiology, physiology, subjective experience, affect, and cognition relative to placebo." They also stated that there have not yet been enough adequately controlled trials with large enough sample sizes to determine if these effects are due to psilocybin or to the placebo effect and that further research is warranted.[151]

One of the largest studies included in this review is of particular interest to us because it included an investigation of the effect of including Lion's Mane extract in a microdosing protocol known as the Stamets Stack, after famous mycologist Paul Stamets. This is a combination of psilocybin with Lion's Mane extract and niacin (vitamin B3). Microdosers who reported initial depression showed a decrease in depression symptoms over a one-month period. There was no effect of microdosing on cognitive performance assessed by processing speed and spatial memory, but a positive effect was found on psychomotor function.

This improvement in psychomotor functioning was present only for participants over the age of fifty-five who microdosed in combination with Lion's Mane and niacin. The review authors point out that these findings are very preliminary and more work is needed, but that they suggest the combination of psilocybin and Lion's Mane could benefit possible neurological disorders.[152]

Most trials tend to focus on measuring participants' experience with standardized questionnaires or cognitive tests and then analyze the result for the entire group. This is the methodology employed by the majority of clinical trials. However, these methods easily miss the *experience* of the humans participating in the study. This experience, unique to each person who takes psilocybin, turns out to be crucial to the effects the mushroom can have.

In a British study, eight of twelve participants reported that they started microdosing because of mental health challenges (including ADHD, depression, anxiety and PTSD).[153] Four of those participants reported "phenomenal breakthroughs" that they attributed to the microdosing. One participant described that it had worked by bringing to the surface previously suppressed painful memories and emotions that she now had the chance to work through. Another participant reported that the microdosing had made their symptoms worse. This person cautioned that microdosing can bring up feelings one may not be prepared to deal with alone.

Many of the participants talked about experiencing a sense of connection: connection to others, to something "bigger than myself," to their spiritual practice, to nature, and to their own life challenges. Such connections have been shown to be supportive in improving mental health, and microdosing may make this sense of connection and belonging more available for some.

DEPRESSION

More than one meta-analysis has been performed on studies of the effects of psilocybin on depression. The results of the most recent meta-analysis at the time of writing show favorable effects of psilocybin for depression compared to placebo.[154] (We note that these clinical trials were conducted using synthetic psilocybin, not the full mushroom.) Reviewers found three factors that tended to lead to the most favorable results. First, that the depression was the result of having a serious or terminal illness (secondary depression). Second, that participants self-reported their levels of depression rather than being observed by a clinician. And thirdly, those who had previously used some type of psychedelic tended to respond more to this treatment.

Trials of psychoactive doses (usually 25 mg, 10 mg, and 1 mg) of psilocybin in the context of ongoing psychotherapy have shown significant reductions in depression symptoms, reductions that persist for six and twelve months.[155] One study looked directly at the effects of psilocybin-assisted therapy in comparison to therapy accompanied by a pharmaceutical antidepressant. Both treatments reduced symptoms of depression over an intensive six weeks; those taking psilocybin showed significantly improved scores in functioning, connectedness, and meaning in life.[156]

Encouraged by this success, some researchers have attempted to use a single dose (25 mg) with minimal psychological support. Three weeks after the session, they observed significant reductions in depression.[157] However, after twelve weeks, only 20 percent of the high-dose group maintained these improvements, suggesting the ongoing support of a therapist is crucial to integrating the experience into daily life. A large proportion of participants, 77 percent overall, experienced adverse effects such as nausea, dizziness, headache, suicidal ideation, or active self-harm. These are significant and concerning adverse effects that are unexpected, especially at the 1 mg level. The authors concluded that larger and longer trials are needed.

This highly publicized study is part of the research base that is pushing for FDA approval of synthetic psilocybin. We feel it is important to fully understand this research, rather than simply accepting the polarized view of it often presented in the media. The rush for FDA approval is driven by for-profit companies. The result is that we are not always treating vulnerable people well—but this is not being presented in the mainstream narrative about this research.

A later study interviewed eleven of the participants from the trial reported above.[158] Even with such a small sample, the interviews made it clear that participants had a wide range of experiences. One of the most prominent themes described by participants was a mistrust in the mental health system, although not in the therapists who accompanied them on their psychedelic journey. Trust is a prerequisite for the ability to surrender into a situation, which is what the psilocybin experience asks for.

Other key themes were challenges in navigating the experience and not feeling adequately prepared for it. Some of the participants had profound experiences that significantly changed their daily life afterward. Some people had very distressing psychedelic experiences that they described as adding trauma to the load they were already carrying. Some expressed that laying down for eight hours with two people observing them was uncomfortable and that the music, which they didn't get to choose, had a large impact on their experience. The authors of this study question the ethics of doing trials that adhere to such rigid protocols and cannot be customized for the needs of the individual.

DEPRESSION AND ANXIETY IN TERMINAL ILLNESS

People facing death from aggressive cancers can, understandably, experience high levels of depression and anxiety. There is no standard treatment for this distressing experience other than attempts to manage physical pain and the use of antidepressants (which are minimally effective). A group from Portugal sifted through the published literature to find the six most rigorous studies of effects of psilocybin on cancer patients; in total this covered ninety-two patients. Patients who received psilocybin showed highly significant reductions in measures of both depression and anxiety, without notable adverse reactions, and these changes persisted long after the psychedelic experience. Patients reported feeling much less anxiety, reconciling with death, feeling more emotionally unattached to their cancer, experiencing spiritual or religious phenomena, and a reconnection to life.

Analysis in one study using the Mysticism Scale (a research tool used as a predictor of self-rated spirituality) revealed that patients who reported having a profound mystical experience received the most benefits in terms of reduced anxiety and depression along with increased quality of life.[159] The Mysticism Scale includes experiences such as unity consciousness, infinite space and time, encountering objective truth, sacredness, deep peace and joy, and the sense that none of it can adequately be put into words.[160]

POST-TRAUMATIC STRESS DISORDER (PTSD)

There have not been enough well-controlled studies of psilocybin effects on people suffering from PTSD to draw conclusions. Given the challenges described by people with treatment-resistant depression, this is tender territory. High-dose psilocybin is an intense experience and can bring up distressing material.

In a 2024 study with thirty medical staff who provided frontline care during the COVID-19 epidemic in the United States, researchers administered a single high dose (25 mg) of psilocybin in a placebo-controlled trial. None of these participants had mental health concerns before the pandemic. Twenty-eight days after taking psilocybin, they showed a statistically significant reduction in depression scores. Scores assessing burnout and PTSD symptoms trended in the positive direction but did not reach statistical significance. The authors conclude that more research is warranted to better understand the role of psilocybin in the treatment of PTSD.[161]

ADDICTION

A recent (2024) review found four studies of the use of psilocybin in treating addiction (to alcohol or tobacco). The results of all four studies were positive in favor of the use of psilocybin, in combination with therapy, for reduction in substance use.[162]

TRAUMATIC BRAIN INJURY (TBI)

Psilocybin is of interest to those studying brain injuries because it is known to promote neuroplasticity (the brain's ability to rewire itself) and neurogenesis (the growth of new neurons) and to reduce inflammation throughout the body.[163] This is a growing area of research but with no conclusive results.

CHRONIC PAIN

Psilocybin has been investigated for relief for those suffering from chronic pain, including phantom limb pain in amputees, cluster headaches, and neuropathic pain. A small, randomized, placebo-controlled trial with a low dose of psilocybin showed a significant reduction in headache frequency.[164] A follow-up study with people who reported frequent headaches found that a repeated dose six months later had an additional positive effect, even in those who hadn't seen a result from the first dose.[165] This work is ongoing.

IMMUNE SYSTEM

Healthy volunteers who received a moderate dose of psilocybin (0.17 mg per kg of body weight) showed a significant, immediate decrease in one specific proinflammatory marker, and no change in others. However, testing seven days after dosing showed a significant reduction in other biomarkers associated with inflammation. This suggests that psilocybin can have a positive, and persistent, effect on the immune system of healthy people. The degree of reduction in inflammatory markers was correlated with improved mood as reported by the participants. No significant adverse effects were reported.[166]

Role in Holistic Healing

The challenges facing people in the modern industrialized age are different from the challenges our ancestors faced. Instead of isolated high-stress moments where moving quickly was imperative to evade predators or stampeding megafauna, most of us face continual daily stress: deadlines, social pressures, social media overload, driving in high-volume traffic, juggling work and family demands, and so on, all while attempting to flourish on food that lacks nutrients and is likely burdened by toxins. A sense of isolation and lack of a supportive community also contribute to decline in well-being, mood, satisfaction of life, and creativity.

Psychedelic fungi offer the gift of peeling away the social programming that traps us in the daily grind. This gift can involve an overwhelming feeling that everything is special and beautiful. It can be paralyzing, to the point that we may not know how to move forward for some time, until a sense of normalcy has returned. A feeling of happiness and other positive emotions can persist for months afterward.

P. cubensis is one of the most powerful fungi to facilitate change in our modern lives. In a culture that fears death and denies the truth of the harmful effects of modern living, experiencing *P. cubensis* has the potential to be life altering. It can give people a new perspective on their lives and help them avoid getting wrapped up in fears that hold them back from progress or from dealing with traumas. For people suffering from a terminal illness, nearing death, and afraid of what they may face next, psilocybin can be a powerful ally in gracefully accepting the final decline—which will happen to all of us eventually.

With hopefulness, not despair, I ask you to realize we all deal with death on a consistent basis. I am not speaking of the death of a loved one but rather what I regard as tiny deaths. The death of the things that no longer serve us. The parts of our psyche that are holding us back from moving toward what life wants to offer us—those parts need to be transformed. These small impediments need to be clipped away, just as trees shed limbs that are too shaded and not photo-synthesizing enough to contribute to the tree's well-being. This is the natural order. We can use the fungi that naturally make psilocybin to free ourselves from our own adopted or self-imposed chains. Trim that dead wood so it doesn't become a hazard in our lives!

Everyone has suffered some type of trauma. For some, it dictates their lives. And sometimes traumas are best dealt with in a setting where trained profes-sionals can help. But in capitalist societies, professional psychedelic-assisted sessions with a psychotherapist are usually very expensive. People in marginal-ized communities cannot afford these types of treatments, even though they are the very people that need it the most. In these communities, support for those suffering is limited. There is often inadequate care following psychedelic expe-riences. This is a serious concern to us—that this sacred medicine, psilocybin, will be absorbed into the for-profit medicine monster and become inaccessible to all but the few who can afford its high price tag.

This would not happen in a decentralized model of medical care or in tra-ditional communities of people. The people conducting traditional medicine ceremonies would likely have known you since childhood. They would, there-fore, care about your well-being because you are a part of a larger extended family or village or community. This is the context that humans have existed in ever since before we were *Homo sapiens*, and it is the type of connection many crave and turn to the mushrooms for. Ultimately, we must heal our relation-ships with each other and our beyond-human kin to remember that we belong to this world. One mushroom journey isn't going to do it.

Cultivation Notes

Note: The cultivation of *Psilocybe* species is still illegal in many states. Please check with your state laws.

Because *Psilocybe* mushrooms are secondary decomposers it is easy to understand that they love higher-nitrogen substrates and will grow in substrates that thermophiles (organisms that live in high-heat environments) have heated up to pasteurization temperatures. For this reason, pasteurized substrates of sawdust to composted manure in a one-to-one ratio is ideal. One of the most common methods is to pasteurize the substrate for 90 minutes and then inoculate with grain spawn after the substrate has cooled. Sometimes cultures are not available for legal reasons. In that case, spores can be introduced into sterilized grain to expand the mycelium. Once colonized, the grain is used to inoculate the pasteurized manure and sawdust bulk substrate as described above. Chapters 4 and 5 cover details of grain spawn production.

Ethical Wild Harvesting

The wild harvesting of psilocybin-containing mushrooms varies from one part of the world to another. In nature, these mushrooms occupy piles of manure from megafauna. Such manure piles can be found on cattle farms in the southern United States and in tropical regions around the world. Some *Psilocybe* species are wood loving and can thrive on wood chips or mulch beds. These mushrooms can be prolific; it is usually safe to take what you need for medicine. If one is overharvesting and overusing these sacred mushrooms, the mushrooms will let them know.

Psilocybe species are often small and delicate. When harvesting, we choose the ones with their caps still attached to the stem. This button stage contains the highest concentration of medicinal compounds. When the caps open, then the spores have already started to disperse and are in the process of distributing for the next generation. We pass these by so that they continue expanding in number and providing medicine. This sacred medicine is not to be abused by overharvesting.

Schizophyllum commune

SPLIT GILL

Schizophyllum commune is a modest mushroom that is widely available from the mountains of the far East to the jungles of the Congo to the West Coast of the Americas. The benefits it offers for human health and planet Earth are emerging into modern awareness. We hope more research will be carried out on this fungus and others that coexist beside us on our wonderful and wild planet in the near future.

Most people know little about *S. commune,* better known as the Split Gill mushroom, unless to use in traditional foods. One look at this mushroom makes it clear where the name Split Gill comes from—*S. commune* have gills that appear to divide many times. Viewing this mushroom from above, the cluster of caps reminds me of cumulus clouds on the horizon. However, upon further inspection of the hymenium, we see that the spore-producing surface of this mushroom is not made up of gills. Instead, the surface has rippled folds with splits arising on top of the folds. This sight also brings up images of clouds, rolling in and rippling across the sky. This fungus is saprotrophic and only occasionally grows on living trees. It is reported to be sometimes parasitic, but we have never witnessed this. I suspect that it may grow as a parasite when plants are stressed by adverse environmental conditions such as drought, a sudden freeze, or extreme heat or cold.

S. commune will grow on a variety of types of wood and in a variety of environments. It is distributed across all continents, except Antarctica, and it is commonly found in polluted areas deep in the square jungles of cityscapes. I have seen it deep in the shade of the forest here on our farm, but it can also grow in full sun. We recently witnessed it growing from a huge, freshly cut poison ivy vine that we had dropped into the field so our goats could eat the leaves. The denuded vine had lain in the field for over a year, and then *S. commune* started fruiting on it. The fungus had thrived even in those exposed, completely unshaded conditions.

Split Gill is a tough little fungus, similar to *Auricularia* spp. (Wood Ears), in that they both have the ability to withstand drought. We often observe that these mushrooms can dry up and go dormant, waiting for the next rain, when they will swell with moisture, grow, and produce more spores. Another amazing

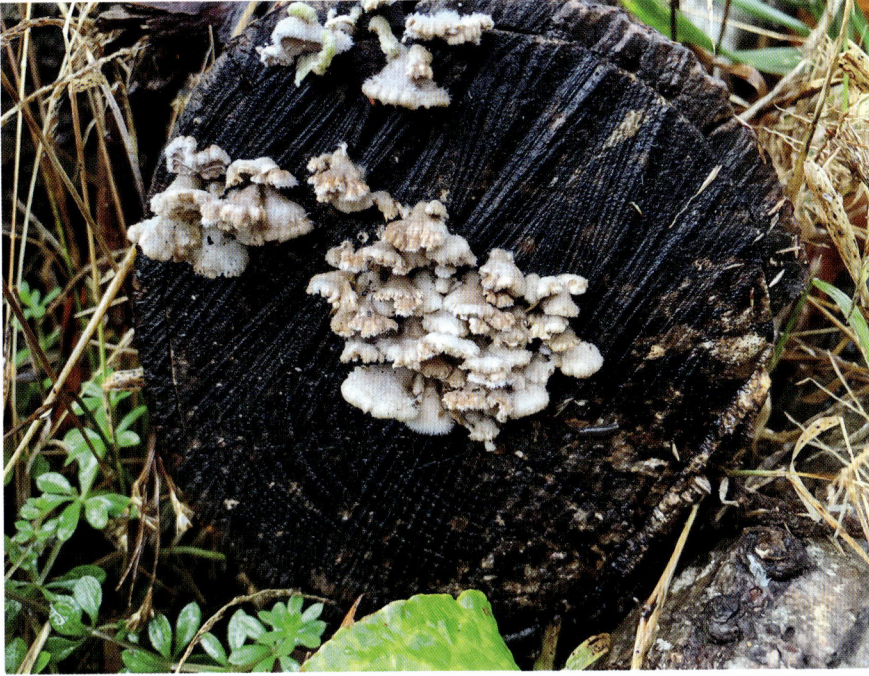

Figure 7.44. Young wild *Schizophyllum commune*.

fact about *S. commune*: it is said to have 28,000 sexes. This is the world record for the greatest number of sexes.

It is not a common occurrence, but *S. commune* can cause human infections of skin, mucous membranes, sinuses, lungs, and the brain. It is often difficult to treat fungal infections—they have a knack for being persistent, given that they have been successful in perpetuating themselves across time on the planet for nearly a billion years. I would caution anyone with compromised health or lungs in starting a venture of growing *S. commune* on a commercial scale. I discuss this potential for infection in more detail in "Role in Holistic Healing" on page 245.

Traditional Uses

Across cultures and continents, Split Gill fungi have been used as a food source and medicine. In Gastón Guzmán's *Diversity and Use of Traditional Mexican Medicinal Fungi*, he notes that *S. commune* was used for headache, indigestion, inflammation, intestinal pain, obesity, rheumatism and weakness. "Among the medicinal mushrooms *Ustilago maydis*, *Schizophyllum commune*, and *Pleurotus* spp. are most essential for treating numerous illnesses and health problems."[167]

Traditional peoples in Asia have used this mushroom as food and medicine. In Africa, members of six different ethnic communities in the Congo were interviewed in 2018. The Ngando had the most mycological prowess, revealing extensive knowledge, and they reported *S. commune* was mainly used as a food source.[168] In parts of Nigeria it is used as a health food and as a medicine for diabetes.[169]

Research on Human Health Effects

S. commune is an underutilized mushroom in the area of human health. As preclinical research becomes more frequent, and evidence about the safety of this mushroom becomes closer to conclusive, the doors will be opened for more clinical trials. There is potential to pair *S. commune* with other more popular fungi to create blends tailored to treat a variety of diseases.

S. commune is also receiving more attention from researchers in industries including food, fuel, hazardous waste cleanup, and pharmaceutical.

CANCER

We found only one clinical trial, published in Japan in 1986, that investigated the effects of *S. commune* (most importantly the polysaccharide schizophyllan) as an antitumor treatment. A hot-water extract was administered intramuscularly, once or twice a week, at the dose of 40 mg. The tumor response was found to be higher in the Split Gill group compared to the control group. The survival of the Split Gill group was also longer than the control group.[170]

GUT HEALTH

Some preclinical trials have shown that β-glucans from Split Gill mushroom improve gut motility and gut microbiota as well as intestinal atrophy. A 2023 trial asked patients to take two 80 mg doses of the β-glucans daily for eight weeks. Results indicate that taking *S. commune*–derived β-glucan increased beneficial lactobacillus bacteria in the digestive system, which corresponded with patients reporting of relieved constipation.[171]

ANTIVIRAL AND ANTIBACTERIAL EFFECTS

Studies in the lab and with animals have found some Split Gill preparations to be antiviral, including against the dengue virus and SARS-CoV-2 in mice.[172]

Lab-based studies have found *S. commune* to reduce the growth of various bacteria. One study from the Philippines found that *S. commune* mycelia grown in coconut water could be mass produced, and that certain extracts from this mycelium showed high antibacterial activity against common pathogens.[173]

Role in Holistic Healing

S. commune has the potential to become a major medicinal mushroom in the everyday lives of those seeking better health. The Split Gill mushroom also has some potentially valuable applications in industrial processes. This versatile mushroom can be cultivated worldwide on a variety of substrates, making it a candidate for use by emerging economies or by those who seek better health without resorting to use of pharmaceuticals. Here, we give some examples of possible uses in industrial processes.

Biosorption is the process in which biological material is used to accumulate substances from a solution. The materials recovered can be toxins or undesirable compounds, such as pharmaceuticals or heavy metals. *S. commune* has been investigated for its biosorption capacity for several positively charged metals that are used in electroplating processes. The effluents of these applications are toxic. In one study, the authors conclude that *S. commune* can be classified as an efficient biosorbent on the basis of rapid kinetics, remarkable biosorption capacity, and selective removal of metal ions from electroplating effluents.[174]

Azo dyes, synthetic organic compounds, are problematic when released into waterways after the dyeing process. They block light in water, which reduces aquatic plant life and upsets the natural balance. Additionally, azo dyes are known to cause mutagenic, carcinogenic, and reproductive harm in many organisms, including humans, further down the food chain. *S. commune* may offer cost effective and safe treatment.

Three enzymes—manganese peroxidase, laccase, and lignin peroxidase—produced by *S. commune* have been tested to determine their decolorization capabilities. Three different azo dyes were tested with these enzymes, and unrefined manganese peroxidase played a major role in their decolorization. These *S. commune*–produced enzymes could be a low-cost, large-scale, and safe option for treatment of azo dye effluents with a positive impact on our aquatic ecosystems.[175]

The polysaccharide xylan is a major constituent of plant material, and *S. commune* produces xylanase enzymes. Unlike other types of enzymes, the xylanases that *S. commune* produces hold promise for future roles in safe and effective industrial biobleaching of cellulose, but further studies are required.[176]

S. commune is known to produce more than 350 carbohydrate-active enzymes. Of these enzymes, more than one hundred are thought to be involved in plant polysaccharide disintegration. Some of these enzymes have the ability to reduce the integrity of other fungi, which would effectively keep those fungi in check. This seems to hold promise as an environmentally safe way to manage fungi that attack crop plants.

A group in Malaysia is testing a product using β-glucans from Split Gill mushrooms along with discarded cooking oil to make a solid dishwashing soap. This product is called SchizoComm, and questionnaire results show that people preferred it over other dishwashing soaps.[177] In this way Split Gills have the potential to make hands smoother and be part of a human–fungi collaboration to keep water clean and reuse precious resources.

S. commune does have the potential to cause health issues for those who cultivate it. Just as the commercial cultivation of Oyster mushrooms poses the risk of allergic reaction (as described in the *Pleurotus* profile on page 228), *S. commune* can also lead to an allergic response. The first case of Split Gill infection was reported in 1950. A thirty-two-year-old female was diagnosed after a lung biopsy that found *S. commune*. She was treated with two pharmaceutical antifungals and made a recovery even though the recovery was an uncomfortable one.

We as humans have made some major mistakes, and fungi can offer solutions to some of the problems we face—if we can slow down enough to study what is already going on around us. If you decide to pursue commercial cultivation of *S. commune,* I recommend providing protective gear for employees. It will be very important to have safety protocols in place and proper equipment to remove as many spores from the working environment as possible. The commercial cultivation of *S. commune,* providing that these health risks can be surmounted, should launch this humble fungus onto the world stage to become a major medicinal mushroom.

The research work done with *S. commune* shows that it has a role in healing our bodies and helping us heal our planet from the toxins we have produced during our continued experimental existence on Earth. We are inspired by the potential for using Split Gills to help break down synthetic dyes and create soaps that are healthier for people and planet. Looking to the future, we are sure these are just two of the many ways we will be employing these mushrooms in our daily lives.

Cultivation Notes

The cultivation of Split Gill is similar to other wood-loving species. As explained in "Role in Holistic Healing" previously, outdoor cultivation is the only method we recommend because of the potential for *S. commune* to parasitize humans and have serious impact on lung health. Outdoor cultivation on plant matter is possible, and it is easy to cultivate mycelium on grain and sawdust to then inoculate substrate for outdoor cultivation. We have found this mushroom on many invasive plant species here in the Southern Appalachians. This would potentially be a worthy use of some invasive species, such as Tree of Heaven (*Ailanthus altissima*), Oriental Bittersweet (*Celastrus orbiculatus*), and kudzu (*Pueraria* spp.).

Ethical Wild Harvesting

S. commune is a cosmopolitan species found in many types of landscapes, and overharvesting of this species seems to be of least concern. Not many people are aware of its benefits and therefore do not harvest it. We mostly harvest this fungus from "contaminated" logs that we were cultivating other species on. We have found that if we harvest all of the fruit from our logs, they will easily grow back the next season and for several years in a row. Of course, never harvest all of any mushroom. Leave some behind for spore distribution.

Trametes versicolor

TURKEY TAIL

Turkey Tail (*Trametes versicolor*) is one of the most widespread macrofungi on Earth. This cosmopolitan species is a polypore that has made its way across every continent (with the exception of Antarctica). *Tram-* means "thin" and *-etes* means "one who is"; *versicolor* is "many colors" or "various colors." One who is thin and has varying colors is the ideal description of this medicinal powerhouse. Some older or synonymous scientific names for Turkey Tail are *Polyporus versicolor*, *Coriolus versicolor*, or *Polystictus versicolor*. Traditional Chinese Medicine practitioners call Turkey Tail by the name *Yun Zhi*. The Japanese call it *Kawaratake*. *Kawara* means "tile" or "roof tile"—thus Roof Tile Mushroom. Turkey Tail is suited to this descriptive name, too, because of the curving shape of the fruiting bodies and their slate-like colors. Slate is "versicolored" just like Turkey Tail, in shades of gray, tan, steel blue, brick red, and sometimes even gray-green.

T. versicolor appears on dead wood as thin, overlapping fruiting bodies. Sometimes when it is on small branches lying on the forest floor, it produces only a single layer. In fact, this is the perfect opportunity to harvest Turkey Tail, during the fall fruiting season, with a walk in the forest right after a good rain and some strong winds. When fresh they are flexible, pliable and somewhat like thin leather. The hymenium consists of tiny, tightly packed, irregular pores. If you have good eyesight, you can distinguish the individual pores. To the touch the hymenium surface feels slightly rough compared to the smooth, almost glass like feeling of the look-alike fungus called False Turkey Tail (*Stereum ostrea*).

The cap is zonate with differing colors; the number of color combinations as one of the identifying characteristics of Turkey Tail is

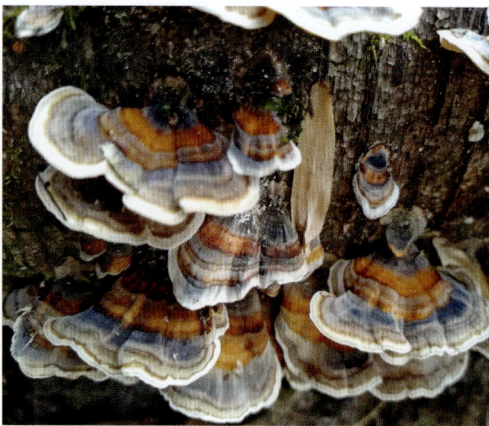

Figure 7.45. Turkey Tail showing its colors.

fascinating to say the least. The cap has a slight velvety surface, which tends to become fuzzier as the specimens age. Budding mycologists may easily confuse *T. versicolor* with *T. hirsuta* (Hairy Turkey Tail), which has a lighter colored cap with more pronounced fuzziness, as well as a much thicker fruiting body with a cork-like texture.

Turkey Tail occurs en masse on fallen or dead standing trees in the forests and ones that fall in open spaces as well. This species doesn't seem to mind fruiting in the full sun, although it is more at home in the shaded forest. Despite the thinness of the fruiting bodies, Turkey Tail is tenacious and persistent. In the lab, *T. versicolor* has some of the most aggressive mycelial growth. In the wild it adapts well to hostile environments.

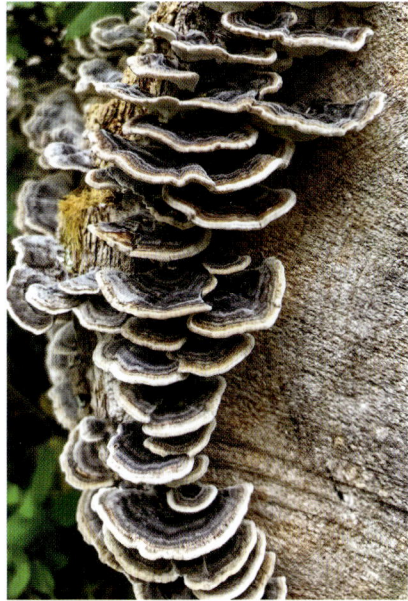

Figure 7.46. Turkey Tail overlapping fruitbodies.

With this mushroom being so prevalent and so ready to use many things, including toxic compounds, as a food source, it only makes sense to explore its potential for enhancing the health of humans, animals, and our Earth. On our farm we find beautiful specimens with pale blue bands alternating with deep blues and steel grays. We have also come across clusters that are light tan alternating with deeper shades of browns. Occasionally all of the color combinations will show up in a single cluster.

Turkey Tail can be found year-round, but the fruiting bodies are not good to harvest for use as medicine or in healing broths in all seasons. We find that in the Southern Appalachians, most wild Turkey Tail start producing in late August and early September (late summer and early fall), and that's when we harvest the majority. Judging harvest time correctly is important. Because these mushrooms are so thin and lightweight, it's best to let them grow as much as possible before harvesting. It typically takes a couple of weeks for Turkey Tail to reach maturity. The color of the margin (edge of the cap) will change from fresh white to one of the many possible mature colors.

The key thing to look for when harvesting is that the spore-producing surface is still a bright and clean white color. If it is turning brown, do not use it. Most of the time you will notice that the hymenium has lost the clean white surface and has started to become mottled or spotted dark brown. These specimens are not to be used.

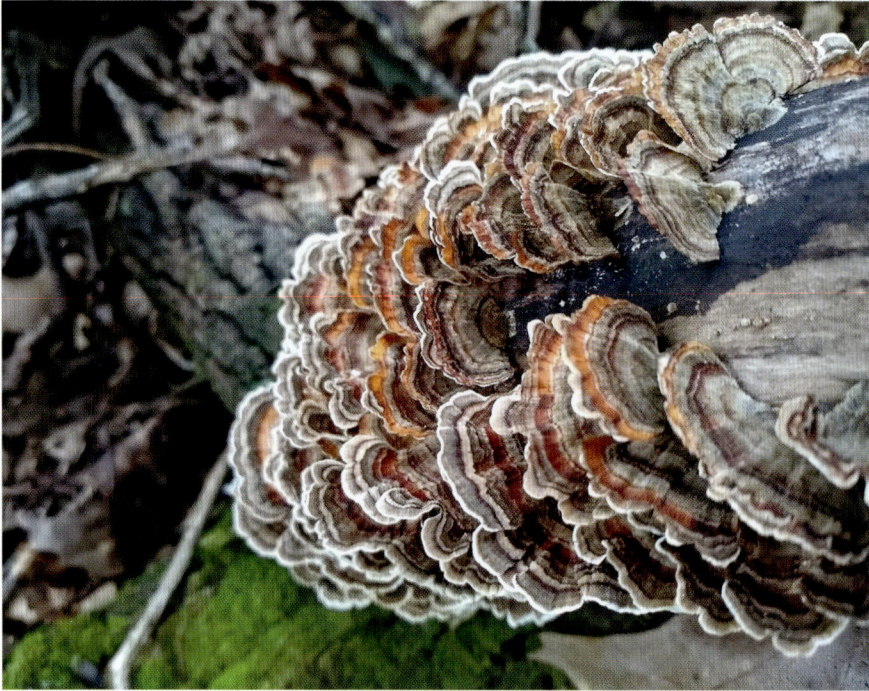

Figure 7.47. Turkey Tail with brick red colors.

In rare instances, we find dried-up fruiting bodies on logs that could still be used for medicine. Occasionally you may find spring or early summer flushes of *T. versicolor*; they are the exception in our region. Check with a local mycologist or forager to understand the best times to find Turkey Tail in your area.

Traditional Uses

The oldest written records of traditional uses of *T. versicolor* come to us from the far East. The Chinese have been using this mushroom for medicinal purposes for over two thousand years. We agree with some mycologists who hold the view that these mushrooms were being used well before they were first mentioned in writings. Turkey Tail is mentioned in the *Chinese Compendium of Materia Medica*, written during the fifteenth century.

In TCM, Yun Zhi's action is to restore qi and essence as well as regulate immune functions. Traditional functions are restoring spleen and removing dampness. It has been used for lack of appetite, diarrhea, and general debility. Modern TCM practitioners use it to treat liver cirrhosis, rheumatoid arthritis, and hepatitis, along with chronic cough and asthma. Yun Zhi has been known to be effective for those suffering from chronic fatigue syndrome (CFS) or the

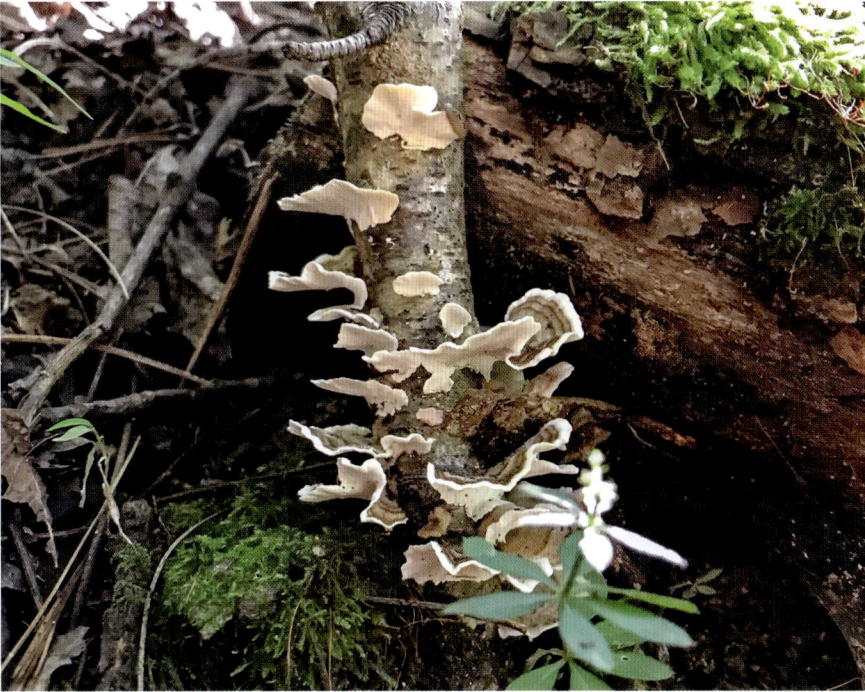

Figure 7.48. Turkey Tail on smaller fallen branch near a creek.

effects of chemotherapy, and in general for improving the quality of life for those battling cancer.

There are reports from Mexico of Indigenous people using Turkey Tail in combination with other mushrooms as a remedy for warts or scalp ringworm.[178] In South Kashmir, in the mountains of India, *T. versicolor* was included in various ethnomedical formulas for the treatment of many diseases such as skin diseases, diabetes, and cardiac issues. In India and Nigeria, Turkey Tail is used as a fever-reducing medicine.[179]

Research on Human Health Effects

Scientific research on Turkey Tail as a medicine has been ongoing since at least 1990. This research reveals a strong effect on certain types of cancer and so this area of human health has received the most research attention. Turkey Tail is also being investigated for its antimicrobial effects and its ability to modulate the immune system and improve gut health.

CANCER

Turkey Tail has been applied to human cancers as an agent that is directly toxic to cancer cells, and also as an immunomodulator that increases the

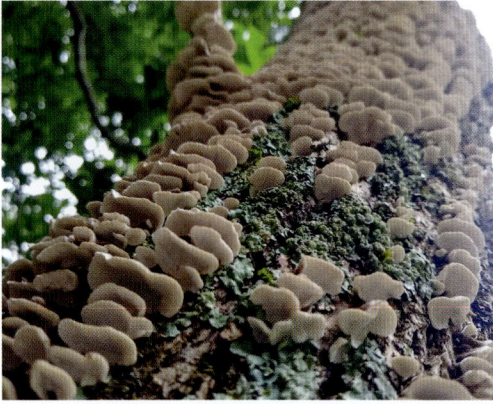

Figure 7.49. Young Turkey Tail stage.

body's natural ability to regulate the cancer cells. Research began in the 1990s, and in the 2000s turned to human clinical trials with cancer patients. A 2012 meta-analysis reviewed thirteen published, peer-reviewed clinical trials on Turkey Tail's effects on various types of cancer. The reviewers concluded that patients who received Turkey Tail had a significantly higher five-year survival rate than those who received only conventional cancer treatment. The survival rate was especially high in those with breast, gastric, or colorectal cancers.[180]

Research on the immunomodulatory effects of Turkey Tail has been going on since the 1970s. Both in the lab and in animals, Turkey Tail extracts have been shown to enhance a wide variety of biomarkers for a healthy, cancer-fighting immune system. They appear to have a generally stimulating effect on the immune system, activating, through various mechanisms, the body's innate ability to destroy cancer cells. Researchers looking at this immunostimulatory role of Turkey Tail in cancer have tended to use the mushroom alongside chemotherapy and radiotherapy, as both these conventional treatments are known to suppress the immune system. In Japan, Turkey Tail treatment is covered by insurance as an adjunct treatment for various types of cancer as it has been shown to significantly improve survival rates.[181]

Some studies have investigated the preventative role of Turkey Tail in breast cancer.[182] One study in women with breast cancer found that taking 6 g and 9 g (but not 3 g) of freeze-dried Turkey Tail mycelial powder daily safely produced increased immune functioning, measured by lymphocyte and natural killer cell counts.[183]

VIRAL AND BACTERIAL INFECTIONS

It is well established that Turkey Tail extracts are antibacterial and antiviral and show strong effects against widespread pathogens including *E. coli*, candida, listeria, and streptococcus in the lab and the H1N1 influenza strain in animals.[184] But what about in humans? We found two clinical trials of note, both on oral human papillomavirus (HPV). The first used a combination of Turkey Tail and Reishi (*Ganoderma lucidum*) mushrooms. After two months, 88 percent of the patients who had been taking the combination were clear of HPV, compared to 5 percent in the control group (who were taking Chicken-of-the-Woods [*Laetiporus sulphureus*], a mushroom that is delicious but not a strong antiviral).[185]

Cervical lesions associated with HPV can be, in a small number of cases, a precursor to cervical cancer and thus a source of worry for HPV-infected women.[186] The second study tested the efficacy of a commercial vaginal gel based on Turkey Tail in clearing the lesions. After three and six months of treatment, women using the gel were significantly more likely to have a normal Pap smear result showing no cervical lesions than those in the control group. After six months, more women using the gel than those not using the gel, had entirely cleared the HPV. Women reported feeling significantly less stressed when using the gel.

IMMUNE SYSTEM MODULATION

Some of the cancer studies described above also showed that Turkey Tail has beneficial effects on immune system function.

Another study tested the immunomodulatory effects of Turkey Tail combined with Red Sage (*Salvia miltiorrhiz*, an herb used often in TCM to increase circulatory system function) in healthy volunteers for four months.[187] The treatment resulted in improved immune system functioning and changed gene expression to support more effective immune function. Additionally, no adverse effects were reported, and tests showed no harm to liver, kidney, or bone function.

GUT HEALTH

A study in Boston was the first to look at the impacts of polysaccharides from Turkey Tail in the human gut.[188] Participants received 1,200 mg three times a day of polysaccharide peptide (PSP) for fourteen days. Previous work in the lab and with animals had suggested that Turkey Tail extracts would have a prebiotic effect. The researchers found that a pharmaceutical antibiotic significantly impacted the microbiome in ways that are known to increase risk for various disorders. This impact lasted for at least forty-two days after the end of the antibiotic treatment period. They found that the microbiota of the group taking the Turkey Tail was more able to promote the growth of beneficial bacteria in the gut.

Role in Holistic Healing

T. versicolor has been shown to be an invaluable ally for human and planetary health that gets its share of the limelight for good reason. This mushroom has been used by people worldwide. It has a voracious appetite for anything that contains cellulose, from straw to wood, and even for toxic petroleum-based compounds. Not nearly enough of this mushroom is intentionally cultivated. It is our job to advocate for all communities to cultivate this versatile mushroom for the benefits it provides to us humans, animals, waterways, air, and soil. New ways to use this fungus are just waiting on us to be more curious. Let us give this species the opportunity to shine brighter and help us solve some of the problems we face of our own doing.

In the 1960s, Japanese researchers identified Krestin (polysaccharide-K, or PSK) from Turkey Tail. PSK has been used as a successful adjunct therapy for cancer treatment. It is known for increasing life spans as well as improving quality of life for those undergoing cancer treatments. A few decades later, PSP from Turkey Tail was studied by Chinese researchers. PSP and PSK were found through research and clinical trials to be effective; their use is encouraged because of minimal side effects, immune system stimulation, and anticancer properties. These two compounds are soluble in water and thus are easily accessible. Simply put Turkey Tail in a stockpot with water and heat it all up.

As a child growing up in various parts of the Southern Appalachians, I spent time in Rutherford County, North Carolina, which straddles the foothills and the mountains. This county was a textile giant. In fact, North Carolina was the heart of the textile industry in the United States for a while. With textile production comes problematic long-term environmental pollution. The various textile companies dumped their effluent into the creeks and rivers. In fact, it seemed a requirement to locate textile plants where the dyeing process took place close to rivers or streams as a way to easily get rid of waste. The Second Broad River was subjected to these toxic sludges even up until the 2000s. I remember seeing the water look purplish and brown, sometimes with tinges of red. Now environmental regulations require companies to decolorize the dye effluent, but the decolorizing process also relies on chemicals and can be expensive. Turkey Tail could provide an economical solution. Experiments

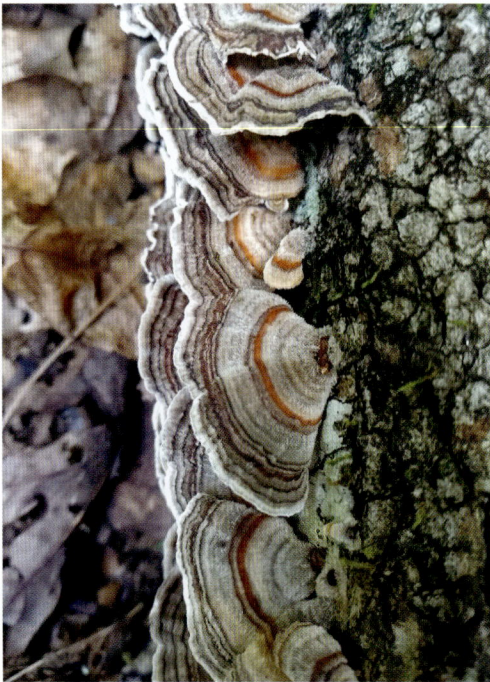

Figure 7.50. Beautiful wild tan-colored Turkey Tail.

have shown the *T. versicolor* mycelium can degrade dyes, reducing coloring by 90 percent of initial dye concentration.[189] Toxins in holding ponds or waterways are a pollution problem in all textile-dominated regions of the world. *T. versicolor* could provide solutions to protect those waterways and their aquatic life.

Phenanthrene (Phe) is a polycyclic, aromatic, petroleum-based hydrocarbon. This compound is a result of incomplete combustion of fossil fuels. It is cardiotoxic to fish. Phe is absorbed into both particulate matter and into the gas phase of air pollution. It is also found in rainwater. *T. versicolor* culture has been shown to degrade Phe most effectively at a pH of 6. The higher the concentration of fungal culture, the higher the rate of pollution breakdown.[190]

In our modern medicalized era, there is still a lot for us to learn from the natural world. Chitin is a compound found in the cell walls of all mushrooms; from it we can derive chitosan, which has been studied as a wound dressing. One study found that using chitosan with polyvinal alcohol (PVA) nanofiber dressing inhibited bacterial growth by 57.5 to 93 percent and rapidly accelerated the wound healing rate. The combination of the chitosan and nanofibers allowed fibroblast cells to adhere and exchange oxygen and moisture. The healing process was therefore accelerated.[191]

That experiment was run in a lab, but we know a similar outcome can be achieved by simply grinding Turkey Tail into a powder. This powder will not be the texture of flour; it will be fluffy and cottony. The fibers that are produced in the processing can be used in wound dressings. We have used this method successfully in treating hard-to-heal and infected wounds. The results are remarkable. We have watched wounds transform from red and swollen to having little inflammation, to having color return to normal within the first wound dressing. The dressing of powdered Turkey Tail, in our experience, is changed twice a day, morning and before bed. This method has produced results of complete healing within five to seven days on average.

Another study on wound healing in mice with a polysaccharide extract found that the healing was enhanced after only 0.01 g of extract was used. The skin thickness, collagen fiber, and number of fibroblasts were all increased up to three-fold in the treated mice compared to those left untreated. 100 percent of mice treated healed within fourteen days and 60 percent of untreated mice healed in the fourteen-day period.[192] This study once again shows the promise of *T. versicolor* as a wound healer and a natural alternative to chemical-based wound treatments.

We all know that we are tempted to eat way too many processed foods. Because of this, we are not getting the beneficial microbes nor the prebiotics through our diet that our ancestors once did. This has resulted in many digestive health issues. Reaping the health benefits for our digestive system has been one of the uses of Turkey Tail in TCM. A study from just over a decade ago found that *T. versicolor* and PSP have the ability to alter the microbial community in our gut. Levels of beneficial bifidobacterium and lactobacillus were increased while disadvantageous organisms such as clostridia, enterococci, and staphylococci were reduced.[193]

When certain aspergilli infect nut, seed, and grain crops, they can produce aflatoxin B1 (AFB1), a common carcinogenic mycotoxin. Researchers have experimented with growing Turkey Tail mycelium on corn and found that this degraded the AFB1 by 93 percent and increased the beneficial lysine content in the corn.[194]

Cultivation Notes

Turkey tail is not commonly cultivated indoors, but sawdust substrate for general indoor growing is sufficient. The most important aspect is to top fruit the mushroom from sawdust. An alternate approach is a series of twelve to sixteen horizontal cuts along the sides of substrate blocks; this will result in nicely thin fruiting bodies.

Outdoor cultivation can happen on a range of softwoods and hardwoods. We recommend using logs that are smaller than the usual size for Shiitake, Lion's Mane, Oyster, or other fungi that benefit from more substrate. See the Turkey Tail profile on page 43 for details on log cultivation of Turkey Tail.

Ethical Wild Harvesting

Wild harvesting is the most common way to collect Turkey Tail mushrooms. The fruitings tend to be en masse. Even though we find huge flushes of this mushroom, we harvest only a small percentage—the amount we know we can use up within about six months. In our region we tend to get smaller spring flushes, and in early fall are the more substantial flushes. On our farm there are so many wild Turkey Tail we have not had to grow any in the last five years. If there are very little Turkey Tail in your region, consider inoculating logs to establish Turkey Tail in the forest nearby.

Acknowledgments

I would like to acknowledge the following with the deepest love, gratitude, and appreciation: My parents, Angela Chapman and Eddie Parker, for raising me in the way they did.

My grandparents, for their knowledge of the natural world, encouraging it in me and keeping that fire burning for me to pass on to my children.

My great grandparents, with their wisdom and connection to the past.

All the students I have had, with the questions that sparked my curiosity in many different directions.

I thank all the previous authors of mycology books who gifted me their knowledge. Most especially Paul Stamets for his wisdom and curiosity; he has done more for mycology than any single person.

I acknowledge and appreciate the tenacity and adaptability of my Cherokee ancestors, who resisted the removal and remained in our homeland.

We acknowledge the spirits of this land, who provide an abundant bounty of food and medicine and protect our mountain home.

We acknowledge and thank the spirits of the mushrooms for teaching us and opening our awareness.

We acknowledge the too-many-to-list people who have shaped who we are as people.

We acknowledge the editing and design team at Chelsea Green for expertly shepherding the writing process.

Wood Species for Outdoor Cultivation

TABLE 1. Log Fruiting Times and Wood Choices for Medicinal Species

Mushroom Species	Time to Fruiting from Plugging	Results with Small Logs (2- to 6-inch diameter)	Results with Large Logs (6-inch diameter or larger)
Shiitake	*Small logs:* 6 months *Large logs:* Less than 12 months	Flush in spring and fall for 2–6 years	Flush in spring and fall for 6+ years
Oyster	Within 6 months	Flush in spring and fall for 2 years	Flush in spring and fall for 3–4 years
Reishi	Possible within 6 months; likely within 12 months	Flush in summer for 3–4 years	Not recommended
Lion's Mane	*Softwood:* 1–2 years *Hardwood:* 2+ years	Produces for 1–3 years	Can produce for 8–10 years on hardwoods
Chicken-of-the-Woods	1–2 years	Not recommended	Flush in summer

Type of Wood for Plugging		Notes
oak Wild Cherry Sweetgum	American Beech Paper Birch Black Birch alder	
Tulip Poplar maple willow beech	birch Paulownia Tree of Heaven	Larger logs = larger flushes
oak Red Maple	Southern Magnolia gum trees	Summer flush only
For short-term production: maple, willow, Paulownia, Tree of Heaven, beech, birch *For long-term production:* elm, oak, chestnut, Black Walnut		Fall flush only. Plugging short-term wood will produce mushrooms more quickly, especially on smaller logs, but not last as long. Plugging long-term wood will take longer to produce but will produce longer, especially with larger diameter logs
Any hardwood (except locusts) and most softwoods		Use logs 12+ inches in diameter

Medicinal Compounds Found in Mushrooms

The medicinal mushroom species covered in chapter 7 are the source of a wide range of medicinal compounds. The lists below are not meant to be exhaustive but are ample enough to give beginning mycologists an introduction to the names of significant medicinal compounds and to help seasoned mycologists deepen their relationship with and understanding of these fungi. Some of the compounds listed below are discussed in the mushroom profiles or other chapters, but many are not. Some are well-known and others are just recently uncovered by scientists. Inevitably, more medicinal compounds will be identified in these mushroom species in the near future as mycology continues to rise in popularity with researchers and citizen scientists.

CORDYCEPS SPP.

alanine
arginine
campesterol
cerevisterol
chitin
cholesteryl palmitate
cordycepic acid
cordycepin
cyclic peptides

daucosterol
ergosterol
ergosterol peroxide
glucogalactomannans
glutamic acid
glycine
heteropolysaccharides
histidine
leucine

lysine
methionine
proline
serine
threonine
tryptophan
valine
β-sitosterol

FOMES FOMENTARIUS

betulin
betulin 28-o-acetate
chitin
daphnetin

ergosterol
fomentaric acid
fomentariol
phenols

polysaccharides
β-glucans

FOMITOPSIS BETULINA

betulinic acid
carboxylic acids
chitin
chitosan
ergosterol peroxide
lycopene

mannitol
piptamine
polyporenic acids
sesquiterpenes
stigmasterol
terpenes

trehalose
triterpenoids
ungalinic acid
α-glucans
β-carotene
β-d-glucans

GANODERMA SPP.

alkaloids
ergosterols
lipids
phenols

polyphenols
polysaccharides
steroids
sterols

terpenoids
triterpenes
β-glucans

GRIFOLA FRONDOSA

aspartic acid
chitin
D-fraction
ergosterol
glutamic acid
grifolan

heteroglycans
linoleic acid
oleic acid
phenolic acids
polysaccharides
sterols

SX-fraction
triterpenes
X-fraction
β-glucans

HERICIUM SPP.

3-hydroxyhericenone F
amino acids
arabitol
erinacerin A and G

erinacine A
hericenones
herierin III and IV
mannitol

polysaccharides
trehalose
β-glucans

INONOTUS OBLIQUUS

antioxidants
betulin
betulinic acid
chitin
ergosterol
galactose
glucose

inositol
inotodiol
mannose
melanin
oxalic acid
polyphenols
polysaccharides

rhamnose
triterpenes
xylose
α-glucans
β-glucans

LACTARIUS AND LACTIFLUUS SPP.

caryophyllene
chitin
drimane

isolactarorufin
lactaroviolin
mannitol

phenols
polysaccharides
sesquiterpenoids

261

sterols
terpenes

trehalose
tryptophan

volemolide
β-glucans

LENTINULA EDODES

arabinoses
chitin-rich heteroglycan
ergosterol
eritadenine
glycerol
lentinan

linoleic acid
mannitol
mannose
myristic acid
oleic acid
palmitic acid

stearic acid
trehalose
xyloglucan
β-glucans

PENICILLIUM SPP.

compactin
conidiogenone B

coniochaetones
palitantin

penicillin

PLEUROTUS SPP.

carotenoids
chitin
chrysin

ergosterol
ergothioneine
lovastatin

mannogalactans
tricholomic acid
β-glucans

PSILOCYBE SPP.

aeruginasin
baeocystin

indole alkaloids
norbaeocystin

psilocin
psilocybin

SCHIZOPHYLLUM COMMUNE

adenosine
amino acids
chitin
ergosterol
ethanol

exopolysaccharides
hydroxybenzoic acid
iminolactones
phenols
protocatechuic acid

schizophyllan
terpenoids
tocopherol
β-glucans

TRAMETES VERSICOLOR

amino acids
chitin
chitosan
ergosterol
fungisterol
hydroxybenzoic acid
lectins
linoleic acid

melanin
oleic acid
palmitic acid
phenols
polysaccharide krestin
polysaccharide peptide
protocatechuic acid
statins

stearic acid
terpenoids
triterpenoids
vanillic acid
β-glucans
β-sitosterol

Glossary

Agar. A phycocolloid (a type of polysaccharide) produced by some species of red algae in the genus *Gelidium*; used to solidify culture media used in mycology and bacteriology.

Arbuscular mycorrhizal fungi (AMF). A type of soilborne fungi that have a symbiotic relationship with plant roots, providing nutrient and water exchange. AMF are key for the survival of the vast majority of plants on Earth.

Arbuscules. Extensively branching modified organs in fungi that resemble tree-like structures; they occur within root cells of plants.

Autoclave. A robust container that can withstand high pressure, used to sterilize equipment and tools.

Conk. A shelf- or bracket-type fungus; also, the reproductive fruitbody of such fungi. They are produced by wood-decaying species of fungi and can be annual or perennial species.

Contamination. A process of infection by undesired foreign organisms (contaminants) in a growing medium. Contamination often occurs due to insufficient sterilization or pasteurization, or from improper sterile technique.

Culture. Fungal mycelium growing on a medium such as agar. Culture is also used interchangeably with strain. (See Strain definition below.)

Ectomycorrhizal fungi. Soilborne fungi that develop a symbiotic relationship with plant roots by connecting primarily with the outside of the root system, creating what is referred to as a sheath or mantle.

Endomycorrhizal fungi. Soilborne fungi that develop a symbiotic relationship with plant roots by incorporating into the cell walls of the plant. Over 85 percent of plants on Earth are supported by relationships with this type of fungi.

Flush. A sudden development of many fruiting bodies at the same time. Usually there is a resting period between flushes.

Fruiting body or fruitbody. The reproductive structure of fungi. When we consume mushrooms, we are eating fruitbodies.

Fruiting. The formation of the edible fruiting bodies of a fungus—that is, the mushrooms.

Heartwood. Older, dark-colored portion of the wood in the center of a tree trunk or limb.

Hymenium. The spore-bearing or spore-producing surface of all higher fungi.

Hyphae. Single strands of mycelium.

Imperfect fungi. A large group of fungi that reproduce by asexual spores. Often but not always observed as molds.

Incubation. The time after inoculation and before mycelium has fully colonized a substrate. This stage of the cloning process is done in a sterile environment to prevent/reduce contamination. When logs are inoculated, incubation is simply the period during which the logs are maintained under conditions favorable for the mycelium to grow throughout the sapwood.

Inoculation. The process of introducing spores or mycelium culture into wood or another substrate.

Lignocellulose. The essential part of woody material that contains cellulose, lignin, and hemicellulose. Lignocellulose imparts rigidity to plants and provides a food source for wood-decaying species of fungi.

Liquid culture. A myceliated product in which mycelium has been propagated in a mixture of sterilized water and sugar to obtain a pure culture. Usually injected into a substrate via needle and syringe. Occasionally other nutrients are added to a liquid culture to assist mycelial growth. "Liquid culture" is used interchangeably as a method and a product.

Macrofungi. Fungal species that produce large, easily visible fruitbodies. The mushrooms most commonly hunted, cultivated, and consumed are all macrofungi.

Mycelium. The vegetative part of a fungus, consisting of many fine white filaments called hyphae.

Mycorrhiza. A symbiotic association between a plant root and fungal hyphae.

Parasitic mushrooms. Fungi that survive by attacking and consuming other living organisms.

Pasteurization. Heat treatment applied to a substrate to destroy unwanted organisms but allowing favorable organisms to survive. The temperature range for pasteurization is 140°F to 175°F (60°C to 80°C). Pasteurization is different from sterilization, which aims at destroying all organisms in a substrate.

Pilot study. A trial-run study that is preliminary to larger studies to develop more refined methodologies and larger sample sizes.

Pinning. The process of forming primordia.

Polypore fungi. Polypores (including shelf polypore and bracket polypore) are fungi that have a spore producing surface that consists of pores.

Primordia. Tiny fruiting mushrooms, also called pins or pinheads, that are roughly ⅛- to ¼-inch in diameter.

Randomized controlled trial (RCT). A scientific study conducted with participants randomly assigned to groups, often using computer-generated randomization, to study the effectiveness of a drug or other type of medical treatment.

GLOSSARY

Saprotrophic fungi. Mushrooms or fungi that live on dead or decaying organic material.

Sapwood. Young, light-colored portion of the wood near the outside of a log.

Sawdust plunger. A tool for injecting sawdust into holes in a log.

Spawn. Substrate that is completely colonized by mycelium; used to inoculate a bulk substrate. Rye, wheat, millet, other grains, and sawdust are all used as spawn. Cardboard can also be used for spawn, according to the intended use.

Spawn run. The incubation period during which the vegetative stage of the mycelium grows throughout the sapwood of a log.

Spores. Tiny reproductive units. Mushroom spores are produced on the hymenium of the fruitbody. They are similar to seeds of higher plant life but are microscopic. After being released into the air from the spore-producing surface or carried by insects and animals, spores find a new home and germinate.

Sterilization. A treatment that completely destroys all microorganisms present by exposure to heat (as in an autoclave or pressure cooker) or chemicals.

Strain. A selected variety of a fungus, bacterium, plant, etc.

Substrate. A material on which mushrooms live and grow. Some examples are compost, wood, sawdust, and hay. The choice of substrate varies depending on the type of mushroom.

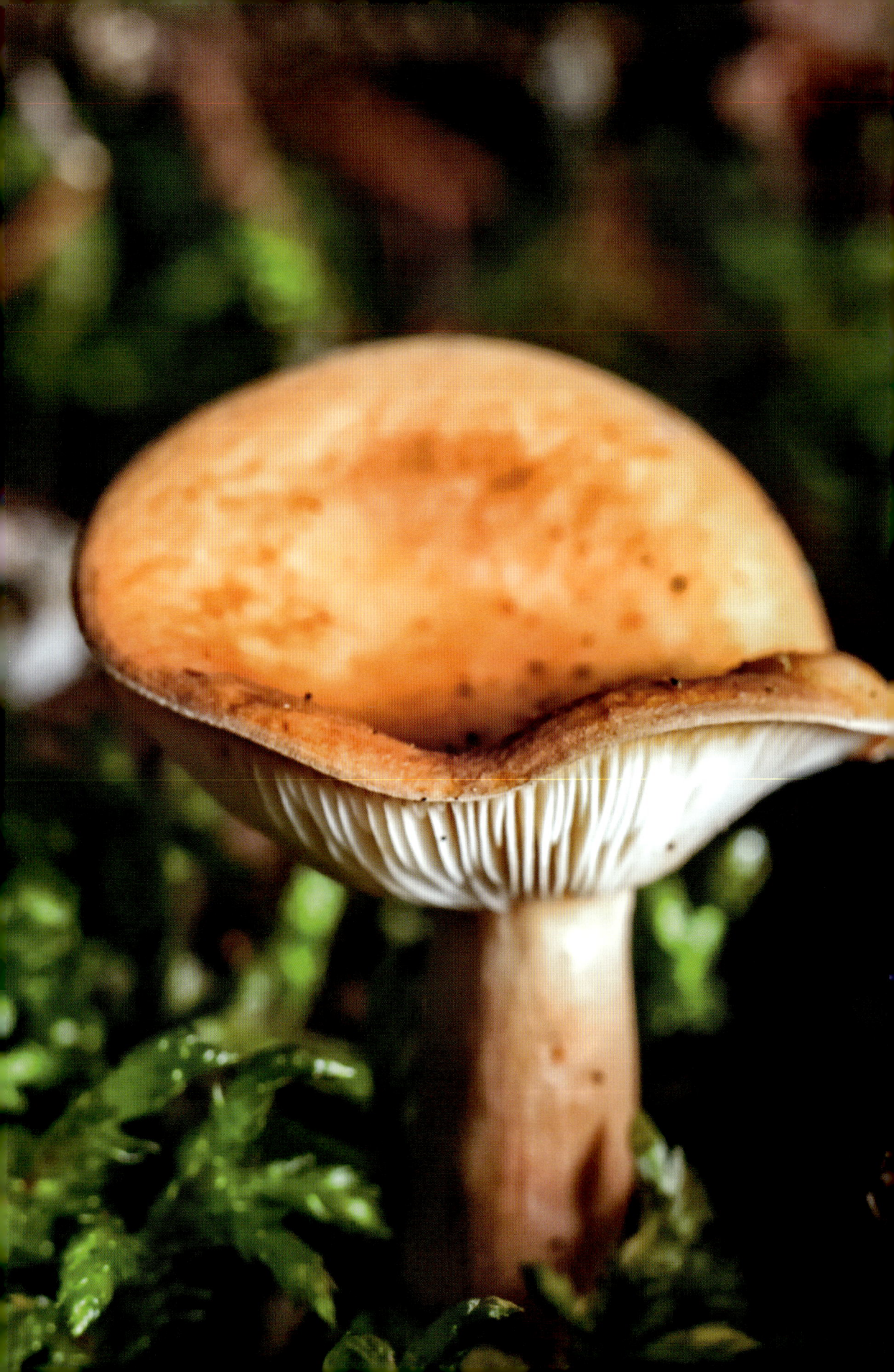

Notes

CHAPTER 1. THE WORLD ACCORDING TO FUNGI

1. Chayanard Phukhamsakda et al., "The Numbers of Fungi: Contributions from Traditional Taxonomic Studies and Challenges of Metabarcoding," *Fungal Diversity* 114 (April 2022): 327–86, https://doi.org/10.1007/s1322 5-022-00502-3.

2. S. Bonneville et al., "Molecular Identification of Fungi Microfossils in a Neoproterozoic Shale Rock," *Science Advances* 6, no. 4 (January 2020): eaax7599, https://doi.org/10.1126 /sciadv.aax7599.

3. Charles H. Wellman, "Origin, Function and Development of the Spore Wall in Early Land Plants," in *The Evolution of Plant Physiology*, ed. Alan R. Hemsley and Imogen Poole (Cambridge, MA: Academic Press, 2004), 43–63, https://doi.org/10.1016/B978-012339552 -8/50004-4.

4. Marc-André Selosse et al., "Plants, Fungi and Oomycetes: A 400-Million Year Affair That Shapes the Biosphere," *New Phytologist* 206, no. 2 (April 2015): 501–6, https://doi.org /10.1111/nph.13371.

5. Matthew P. Nelsen and C. Kevin Boyce, "What to Do with *Prototaxites*?" in "Tribute to Francis M. Hueber," ed. Christina Caruso et al., special issue, *International Journal of Plant Sciences* 183, no. 6 (July/August 2022): 556–65, https://doi.org/10.1086/720688.

6. Mark C. Brundrett et al., "Fossils of Arbuscular Mycorrhizal Fungi Give Insights into the History of a Successful Partnership with Plants," in *Transformative Paleobotany: Papers to Commemorate the Life and Legacy of Thomas N. Taylor*, ed. Michael Krings et al. (Cambridge, MA: Academic Press, 2018), 461–80, https:// doi.org/10.1016/B978-0-12-813012-4.00019-X.

7. David Kearns, "Irish Bog Butter Proven to be '3500 Years' Past Its Best Before Date," News, University College Dublin, March 14, 2019, https://www.ucd.ie/newsandopinion/ news/2019/march/14/irishbogbutterproven tobe3500yearspastitsbestbeforedate/.

8. Ken Sayers et al., "Blood, Bulbs, and Bunodonts: On Evolutionary Ecology and the Diets of *Ardipithecus*, *Australopithecus*, and Early *Homo*," *The Quarterly Review of Biology* 89, no. 4 (December 2014): 319–57, https:// doi.org/10.1086/678568.

9. Amy M. Hanson, Kathie T. Hodge, and Leila M. Porter, "Mycophagy among Primates," *Mycologist* 17, no. 1 (February 2003): 6–10.

10. Terence McKenna, *Food of the Gods: The Search for the Original Tree of Knowledge: A Radical History of Plants, Drugs, and Human Evolution* (New York: Bantam Books, 1993).

11. José Manuel Rodríguez Arce and Michael James Winkelman, "Psychedelics, Sociality, and Human Evolution," *Frontiers in Psychology* 12 (September 2021): 729425, https://doi.org /10.3389/fpsyg.2021.729425.

12. Yu Fukasawa et al., "Electrical Integrity and Week-Long Oscillation in Fungal Mycelia," *Scientific Reports* 14 (July 2024): 15601, https://doi.org/10.1038/s41598-024-66223-6.

13. Anne Pringle et al., "Mycorrhizal Symbioses and Plant Invasions," *Annual Review of Ecology, Evolution, and Systematics* 40 (December

2009): 699–715, https://doi.org/10.1146
/annurev.ecolsys.39.110707.173454.

14. Martin Pion et al., "Bacterial Farming by the
Fungus *Morchella crassipes*," *Proceedings of the
Royal Society B* 280, no. 1773 (December
2013): 20132242, https://doi.org/10.109
/rspb.2013.2242.

15. Lawrence A. Clayton, Vernon J. Knight, and
Edward C. Moore, *The De Soto Chronicles: The
Expedition of Hernando de Soto to North
America in 1539–1543* (Tuscaloosa: University
of Alabama Press, 1993), https://archive.org
/details/isbn_9780817305932.

CHAPTER 5. INDOOR CULTIVATION

1. For more information about Ryan's company,
visit the Terrestrial Fungi website: https://www
.terrestrialfungi.com.

**CHAPTER 6. MUSHROOMS AS
FOOD AND MEDICINE**

1. John Dighton, Tatyana Tugay, and Nelli
Zhdanova, "Fungi and Ionizing Radiation from
Radionuclides," *FEMS Microbiology Letters*
281, no. 2 (April 2008): 109–20, https://doi
.org/10.1111/j.1574-6968.2008.01076.x.

2. Anusha H. Ekanayaka et al., "A Review of the
Fungi that Degrade Plastic," *Journal of Fungi* 8,
no. 8 (July 2022): 772, https://doi.org/10
.3390/jof8080772.

3. Daniel Elieh Ali Komi, Lokesh Sharma, and
Charles S. Dela Cruz, "Chitin and Its Effects on
Inflammatory and Immune Responses," *Clinical
Reviews in Allergy & Immunology* 54 (April
2018): 213–23, https://doi.org/10.1007
/s12016-017-8600-0.

4. Xujiao Ren et al., "Comparative Studies on
Bioactive Compounds, Ganoderic Acid
Biosynthesis, and Antioxidant Activity of Pileus
and Stipes of Lingzhi or Reishi Medicinal
Mushroom, *Ganoderma lucidum* (Agaricomy-
cetes) Fruiting Body at Different Growth
Stages," *International Journal of Medicinal
Mushrooms* 22, no. 2 (March 2020): 133–44,
https://doi.org/10.1615/intjmedmushrooms
.2020033683.

5. Surya Sudheer et al., "Development of Antler-
Type Fruiting Bodies of *Ganoderma lucidum*
and Determination of Its Biochemical
Properties," *Fungal Biology* 122, no. 5 (May
2018): 293–301, https://doi.org/10.1016/j
.funbio.2018.01.007.

6. Ha Thi Hoa, Chun-Li Wang, and Chong-Ho
Wang, "The Effects of Different Substrates on
the Growth, Yield, and Nutritional Composition of Two Oyster Mushrooms (*Pleurotus
ostreatus* and *Pleurotus cystidiosus*)," *Mycobiology*
43, no. 4 (December 2015): 423–34, https://
doi.org/10.5941/MYCO.2015.43.4.423.

7. Adrian Zając et al., "Pro-Health and Anti-Cancer
Activity of Fungal Fractions Isolated from
Milk-Supplemented Cultures of *Lentinus* (*Pleurotus*) *Sajor-caju*," *Biomolecules* 11, no. 8 (July
2021): 1089, https://doi.org/10.3390/biom
11081089.

8. Xian-Bing Mao et al., "Optimization of Carbon
Source and Carbon/Nitrogen Ratio for
Cordycepin Production by Submerged
Cultivation of Medicinal Mushroom *Cordyceps
militaris*," *Process Biochemistry* 40, no. 5 (April
2005): 1667–72, https://doi.org/10.1016/j
.procbio.2004.06.046.

9. Chung Duong Dinh, "Cordycepin in the Fruiting
Body of *Cordyceps militaris* cultured from 5
Different Materials in Vietnam: Analysis and
Comparison," *World Journal of Advanced
Research and Reviews* 22, no. 2. (2024):
1255–64, https://doi.org/10.30574/wjarr
.2024.22.2.1521.

10. Dinh, "Cordycepin in the Fruiting Body of
Cordyceps militaris."

11. Taisei Shibata et al., "Isolation and Characterization of a Novel Two-Component Hemolysin,
Erylysin A and B, from an Edible Mushroom,
Pleurotus eryngii," *Toxicon* 56, no. 8 (December
2010): 1436–42, https://doi.org/10.1016/j
.toxicon.2010.08.010.

12. Bela Toth and James Erickson, "Cancer Induction
in Mice by Feeding of the Uncooked Cultivated
Mushroom of Commerce *Agaricus bisporus*,"
Cancer Research 46, no. 8 (August 1986):
4007–11, https://aacrjournals.org/cancerres

/article/46/8/4007/491026/Cancer
-Induction-in-Mice-by-Feeding-of-the; T. Kopp
et al., "Systemic Allergic Contact Dermatitis
Due to Consumption of Raw Shiitake
Mushroom, *Clinical and Experimental
Dermatology* 34, no. 8 (December 2009):
910–13, https://doi.org/10.1111/j.1365
-2230.2009.03681.x.

CHAPTER 7. MEDICINAL
MUSHROOM PROFILES

1. Albert Einstein College of Medicine, "98.6
Degrees Fahrenheit Ideal Temperature for
Keeping Fungi Away and Food at Bay,"
ScienceDaily, December 30, 2010, https://
www.sciencedaily.com/releases/2010
/12/101222121610.htm.

2. "This Mushroom Increases Endurance," *The
Journal of Plant Medicines*, accessed November
15, 2024, https://www.plantmedicines.org
/2022/05/this-mushroom-increases
-endurance.html.

3. William Watson, "An Account of the Insect Called
the Vegetable Fly: By William Watson, M. D. F.
R. S.," *Philosophical Transactions (1683–1775)*
53 (1763): 271–74, http://www.jstor.org
/stable/105733.

4. Robert Rogers, *The Fungal Pharmacy: The
Complete Guide to Medicinal Mushrooms and
Lichens of North America* (North Atlantic
Books, 2011), 117.

5. Yilin Tao et al., "Use of Bailing Capsules (*Cordy-
ceps sinensis*) in the Treatment of Chronic
Kidney Disease: A Meta-Analysis and Network
Pharmacology," *Frontiers in Pharmacology* 15
(April 2024): 1342831, doi.org/10.3389
/fphar.2024.1342831.

6. Canran Wang, Jiawei Wang, and Yuanfu Qi,
"Adjuvant Treatment with *Cordyceps sinensis* for
Lung Cancer: A Systematic Review and
Meta-Analysis of Randomized Controlled
Trials," *Journal of Ethnopharmacology* 327 (June
2024): 118044, https://doi.org/10.1016/j.jep
.2024.118044.

7. Huan Zhang et al., "Efficacy of Jinshuibao as an
Adjuvant Treatment for Chronic Renal Failure

in China: A Meta-Analysis," *Medicine* 102,
no. 32 (August 2023): e34575, https://doi
.org/10.1097/MD.0000000000034575.

8. Wu Liu et al., "Mechanism of *Cordyceps sinensis*
and Its Extracts in the Treatment of Diabetic
Kidney Disease: A Review," *Frontiers in
Pharmacology* 13 (May 2022): 881835, https://
doi.org/10.3389/fphar.2022.881835.

9. Zhong Li et al., "Effects of Bailing Capsule
Combined with Irbesartan on Oxidative Stress,
Inflammatory Response and Immune Function
in Patients with Diabetic Nephropathy," *Journal
of Hainan Medical University* 25, no. 9
(May 2019): 33–36, The Internet Archive.

10. Xuhua Yu et al., "Effectiveness and Safety of Oral
Cordyceps sinensis on Stable COPD of GOLD
Stages 2–3: Systematic Review and Meta-
Analysis," *Evidence-Based Complementary and
Alternative Medicine* (April 2019): 4903671,
https://doi.org/10.1155/2019/4903671.

11. Xinmin Yu, "Analysis on Effect of Jinshuibao
Capsule Combined Treatment on Newly
Diagnosed Pulmonary Tuberculosis," *Advanced
Emergency Medicine* 4, no. 3 (September 2015):
37–39, https://aem.usp-pl.com/index.php
/aem/article/view/12.

12. Fellipe Pinheiro Savioli et al., "Effects of
Cordyceps sinensis Supplementation During 12
Weeks in Amateur Marathoners: A Randomized, Double-Blind Placebo-Controlled Trial,"
Journal of Herbal Medicine 34 (July 2022):
100570, https://doi.org/10.1016/j.hermed
.2022.100570.

13. Luthfia Dewi et al., "*Cordyceps sinensis* Accelerates Stem Cell Recruitment to Human Skeletal
Muscle After Exercise," *Food & Function* 15,
no. 8 (April 2024): 4010–20, https://doi.org
/10.1039/D3FO03770C.

14. Liping Chen et al., "*Cordyceps* Polysaccharides: A
Review of Their Immunomodulatory Effects,"
Molecules 29, no. 21 (October 2024): 5107,
https://doi.org/10.3390/molecules29215107.

15. Atcharaporn Ontawong et al., "A Randomized
Controlled Clinical Trial Examining the Effects
of *Cordyceps militaris* Beverage on the Immune
Response in Healthy Adults," *Scientific Reports*

14 (April 2024): 7994, https://doi.org/10.1038/s41598-024-58742-z.

16. Shao-An Hsieh et al., "The Effects of *Cordyceps militaris* Fruiting Bodies in Micturition and Prostate Size in Benign Prostatic Hyperplasia Patients: A Pilot Study," *Pharmacological Research—Modern Chinese Medicine* 4 (September 2022): 100143, https://doi.org/10.1016/j.prmcm.2022.100143.

17. Kam Ming Ko and Hoi Yan Leung, "Enhancement of ATP Generation Capacity, Antioxidant Activity and Immunomodulatory Activities by Chinese Yang and Yin Tonifying Herbs," *Chinese Medicine* 2, no. 3 (March 2007), https://doi.org/10.1186/1749-8546-2-3.

18. Siddharth Dubhashi et al., "Early Trends to Show the Efficacy of *Cordyceps militaris* in Mild to Moderate COVID Inflammation," *Cureus* 15, no. 8 (August 2023): e43731, https://doi.org/10.7759/cureus.43731; Mehmet A. Kaymakci and Eray M. Guler, "Promising Potential Pharmaceuticals from the Genus *Cordyceps* for COVID-19 Treatment: A Review Study," *Bezmialem Science* 8, no. 3 (December 2020):140–44, https://doi.org/10.14235/bas.galenos.2020.4532; Jing Du et al., "Interactions Between Adenosine Receptors and Cordycepin (3-Deoxyadenosine) from *Cordyceps militaris*: Possible Pharmacological Mechanisms for Protection of the Brain and the Amelioration of Covid-19 Pneumonia," *Journal of Biotechnology and Biomedicine* 4 (June 2021): 26–62, https://doi.org/10.26502/jbb.2642-91280035.

19. Jun He, "Harvest and Trade of Caterpillar Mushroom (*Ophiocordyceps sinensis)* and the Implications for Sustainable Use in the Tibet Region of Southwest China," *Journal of Ethnopharmacology* 221 (July 2018): 86–90, https://doi.org/10.1016/j.jep.2018.04.022.

20. Robert Pylkkänen et al., "The Complex Structure of *Fomes fomentarius* Represents an Architectural Design for High-Performance Ultralightweight Materials," *Science Advances* 9, no. 8 (February 2023): eade5417, https://doi.org/10.1126/sciadv.ade5417.

21. Ingvar Svanberg, "Ethnomycological Notes on *Haploporus odorus* and Other Polypores in Northern Fennoscandia," *Journal of Northern Studies* 12, no. 1 (September 2018): 73–91, https://doi.org/10.36368/jns.v12i1.900.

22. Nóra Papp et al., "Ethnomycological Use of *Fomes fomentarius* (L.) Fr. and *Piptoporus betulinus* (Bull.) P. Karst. in Transylvania, Romania," *Genetic Resources and Crop Evolution* 64, no.1 (January 2017): 101–11, https://doi.org/10.1007/s10722-015-0335-2.

23. Ulrike Grienke et al., "European Medicinal Polypores—A Modern View on Traditional Uses," *Journal of Ethnopharmacology* 154, no. 3 (July 2014): 564–83, https://doi.org/10.1016/j.jep.2014.04.030.

24. Győző Zsigmond, "The *Amanitaceae* in Hungarian Folk Tradition," *Moeszia Erdélyi Gombász* 1 (2003): 55–68, https://www.samorini.it/doc1/alt_aut/sz/zsigmond-the-amanitaceae-in-hungarian-folk-tradition.pdf.

25. Joachim Storsberg, Anne Krüger-Genge, and Liudmila Kalitukha, "In Vitro Cytotoxic Activity of an Aqueous Alkali Extract of the Tinder Conk Mushroom, *Fomes fomentarius* (Agaricomycetes), on Murine Fibroblasts, Human Colorectal Adenocarcinoma, and Cutaneous Melanoma Cells," *International Journal of Medicinal Mushrooms* 24, no. 9 (July 2022): 1–13, https://doi.org/10.1615/IntJMedMushrooms.2022044657.

26. Matjaž Ravnikar et al., "Fomentariol, a *Fomes fomentarius* Compound, Exhibits Anti-Diabetic Effects in Fungal Material: An In Vitro Analysis," *Nutraceuticals* 4, no. 2 (May 2024): 273–82, https://doi.org/10.3390/nutraceuticals4020017.

27. Marina Kolundžić et al., "Antibacterial and Cytotoxic Activities of Wild Mushroom *Fomes fomentarius* (L.) Fr., Polyporaceae," *Industrial Crops and Products* 79 (January 2016): 110–15, https://doi.org/10.1016/j.indcrop.2015.10.030.

28. Gülşah Gedik et al., "The Antimicrobial Effect of Various Formulations Obtained from *Fomes Fomentarius* Against Hospital Isolates," *Mantar*

Dergisi 10, no. 2 (October 2019): 103–9, https://doi.org/10.30708/mantar.535994.

29. Małgorzata Pleszczyńska et al., "*Fomitopsis betulina* (Formerly *Piptoporus betulinus*): The Iceman's Polypore Fungus with Modern Biotechnological Potential," *World Journal of Microbiology and Biotechnology* 33, no. 5 (May 2017): 83, https://doi.org/10.1007/s11274-017-2247-0.

30. Pleszczyńska et al., "*Fomitopsis betulina.*"

31. Pleszczyńska et al., "*Fomitopsis betulina.*"

32. Justyna Bożek et al., "Effects of *Piptoporus betulinus* Ethanolic Extract on the Proliferation and Viability of Melanoma Cells and Models of Their Cell Membranes," *International Journal of Molecular Sciences* 23, no. 22 (November 2022): 13907, https://doi.org/10.3390/ijms232213907.

33. Marta Kinga Lemieszek et al., "Anticancer Effect of Fraction Isolated from Medicinal Birch Polypore Mushroom, *Piptoporus betulinus* (Bull.: Fr.) P. Karst. (Aphyllophoromycetideae): *In Vitro* Studies," *International Journal of Medicinal Mushrooms* 11, no. 4 (2009): 351–64, https://doi.org/10.1615/IntJMedMushr.v11.i4.20.

34. Katarzyna Sułkowska-Ziaja et al., "Chemical Composition and Biological Activity of Extracts from Fruiting Bodies and Mycelial Cultures of *Fomitopsis betulina*," *Molecular Biology Reports* 45 (October 2018): 2535–44, https://doi.org/10.1007/s11033-018-4420-4.

35. Philipp Dresch et al., "Fungal Strain Matters: Colony Growth and Bioactivity of the European Medicinal Polypores *Fomes fomentarius*, *Fomitopsis pinicola* and *Piptoporus betulinus*," *AMB Express* 5, no. 1 (January 2015): 4, https://doi.org/10.1186/s13568-014-0093-0.

36. Ingvar Svanberg and Isak Lidström, "Viking Games and Sámi Pastimes: Making Balls of *Fomitopsis betulina*," *Ethnobiology Letters* 10, no. 1 (November 2019): 86–96, https://doi.org/10.14237/ebl.10.1.2019.1565.

37. Pleszczyńska et al., "*Fomitopsis betulina.*"

38. Reyes Sierra-Alvarez, "Fungal Bioleaching of Metals in Preservative-Treated Wood," *Process Biochemistry* 42, no. 5 (May 2007): 798–804, https://doi.org/10.1016/j.procbio.2007.01.019.

39. Mark Button et al., "Arsenic Speciation in the Bracket Fungus *Fomitopsis betulina* from Contaminated and Pristine Sites," *Environmental Geochemistry and Health* 42 (September 2020): 2723–32, https://doi.org/10.1007/s10653-019-00506-0.

40. The Business Research Company, *Reishi Mushroom Global Market Report 2025*, January 2025, https://www.thebusinessresearchcompany.com/report/reishi-mushroom-global-market-report.

41. *The Divine Farmer's Materia Medica: A Translation of the Shen Nong Ben Cao Jing*, trans. Yang Shou-zhong, (Boulder: Blue Poppy Press, 1998), 17–18, https://komornlaw.com/wp-content/uploads/2018/04/The_Divine_Farmers_Materia_Medica-Shen-Nong-Ben-Cao-Jing.pdf.

42. Xingzhong Jin et al., "*Ganoderma lucidum* (Reishi Mushroom) for Cancer Treatment," *Cochrane Database of Systematic Reviews* 2016, no. 4 (April 2016): CD007731, https://doi.org/10.1002/14651858.CD007731.pub3.

43. Yihuai Gao et al., "A Randomized, Placebo-Controlled, Multicenter Study of *Ganoderma lucidum* (W.Curt.:Fr.) Lloyd (Aphyllophoromycetideae) Polysaccharides (Ganopoly®) in Patients with Advanced Lung Cancer," *International Journal of Medicinal Mushrooms* 5, no. 4 (2003): 369–382, https://doi.org/10.1615/InterJMedicMush.v5.i4.40.

44. Shiro Oka et al., "A Water-Soluble Extract from Culture Medium of *Ganoderma lucidum* Mycelia Suppresses the Development of Colorectal Adenomas," *Hiroshima Journal of Medical Sciences* 59, no. 1 (March 2010): 1–6, https://www.researchgate.net/publication/44644903.

45. Hong Zhao et al., "Spore Powder of *Ganoderma lucidum* Improves Cancer-Related Fatigue in Breast Cancer Patients Undergoing Endocrine Therapy: A Pilot Clinical Trial," *Evidence-Based Complementary and Alternative Medicine* 2012 (January 2012): 809614, https://doi.org/10.1155/2012/809614.

46. Sandra L. Duque Henao et al., "Randomized Clinical Trial for the Evaluation of Immune

Modulation by Yogurt Enriched with β-Glucans from Lingzhi or Reishi Medicinal Mushroom, *Ganoderma lucidum* (Agaricomycetes), in Children from Medellin, Colombia," *International Journal of Medicinal Mushrooms* 20, no. 8 (August 2018): 705–16, https://doi.org/10.1615/intjmedmushrooms.2018026986.

47. Shiu-Nan Chen et al., "Evaluation of Immune Modulation by β-1,3; 1,6 D-Glucan Derived from *Ganoderma lucidum* in Healthy Adult Volunteers, A Randomized Controlled Trial," *Foods* 12, no. 3 (February 2023): 659, https://doi.org/10.3390/foods12030659.

48. Djanggan Sargowo et al., "The Role of Polysaccharide Peptides of Miselia Ganoderma Lucidum Extracts on IL-1, IL-6, HSCRP and No in Dislipidemic Patients with or without Hypertension in STEMI and NSTEMI Patients," *AIP Conference Proceedings* 2108, no. 1 (June 2019): 020027, https://doi.org/10.1063/1.5110002.

49. Ardian Rizal et al., "*Ganoderma lucidum* Polysaccharide Peptide Reduce Inflammation and Oxidative Stress in Patient with Atrial Fibrillation," *The Indonesian Biomedical Journal* 12, no. 4 (October 2020): 384–9, https://doi.org/10.18585/inabj.v12i4.1244.

50. Yihuai Gao et al., "A Phase I/II Study of Ling Zhi Mushroom *Ganoderma lucidum* (W.Curt.:Fr.) Lloyd (Aphyllophoromycetideae) Extract in Patients with Coronary Heart Disease," *International Journal of Medicinal Mushrooms* 6, no. 4 (2004): 327–34, https://doi.org/10.1615/IntJMedMushr.v6.i4.30.

51. Tanya T. W. Chu et al., "Study of Potential Cardioprotective Effects of *Ganoderma lucidum* (Lingzhi): Results of a Controlled Human Intervention Trial," *British Journal of Nutrition* 107, no. 7 (April 2012): 1017–27, https://doi.org/10.1017/S0007114511003795.

52. Yihuai Gao et al., "A Phase I/II Study of Ling Zhi Mushroom *Ganoderma lucidum* (W.Curt.:Fr.) Lloyd (Aphyllophoromycetideae) Extract in Patients with Type II Diabetes Mellitus," *International Journal of Medicinal Mushrooms* 6, no. 1 (2004): 33–40, https://doi.org/10.1615/IntJMedMushr.v6.i1.30.

53. Nerida L. Klupp et al., "A Double-Blind, Randomised, Placebo-Controlled Trial of *Ganoderma lucidum* for the Treatment of Cardiovascular Risk Factors of Metabolic Syndrome," *Scientific Reports* 6 (August 2016): 29540, https://doi.org/10.1038/srep29540.

54. Francesco Pazzi et al., "*Ganoderma lucidum* Effects on Mood and Health-Related Quality of Life in Women with Fibromyalgia," *Healthcare* 8, no. 4 (November 2020): 520, https://doi.org/10.3390/healthcare8040520.

55. Gaétan Chevalier et al., "Earthing (Grounding) the Human Body Reduces Blood Viscosity—a Major Factor in Cardiovascular Disease," *Journal of Alternative and Complementary Medicine* 19, no. 2 (February 2013): 102–110, https://doi.org/10.1089/acm.2011.0820.

56. Qing Shen, David M. Geiser, and Daniel J. Royse, "Molecular Phylogenetic Analysis of *Grifola frondosa* (Maitake) Reveals a Species Partition Separating Eastern North American and Asian Isolates," *Mycologica* 94, no. 3 (May 2002): 472–82, https://doi.org/10.2307/3761781.

57. Jian-Yong Wu, Ka-Chai Siu, and Ping Geng, "Bioactive Ingredients and Medicinal Values of *Grifola frondosa* (Maitake)," *Foods* 10, no. 1 (January 2021): 95, https://doi.org/10.3390/foods10010095.

58. Gary Deng et al., "A Phase I/II Trial of a Polysaccharide Extract from *Grifola frondosa* (Maitake mushroom) in Breast Cancer Patients: Immunological Effects," *Journal of Cancer Research and Clinical Oncology* 135, no. 9 (September 2009): 1215–21, https://doi.org/10.1007/s00432-009-0562-z.

59. Noriko Kodama, Kiyoshi Komuta, and Hiroaki Nanba, "Effect of Maitake (*Grifola frondosa*) D-Fraction on the Activation of NK Cells in Cancer Patients," *Journal of Medicinal Food* 6, no. 4 (December 2003): 371–77, https://doi.org/10.1089/109662003772519949.

60. Jun Nishihira et al., "Maitake Mushrooms (*Grifola frondosa*) Enhances Antibody Production in Response to Influenza Vaccination in Healthy Adult Volunteers Concurrent with Alleviation of Common Cold Symptoms," *Functional Foods in*

Health and Disease 7, no. 7 (July 2017): 462–82, https://doi.org/10.31989/ffhd.v7i7.363.

61. Sensuke Konno, "SX-Fraction: Promise for Novel Treatment of Type 2 Diabetes," *World Journal of Diabetes* 11, no. 12 (December 2020): 572–83, https://doi.org/10.4239/wjd.v1 1.i12.572.

62. Jui-Tung Chen, "Maitake Mushroom (*Grifola frondosa*) Extract Induces Ovulation in Patients with Polycystic Ovary Syndrome: A Possible Monotherapy and a Combination Therapy after Failure with First-Line Clomiphene Citrate," *Journal of Alternative and Complementary Medicine* 16, no. 12 (December 2010): 1295–99, https://doi.org/10.1089/acm.2009.0696.

63. Ju-Ha Kim et al., "*Grifola frondosa* Extract Containing Bioactive Components Blocks Skin Fibroblastic Inflammation and Cytotoxicity Caused by Endocrine Disrupting Chemical, Bisphenol A," *Nutrients* 14, no. 18 (September 2022): 3812, https://doi.org/10.3390/nu14 183812.

64. Thitinard Nitheranont et al., "Decolorization of Synthetic Dyes and Biodegradation of Bisphenol A by Laccase from the Edible Mushroom, *Grifola frondosa*," *Bioscience, Biotechnology, and Biochemistry* 75, no. 9 (September 2011): 1845–47, https://doi.org/10.1271/bbb.110329.

65. Masashi Seto et al., "Degradation of Polychlorinated Biphenyls by a 'Maitake' Mushroom, *Grifola frondosa*," *Biotechnology Letters* 21, no. 1 (January 1999): 27–31, https://doi.org/10.1023/A:1005457201291.

66. Mayumi Nagano et al., "Reduction of Depression and Anxiety by 4 Weeks *Hericium erinaceus* Intake," *Biomedical Research* 31, no. 4 (August 2010): 231–37, https://doi.org/10.2220 /biomedres.31.231.

67. Luisella Vigna et al., "*Hericium erinaceus* Improves Mood and Sleep Disorders in Patients Affected by Overweight or Obesity: Could Circulating Pro-BDNF and BDNF Be Potential Biomarkers?," *Evidence-Based Complementary and Alternative Medicine* 2019, no. 1 (January 2019): 7861297, https://doi .org/10.1155/2019/7861297.

68. Koichiro Mori et al., "Improving Effects of the Mushroom Yamabushitake (*Hericium erinaceus*) on Mild Cognitive Impairment: A Double-Blind Placebo-Controlled Clinical Trial," *Phytotherapy Research* 23, no. 3 (March 2009): 367–72, https://doi.org/10.1002 /ptr.2634.

69. Yin-Ching Chan et al., "Effects of Erinacine A-Enriched *Hericium erinaceus* on Elderly Hearing-Impaired Patients: A Double-Blind, Randomized, Placebo-Controlled Clinical Trial," *Journal of Functional Foods* 97 (October 2022): 105220, https://doi.org/10.1016/j .jff.2022.105220.

70. I-Chen Li et al., "Prevention of Early Alzheimer's Disease by Erinacine A-Enriched *Hericium erinaceus* Mycelia Pilot Double-Blind Placebo-Controlled Study," *Frontiers in Aging Neuroscience* 12 (June 2020): 155, https://doi .org/10.3389/fnagi.2020.00155.

71. Sarah Docherty, Faye L. Doughty, and Ellen F. Smith, "The Acute and Chronic Effects of Lion's Mane Mushroom Supplementation on Cognitive Function, Stress and Mood in Young Adults: A Double-Blind, Parallel Groups, Pilot Study," *Nutrients* 15, no. 22 (November 2023): 4842. https://doi.org/10.3390/nu15224842.

72. Maša Černelič Bizjak et al., "Effect of Erinacine A-Enriched *Hericium erinaceus* Supplementation on Cognition: A Randomized, Double-Blind, Placebo-Controlled Pilot Study," *Journal of Functional Foods* 115 (April 2025): 106120, https://doi.org/10.1016/j.jff.2024 .106120.

73. Xiao-Qian Xie et al., "Influence of Short-Term Consumption of *Hericium erinaceus* on Serum Biochemical Markers and the Changes of the Gut Microbiota: A Pilot Study," *Nutrients* 13, no. 3 (March 2021): 1008, https://doi.org /10.3390/nu13031008.

74. Seul Ki Lee et al., "Characterization of α-Glucosidase Inhibitory Constituents of the Fruiting Body of Lion's Mane Mushroom (*Hericium erinaceus*)," *Journal of Ethnopharmacology* 262 (November 2020): 113197, https://doi.org /10.1016/j.jep.2020.113197.

75. Sirui Zhang et al., "Associations of Sugar Intake, High-Sugar Dietary Pattern, and the Risk of Dementia: A Prospective Cohort Study of 210,832 Participants," *BMC Medicine* 22 (July 2024): 298, https://doi.org/10.1186/s12916-024-03525-6.

76. Antonietta G. Gravina et al., "*Hericium erinaceus*, in Combination with Natural Flavonoid/Alkaloid and B$_3$/B$_8$ Vitamins, Can Improve Inflammatory Burden in Inflammatory Bowel Diseases Tissue: An *Ex Vivo* Study," *Frontiers in Immunology* 14 (July 2023): 1215329, https://doi.org/10.3389/fimmu.2023.1215329.

77. Jing-Yang Wong et al., "Gastroprotective Effects of Lion's Mane Mushroom *Hericium erinaceus* (Bull.:Fr.) Pers. (Aphyllophoromycetideae) Extract against Ethanol-Induced Ulcer in Rats," *Evidence-Based Complementary and Alternative Medicine* 2013 (November 2013): 492976, https://doi.org/10.1155/2013/492976.

78. Antoine Géry et al., "Chaga (*Inonotus obliquus*), a Future Potential Medicinal Fungus in Oncology? A Chemical Study and a Comparison of the Cytotoxicity against Human Lung Adenocarcinoma Cells (A549) and Human Bronchial Epithelial Cells (BEAS-2B)," *Integrative Cancer Therapies* 17, no. 3 (September 2018): 832–43, https://doi.org/10.1177/1534735418757912.

79. Robin Wall Kimmerer, *Braiding Sweetgrass: Indigenous Wisdom, Scientific Knowledge, and the Teachings of Plants* (Milkweed Editions, 2013), 364.

80. Eric Fordjour et al., "Chaga Mushroom: A Super-Fungus with Countless Facets and Untapped Potential," *Frontiers in Pharmacology* 14 (December 2013): 1273786, https://doi.org/10.3389/fphar.2023.1273786.

81. Robin J. Marles et al., *Aboriginal Plant Use in Canada's Northwest Boreal Forest* (Edmonton, AB: Canadian Forest Service, 2000), 13, https://www.cabidigitallibrary.org/doi/full/10.5555/20000311129.

82. Konrad A. Szychowski et al., "*Inonotus obliquus*—from Folk Medicine to Clinical Use," *Journal of Traditional and Complementary Medicine* 11,

no. 4 (July 2021): 293–302, https://doi.org/10.1016/j.jtcme.2020.08.003.

83. Selina Plehn, Sajeev Wagle, and H. P. Vasantha Rupasinghe, "Chaga Mushroom Triterpenoids as Adjuncts to Minimally Invasive Cancer Therapies: A Review," *Current Research in Toxicology* 5 (2023): 100137, https://doi.org/10.1016/j.crtox.2023.100137.

84. Min-Gu Lee et al., "Chaga Mushroom Extract Induces Autophagy via the AMPK-mTOR Signaling Pathway in Breast Cancer Cells," *Journal of Ethnopharmacology* 274 (June 2021): 114081, https://doi.org/10.1016/j.jep.2021.114081.

85. Quentin Frew et al., "Betulin Wound Gel Accelerated Healing of Superficial Partial Thickness Burns: Results of a Randomized, Intra-Individually Controlled, Phase III Trial with 12-Months Follow-Up," *Burns* 45, no. 4 (June 2019): 876–90, https://doi.org/10.1016/j.burns.2018.10.019.

86. Armin Scheffler, "The Wound Healing Properties of Betulin from Birch Bark from Bench to Bedside," *Planta Medica* 85, no. 7 (March 2019): 524–27, https://doi.org/10.1055/a-0850-0224.

87. Tamara V. Teplyakova et al., "Water Extract of the Chaga Medicinal Mushroom, *Inonotus obliquus* (Agaricomycetes), Inhibits SARS-CoV-2 Replication in Vero E6 and Vero Cell Culture Experiments," *International Journal of Medicinal Mushrooms* 24, no. 2 (February 2022): 23–30, https://doi.org/10.1615/IntJMedMushrooms.2021042012.

88. Teplyakova et al., "Water Extract."

89. Jonathan Robins, "Picking Stories, Selling Chaga: How History Helped Make Chaga a Superfood," *The Otter* (blog), NiCHE: Network in Canadian History & Environment, September 7, 2023, https://niche-canada.org/2023/09/07/picking-stories-selling-chaga/.

90. Gastón Guzmán, "Diversity and Use of Traditional Mexican Medicinal Fungi. A Review," *International Journal of Medicinal Mushrooms* 10, no. 3 (2008): 209–17, https://doi.org/10.1615/IntJMedMushr.v10.i3.20.

91. Alejandro R. López et al., "Essential Mineral Content (Fe, Mg, P, Mn, K, Ca, and Na) in Five Wild Edible Species of *Lactarius* Mushrooms from Southern Spain and Northern Morocco: Reference to Daily Intake," in "Edible and Medicinal Macrofungi," ed. Ruilin Zhao, special issue, *Journal of Fungi* 8, no. 12 (December 2022): 1292, https://doi.org/10.3390/jof8121292.

92. Lillian Barros et al., "Effect of Fruiting Body Maturity Stage on Chemical Composition and Antimicrobial Activity of *Lactarius* sp. Mushrooms," *Journal of Agricultural and Food Chemistry* 55, no. 21 (October 2007): 8766–71, https://doi.org/10.1021/jf071435+.

93. Marina Kostić et al., "A Comparative Study of *Lactarius* Mushrooms: Chemical Characterization, Antibacterial, Antibiofilm, Antioxidant and Cytotoxic Activity," in "Mushrooms—Mycotherapy and Mycochemistry 2.0," ed. Jasmina Glamočlija and Dejan Stojković, special issue, *Journal of Fungi* 9, no. 1 (January 2023): 70, https://doi.org/10.3390/jof9010070.

94. Marijana Kosanić et al., "Evaluation of Metal Concentration and Antioxidant, Antimicrobial, and Anticancer Potentials of Two Edible Mushrooms *Lactarius deliciosus* and *Macrolepiota procera*," *Journal of Food and Drug Analysis* 24, no. 3 (July 2016): 477–84, https://doi.org/10.1016/j.jfda.2016.01.008.

95. Murat Şebin, Necmettin Yılmaz, and Ali Aydın, "Some Wild Mushrooms with High Antioxidant Capacity Exhibit Potent Anticancer Activity on Cancer Cells Using the Apoptotic and Antimigration Cell Death Mechanisms," *Anti-Cancer Agents in Medicinal Chemistry* 23, no. 13 (May 2023): 1567–76, https://doi.org/10.2174/1871520623666230331084010.

96. Şebin, Yılmaz, and Aydın, "Some Wild Mushrooms."

97. He Dan, *Records of Longquan County*, n.d., ca. 1209, quoted in "Mushroom Introduction" [in Chinese], Yuwang Jituan, archived February 25, 2017, Internet Archive, https://web.archive.org/web/20170225225742/http://hnywzy.com/news_show.asp?id=1829.

98. "Mushroom Introduction," Yuwang Jituan, archived February 25, 2017, Internet Archive, https://web.archive.org/web/20170225225742/http://hnywzy.com/news_show.asp?id=1829.

99. "Mushroom Introduction," Yuwang Jituan, archived February 25, 2017, Internet Archive, https://web.archive.org/web/20170225225742/http://hnywzy.com/news_show.asp?id=1829.

100. Seerengaraj Vijayaram et al., "Bioactive Immunostimulants as Health-Promoting Feed Additives in Aquaculture: A Review," *Fish & Shellfish Immunology* 130 (November 2022): 294–308, https://doi.org/10.1016/j.fsi.2022.09.011.

101. Selime Semra Erol, Ilgaz Akata, and Ertuğrul Kaya, "Use of Macrofungi in Traditional and Complementary Medicine Practices: Mycotherapy," *International Journal of Traditional and Complementary Medicine Research* 1, no. 2 (August 2020): 70–78, https://dergipark.org.tr/en/pub/ijtcmr/issue/56526/762087.

102. Wangkheirakpam Sujata, Sanjram Nomita Devi, and Subhash C. Mandal, "Phytochemicals and Investigations on Traditionally Used Medicinal Mushrooms," in *Evidence Based Validation of Traditional Medicines: A Comprehensive Approach*, ed. Subhash C. Mandal, Raja Chakraborty, and Saikat Sen (Singapore: Springer Singapore, 2022), 965–84, https://doi.org/10.1007/978-981-15-8127-4_45.

103. Soo Liang Ooi et al., "The Health-Promoting Properties and Clinical Applications of Rice Bran Arabinoxylan Modified with Shiitake Mushroom Enzyme—A Narrative Review," in "Nutraceuticals in Immune Function," ed. Sokcheon Pak and Soo Liang Ooi, special issue, *Molecules* 26, no. 9 (April 2021): 2539, https://doi.org/10.3390/molecules26092539.

104. Mai Hong Bang et al., "Arabinoxylan Rice Bran (MGN-3) Enhances the Effects of Interventional Therapies for the Treatment of Hepatocellular Carcinoma: A Three-Year Randomized Clinical Trial," *Anticancer Research* 30, no. 12 (December 2010): 5145–51, https://ar.iiarjournals.org/content/30/12/5145.

105. Dorothy Faye S. Tan and Jerickson Abbie S. Flores, "The Immunomodulating Effects of Arabinoxylan Rice Bran (Lentin) on Hematologic Profile, Nutritional Status and Quality of Life among Head and Neck Carcinoma Patients Undergoing Radiation Therapy: A Double Blind Randomized Control Trial," *Philippine College of Radiology Journal* 12 (February 2020), 11–15, https://www.biobran.gr/ipdf/MCN-3 _Biobran_2020_Immunomodul_Hematologic _QOL_Carcinoma_Radiation.pdf.

106. Gabriel Petrovics et al., "Controlled Pilot Study for Cancer Patients Suffering from Chronic Fatigue Syndrome Due to Chemotherapy Treated with BioBran (MGN-3-Arabinoxylane) and Targeted Radiofrequency Heat Therapy," in "Supplement Part 2—ECIM Abstracts," *European Journal of Integrative Medicine* 8, no. S2 (September 2016): 29–35, https://doi.org /10.1016/j.eujim.2016.10.004.

107. Hiroaki Maeda et al., "Oral Administration of Hydrolyzed Rice Bran Prevents the Common Cold Syndrome in the Elderly Based on Its Immunomodulatory Action," *BioFactors* 21 (December 2008): 185–87, https://doi.org /10.1002/biof.552210138.

108. Hosny Salama et al., "Arabinoxylan Rice Bran (Biobran) Suppresses the Viremia Level in Patients with Chronic HCV Infection: A Randomized Trial," *International Journal of Immunopathology and Pharmacology* 29, no. 4 (October 2016): 647–53, https://doi.org /10.1177/0394632016674954.

109. Sudhanshu Agrawal, Anshu Agrawal, and Mamdooh Ghoneum, "Biobran/MGN-3, an Arabinoxylan Rice Bran, Exerts Anti-COVID-19 Effects and Boosts Immunity in Human Subjects," *Nutrients* 16, no. 6 (March 2024): 881, https://doi.org/10.3390/nu16060881.

110. John E. Lewis et al., "The Effect of a Hydrolyzed Polysaccharide Dietary Supplement on Biomarkers in Adults with Nonalcoholic Fatty Liver Disease," *Evidence-Based Complementary and Alternative Medicine* 2018 (May 2018): 1751583, https://doi.org/10.1155/2018 /1751583.

111. Takeshi Kamiya et al., "Therapeutic Effects of Biobran, Modified Arabinoxylan Rice Bran, in Improving Symptoms of Diarrhea Predominant or Mixed Type Irritable Bowel Syndrome: A Pilot, Randomized Controlled Study," in "Complementary and Alternative Therapies for Functional Gastrointestinal Diseases," ed. Jiande D. Z. Chen, special issue, *Evidence-Based Complementary and Alternative Medicine* 2014 (November 2014): 828137, https://doi.org /10.1155/2014/828137.

112. J. Avinash et al., "The Unexplored Anticaries Potential of Shiitake Mushroom," *Pharmacognosy Reviews* 10, no. 20 (July–December 2016): 100–4, https://doi.org/10.4103/0973-784 7.194039.

113. S. Tsujiyama, T. Muraoka, and N. Takada, "Biodegradation of 2,4-Dichlorophenol by Shiitake Mushroom (*Lentinula edodes*) Using Vanillin as an Activator," *Biotechnology Letters* 35 (July 2013): 1079–83, https://doi.org/10 .1007/s10529-013-1179-5.

114. C.M. Visagie et al., "Identification and Nomenclature of the Genus *Penicillium*," *Studies in Mycology* 78, no. 1 (June 2014): 343–71, https://doi.org/10.1016/j.simyco.2014.09.001.

115. Frank Matthew Dugan, *Fungi in the Ancient World: How Mushrooms, Mildews, Molds and Yeast Shaped the Early Civilizations of Europe, the Mediterranean and the Near East* (St. Paul, MN: APS Press, 2008), 49.

116. Emory University, "Ancient Brew Masters Tapped Antibiotic Secrets," ScienceDaily, September 2, 2010, www.sciencedaily.com /releases/2010/09/100902094246.htm.

117. Matthew I. Hutchings, Andrew W. Truman, and Barrie Wilkinson, "Antibiotics: Past, Present and Future," *Current Opinion in Microbiology* 51 (October 2019): 72–80, https://doi.org/10 .1016/j.mib.2019.10.008.

118. Charles Fletcher, "First Clinical Use of Penicillin," *British Medical Journal (Clinical Research Edition)* 289, no. 6460 (December 1984): 1721–23, https://doi.org/10.1136/bmj.289.6460.1721.

119. Mayuki Sasaki et al., "Milk-Based Culture of *Penicillium camemberti* and Its Component

Oleamide Affect Cognitive Function in Healthy Elderly Japanese Individuals: A Multi-Arm Randomized, Double-Blind, Placebo-Controlled Study," *Frontiers in Nutrition* 11 (March 2024): 1357920, https://doi.org/10.3389/fnut.2024.1357920.

120. Mohamed S. Mady et al., "The Indole Alkaloid Meleagrin, from the Olive Tree Endophytic Fungus *Penicillium chrysogenum*, as a Novel Lead for the Control of C-Met-Dependent Breast Cancer Proliferation, Migration and Invasion," *Bioorganic & Medicinal Chemistry* 24, no. 2 (January 2016): 113–22, https://doi.org/10.1016/j.bmc.2015.11.038.

121. Qin-Ying Liu et al., "Antitumor Effects and Related Mechanisms of Penicitrinine A, a Novel Alkaloid with a Unique Spiro Skeleton from the Marine Fungus *Penicillium citrinum*," *Marine Drugs* 13, no. 8 (August 2015): 4733–53, https://doi.org/10.3390/md13084733.

122. Aymeric Monteillier et al., "Lung Cancer Chemopreventive Activity of Patulin Isolated from *Penicillium vulpinum*," in "Plant Derived Natural Products and Age Related Diseases," ed. Hermann Stuppner and Alexios Leandros Skaltsounis, special issue, *Molecules* 23, no. 3 (March 2018): 636, https://doi.org/10.3390/molecules23030636.

123. Shahzad Saleem et al., "Identification of Effective and Nonpromiscuous Antidiabetic Drug Molecules from *Penicillium* Species," in "Plant-Derived Bioactive Compounds as an Antidiabetic Agent," ed. Arpita Roy, special issue, *Evidence-Based Complementary and Alternative Medicine* 2022 (August 2022): 7040547, https://doi.org/10.1155/2022/7040547.

124. Neri Azar et al., "Endophytic *Penicillium* Species Secretes Mycophenolic Acid That Inhibits the Growth of Phytopathogenic Fungi," in "End Hunger: Enhancing Crop Yields with Microbes," ed. Patricia Bernal, Davinia Salvachúa, and Juan Luis Ramos, special issue, *Microbial Biotechnology* 16, no. 8 (August 2023): 1629–38, https://doi.org/10.1111/1751-7915.14203.

125. Sarah Remi Ibiang, Kazunori Sakamoto, and Nanami Kuwahara, "Performance of Tomato and Lettuce to Arbuscular Mycorrhizal Fungi and *Penicillium pinophilum* EU0013 Inoculation Varies with Soil, Culture Media of Inoculum, and Fungal Consortium Composition," in "Applications of Agriculturally Important Microorganisms for the Management of Soilborne Phytopathogens," ed. Sina Adl, special issue, *Rhizosphere* 16 (December 2020): 100246, https://doi.org/10.1016/j.rhisph.2020.100246.

126. Georgina Uriarte-Frías et al., "Pre-Hispanic Foods Oyster Mushroom (*Pleurotus ostreatus*), Nopal (*Opuntia ficus-indica*) and Amaranth (*Amaranthus* sp.) as New Alternative Ingredients for Developing Functional Cookies," in "Edible Mushrooms," ed. Monika Gąsecka and Zuzanna Magdziak, special issue, *Journal of Fungi* 7, no. 11 (October 2021): 911, https://doi.org/10.3390/jof7110911.

127. Milos Jesenak et al., "Immunomodulatory Effect of Pleuran (β-Glucan from *Pleurotus ostreatus*) in Children with Recurrent Respiratory Tract Infections," *International Immunopharmacology* 15, no. 2 (February 2013): 395–99, https://doi.org/10.1016/j.intimp.2012.11.020.

128. Ingrid Urbancikova et al., "Efficacy of Pleuran (β-Glucan from *Pleurotus ostreatus*) in the Management of Herpes Simplex Virus Type 1 Infection," *Evidence-Based Complementary and Alternative Medicine* 2020 (April 2020): 8562309, https://doi.org/10.1155/2020/8562309.

129. Khaleda Khatun et al., "Oyster Mushroom Reduced Blood Glucose and Cholesterol in Diabetic Subjects," *Mymensingh Medical Journal* 16, no. 1 (July 2007): 94–99, https://pubmed.ncbi.nlm.nih.gov/17344789.

130. M. Abu Sayeed et al., "Effect of Edible Mushroom (*Pleurotus ostreatus*) on Type-2 Diabetics," *Ibrahim Medical College Journal* 8, no. 1 (April 2015): 6–11, https://doi.org/10.3329/imcj.v8i1.22982.

131. M.B.K. Choudhury et al., "Effects of *Pleurotus ostreatus* on Blood Pressure and Glycemic Status

of Hypertensive Diabetic Male Volunteers," *Bangladesh Journal of Medical Biochemistry* 6, no. 1 (January 2013): 5–10, https://doi.org /10.3329/bjmb.v6i1.13280.

132. Stamatia-Angeliki Kleftaki et al., "A Randomized Controlled Trial on *Pleurotus eryngii* Mushrooms with Antioxidant Compounds and Vitamin D_2 in Managing Metabolic Disorders," *Antioxidants* 11, no. 11 (October 2022): 2113, https://doi.org/10.3390/antiox11112113.

133. Abu Sayeed et al., "Effect of Edible Mushroom."

134. Kleftaki et al., "A Randomized Controlled Trial."

135. Shweta S. Gogavekar et al., "Important Nutritional Constituents, Flavour Components, Antioxidant and Antibacterial Properties of *Pleurotus sajor-caju*," *Journal of Food Science and Technology* 51 (August 2014): 1483–91, https://doi.org/10.1007/s13197-012-0656-5.

136. Daniel Lam-Sidun, Kia M. Peters, and Nica M. Borradaile, "Mushroom-Derived Medicine? Preclinical Studies Suggest Potential Benefits of Ergothioneine for Cardiometabolic Health," *International Journal of Molecular Sciences* 22, no. 6 (March 2021): 3246, https://doi.org /10.3390/ijms22063246.

137. Lam-Sidun, Peters, and Borradaile, "Mushroom-Derived Medicine?"

138. Varsha Satankar et al., "Oyster Mushroom—A Viable Indigenous Food Source for Rural Masses," *International Journal of Agricultural Engineering* 11 (April 2018): 173–78, https:// www.researchgate.net/publication/325267531 _Oyster_mushroom-A_viable_indigenous _food_source_for_rural_masses.

139. Amro Matyori et al., "Statins Utilization Trends and Expenditures in the U.S. Before and After the Implementation of the 2013 ACC/AHA Guidelines," *Saudi Pharmaceutical Journal* 31, no. 6 (June 2023): 795–800, https://doi.org /10.1016/j.jsps.2023.04.002.

140. Curt D. Furberg and Bertram Pitt, "Withdrawal of Cerivastatin from the World Market," *Trials* 2 (September 2001): 205, https://doi.org/10 .1186/cvm-2-5-205.

141. Elena Olmastroni et al., "Statin Use and Risk of Dementia or Alzheimer's Disease: A Systematic Review and Meta-Analysis of Observational Studies, *European Journal of Preventive Cardiology* 29, no. 5 (March 2022): 804–14, https://doi.org/10.1093/eurjpc/zwab208.

142. Gréta Törös et al., "Modulation of the Gut Microbiota with Prebiotics and Antimicrobial Agents from *Pleurotus ostreatus* Mushroom," *Foods* 12, no. 10 (May 2023): 2010, https://doi.org/10.3390/foods12102010.

143. Törös et al., "Modulation of the Gut Microbiota."

144. Satyandra Singh, Bijendra Singh, and A.P. Singh, "Nematodes: A Threat to Sustainability of Agriculture," *Procedia Environmental Sciences* 29 (2015): 215–16, https://doi.org/10.1016/j .proenv.2015.07.270.

145. Lukasz Smigielski et al., "Psilocybin-Assisted Mindfulness Training Modulates Self-Consciousness and Brain Default Mode Network Connectivity with Lasting Effects," *NeuroImage* 196 (August 2019): 207–15, https://doi.org /10.1016/j.neuroimage.2019.04.009.

146. Jahan Khamsehzadeh, *The Psilocybin Connection: Psychedelics, the Transformation of Consciousness, and Evolution of the Planet—An Integral Approach* (Berkeley: North Atlantic Books, 2022).

147. "The Cult of the Mushroom," Ancient Wisdom, accessed March 6, 2025, http://www.ancient -wisdom.com/guatemala.htm.

148. Mark D. Merlin, "Archaeological Evidence for the Tradition of Psychoactive Plant Use in the Old World," *Economic Botany* 57, no. 3 (September 2003): 295–323, https://doi.org/10.1663/0013 -0001(2003)057[0295:AEFTTO]2.0.CO;2.

149. Ahmed M. Abdel-Azeem et al., "The Conservation of Mushroom in Ancient Egypt through the Present" (conference paper, The First International Conference on Fungal Conservation in the Middle East and North of Africa, Ismailia, Egypt, October 18–20, 2016), https:// www.researchgate.net/publication/320991848 _The_Conservation_of_Mushroom_in _Ancient_Egypt_through_the_Present.

150. "The Great Sphinx," Research Highlights, Robert M. Schoch, accessed March 6, 2025, https://www.robertschoch.com/sphinx.html.

151. Vince Polito and Paul Liknaitzky, "Is Microdosing a Placebo? A Rapid Review of Low-Dose LSD and Psilocybin Research," *Journal of Psychopharmacology* 38, no. 8 (June 2024): 701–11, https://doi.org/10.1177/026988 11241254831.

152. Joseph M. Rootman et al., "Psilocybin Microdosers Demonstrate Greater Observed Improvements in Mood and Mental Health at One Month Relative to Non-Microdosing Controls," *Scientific Reports* 12 (June 2022): 11091, https://doi.org/10.1038/s41598 -022-14512-3.

153. Kavita Golia, "Psilocybin as a Healer: A Transcendental Phenomenological Study of Individual Experiences of Microdosing Psilocybin," *Consciousness, Spirituality & Transpersonal Psychology* 3 (2022): 18–34, https://doi.org/10.53074/cstp.2022.37.

154. Athina-Marina Metaxa and Mike Clarke, "Efficacy of Psilocybin for Treating Symptoms of Depression: Systematic Review and Meta-Analysis," *BMJ* 2024, no. 385 (May 2024): e078084, https://doi.org/10.1136 /bmj-2023-078084.

155. R. L. Carhart-Harris et al., "Psilocybin with Psychological Support for Treatment-Resistant Depression: Six-Month Follow-Up," in "Psychedelics and Related Drugs: Therapeutic Possibilities and Pitfalls?," ed. H. Valerie Curran, Harriet de Wit, and David Nutt, special issue, *Psychopharmacology* 235, no. 2 (February 2018): 399–408, https://doi .org/10.1007/s00213-017-4771-x; Natalie Gukasyan et al., "Efficacy and Safety of Psilocybin-Assisted Treatment for Major Depressive Disorder: Prospective 12-Month Follow-Up," *Journal of Psychopharmacology* 36, no. 2 (February 2022): 151–58, https://doi .org/10.1177/02698811211073759.

156. David Erritzoe et al., "Effect of Psilocybin Versus Escitalopram on Depression Symptom Severity in Patients with Moderate-to-Severe Major Depressive Disorder: Observational 6-Month Follow-Up of a Phase 2, Double-Blind, Randomised, Controlled Trial," *eClinicalMedicine* 76 (October 2024): 102799, https://doi.org/10.1016/j.eclinm.2024.102799.

157. Guy M. Goodwin et al., "Single-Dose Psilocybin for a Treatment-Resistant Episode of Major Depression," *New England Journal of Medicine* 387, no. 18 (November 2022): 1637–48, https://doi.org/10.1056/NEJMoa2206443.

158. Joost J. Breeksema et al., "Patient Perspectives and Experiences with Psilocybin Treatment for Treatment-Resistant Depression: A Qualitative Study," *Scientific Reports* 14 (February 2024): 2929, https://doi.org/10.1038/s41598-024 -53188-9.

159. Roland R. Griffiths et al., "Psilocybin Produces Substantial and Sustained Decreases in Depression and Anxiety in Patients with Life-Threatening Cancer: A Randomized Double-Blind Trial," *Journal of Psychopharmacology* 30, no. 12 (December 2016): 1181–97, https://doi.org/10.1177/0269881116675513.

160. Katherine A. MacLean et al., "Factor Analysis of the Mystical Experience Questionnaire: A Study of Experiences Occasioned by the Hallucinogen Psilocybin," *Journal for the Scientific Study of Religion* 51, no. 4 (December 2012): 721–37, https://doi.org/10.1111 /j.1468-5906.2012.01685.x.

161. Anthony L. Back et al., "Psilocybin Therapy for Clinicians with Symptoms of Depression from Frontline Care During the COVID-19 Pandemic: A Randomized Clinical Trial," *JAMA Network Open* 7, no. 12 (December 2024): e2449026, https://doi.org/10.1001 /jamanetworkopen.2024.49026.

162. Pim B. van der Meer et al., "Therapeutic Effect of Psilocybin in Addiction: A Systematic Review," *Frontiers in Psychiatry* 14 (February 2023): 1134454, https://doi.org/10.3389 /fpsyt.2023.1134454.

163. Amy C. Reichelt, Eric Vermetten, and Benjamin T. Dunkley, "Psychedelic and Nutraceutical Interventions as Therapeutic Strategies for Military-Related Mild Traumatic Brain Injuries," *Journal of Military, Veteran and Family Health* 9, no. 5 (October 2023): 28–37, https://doi.org/10.3138/jmvfh-2022-0084.

164. Christopher L Robinson et al., "Scoping Review: The Role of Psychedelics in the Management of Chronic Pain," *Journal of Pain Research* 17 (March 2024): 965–73, https://doi.org/10.2147/JPR.S439348.

165. Emmanuelle A. D. Schindler et al., "Psilocybin Pulse Regimen Reduces Cluster Headache Attack Frequency in the Blinded Extension Phase of a Randomized Controlled Trial," *Journal of the Neurological Sciences* 460 (May 2024): 122993, https://doi.org/10.1016/j.jns.2024.122993.

166. N. L. Mason et al., "Psilocybin Induces Acute and Persisting Alterations in Immune Status in Healthy Volunteers: An Experimental, Placebo-Controlled Study," *Brain, Behavior, and Immunity* 114 (November 2023): 299–310, https://doi.org/10.1016/j.bbi.2023.09.004.

167. Gastón Guzmán, "Diversity and Use of Traditional Mexican Medicinal Fungi. A Review," *International Journal of Medicinal Mushrooms* 10, no. 3 (2008): 209–17, https://doi.org/10.1615/IntJMedMushr.v10.i3.20.

168. Héritier Milenge Kamalebo et al., "Uses and Importance of Wild Fungi: Traditional Knowledge from the Tshopo Province in the Democratic Republic of the Congo," *Journal of Ethnobiology and Ethnomedicine* 14, no. 13 (February 2018): https://doi.org/10.1186/s13002-017-0203-6.

169. Olusegun V. Oyetayo, "Medicinal Uses of Mushrooms in Nigeria: Towards Full and Sustainable Exploitation," *African Journal of Traditional, Complementary and Alternative Medicines* 8, no. 3 (April 2011): 267–74, https://doi.org/10.4314/ajtcam.v8i3.65289.

170. Kunihiro Okamura et al., "Clinical Evaluation of Schizophyllan Combined with Irradiation in Patients with Cervical Cancer," *Cancer* 58, no. 4 (August 1986): 865–72, https://doi.org/10.1002/1097-0142(19860815)58:4%3C865::AID-CNCR2820580411%3E3.0.CO;2-S.

171. Hui-Yeon Jang et al., "TBG-136, a Schizophyllum Commune-Derived β-Glucan Benefits Gut Microbiota and Intestinal Health: A Randomized, Double-Blind, and Placebo-Controlled Clinical Trial," *Journal of Functional Foods* 107 (August 2023): 105668, https://doi.org/10.1016/j.jff.2023.105668.

172. K. Ellan et al., "In Vivo Anti-Dengue Study of Schizophyllum Commune Aqueous Extract in AG129 Mice," in "Abstracts from International Congress on Infectious Diseases 2022, Held in Kuala Lumpur, Malaysia. November 17 - 20, 2022, 'ICID KL 2022'," ed. Shui Shan Lee, supplement, *International Journal of Infectious Diseases* 130, no. S2 (May 2023): S62, https://doi.org/10.1016/j.ijid.2023.04.156; Te-Kai Sun et al., "*Schizophyllum commune* Reduces Expression of the SARS-CoV-2 Receptors ACE2 and TMPRSS2," *International Journal of Molecular Sciences* 23, no. 23 (November 2022): 14766, https://doi.org/10.3390/ijms232314766.

173. Mark Louie S. Torres and Renato G. Reyes, "Antibacterial Potential of Different Crude Extracts of *Schizophyllum commune* Mycelia Grown on Coconut Water," *International Journal of Agricultural and Environmental Research* 6, no. 2 (November 2020): 134–41, https://www.researchgate.net/publication/345305140.

174. Amna Javaid, Rukhsana Bajwa, and Arshad Javaid, "Biosorption of Heavy Metals Using a Dead Macro Fungus *Schizophyllum commune* Fries: Evaluation of Equilibrium and Kinetic Models," *Pakistan Journal of Botany* 42, no. 3 (June 2010): 2105–118, https://www.researchgate.net/publication/236840328.

175. Juntao Yao et al., Rapid Decolorization of Azo Dyes by Crude Manganese Peroxidase from *Schizophyllum* sp. F17 in Solid-State Fermentation," *Biotechnology and Bioprocess Engineering* 18 (September 2013): 868–77, https://doi.org/10.1007/s12257-013-0357-6.

176. Abhishek Walia et al., "Microbial Xylanases and Their Industrial Application in Pulp and Paper Biobleaching: A Review," *3 Biotech* 7 (April 2017): 11, https://doi.org/10.1007/s13205-016-0584-6.

177. Zalina Awang et al., "The Usage of Waste Cooking Oil (Wco) in Production of Solid Dishwashing Soap with Split Gill Mushroom (*Schizophyllum commune*) Extract Addition," *Politeknik & Kolej Komuniti Journal of Social Sciences and Humanities* 7, no. 1 (November 2022): 85–95, https://app.mypolycc.edu.my /journal/index.php/PMJSSH/article/view/225.

178. Guzmán, "Diversity and Use."

179. Asif Hamid Dar et al., "Conspectus of Traditional Ethnomycological Insights Pertaining to Wild Mushrooms of South Kashmir, India," *Phytomedicine Plus* 3, no. 4 (November 2023): 100477, https://doi.org/10.1016/j.phypl u.2023.100477.

180. Wong L.Y. Eliza, Cheng K. Fai and Leung P. Chung, "Efficacy of Yun Zhi (*Coriolus versicolor*) on Survival in Cancer Patients: Systematic Review and Meta-Analysis," *Recent Patents on Inflammation & Allergy Drug Discovery* 6, no. 1 (2012): 78–87, https://doi .org/10.2174/187221312798889310.

181. Gentaro Ito et al., "Correlation Between Efficacy of PSK Postoperative Adjuvant Immunochemotherapy for Gastric Cancer and Expression of MHC Class I," *Experimental and Therapeutic Medicine* 3, no. 6 (June 2012): 925–30, https:// doi.org/10.3892/etm.2012.537.

182. Leanna J Standish et al., "*Trametes versicolor* Mushroom Immune Therapy in Breast Cancer," *Journal of the Society for Integrative Oncology* 6, no. 3 (June 2008): 122–28, https:// pmc.ncbi.nlm.nih.gov/articles/PMC2845472.

183. Carolyn J. Torkelson et al., "Phase 1 Clinical Trial of *Trametes versicolor* in Women with Breast Cancer," *International Scholarly Research Notices* 2012, no. 1 (January 2012): 251632, https://doi.org/10.5402/2012/251632.

184. Emma Camilleri et al., "A Comprehensive Review on the Health Benefits, Phytochemicals, and Enzymatic Constituents for Potential Therapeutic And Industrial Applications of Turkey Tail Mushrooms," *Discover Applied Sciences* 6 (May 2024): 257, https://doi .org/10.1007/s42452-024-05936-9.; Shaohua Shi et al., "β-Glucans from *Trametes*

versicolor (L.) Lloyd Is Effective for Prevention of Influenza Virus Infection," *Viruses* 14, no. 2: 237, https://doi.org/10.3390/v14020237.

185. Bruno Donatini et al., "Control of Oral Human Papillomavirus (HPV) by Medicinal Mushrooms, *Trametes versicolor* and *Ganoderma lucidum*: A Preliminary Clinical Trial," *International Journal of Medicinal Mushrooms* 16, no. 5 (2014): 497–98, https://doi.org /10.1615/IntJMedMushrooms.v16.i5.80.

186. Luis Serrano et al., "Efficacy of a *Coriolus versicolor*–Based Vaginal Gel in Women with Human Papillomavirus–Dependent Cervical Lesions: The PALOMA Study," *Journal of Lower Genital Tract Disease* 25, no. 2 (April 2021): 130–36, https://doi.org/10.1097/LGT .0000000000000596.

187. C. K. Wong et al., "Immunomodulatory Effects of Yun Zhi and Danshen Capsules in Health Subjects—A Randomized, Double-Blind, Placebo-Controlled, Crossover Study," *International Immunopharmacology* 4, no. 2 (February 2004): 201–11, https://doi.org /10.1016/j.intimp.2003.12.003.

188. Kumar Pallav et al., "Effects of Polysaccharopeptide from *Trametes Versicolor* and Amoxicillin on the Gut Microbiome of Healthy Volunteers: A Randomized Clinical Trial," *Gut Microbes* 5, no. 4 (July/August 2014): 458–67, https://doi .org/10.4161/gmic.29558.

189. Sílvia Romero et al., "Different Approaches to Improving the Textile Dye Degradation Capacity of *Trametes versicolor*," *Biochemical Engineering Journal* 31, no. 1 (August 2006): 42–47, https://doi.org/10.1016/j.bej.2006 .05.018.

190. Mun-Jung Han, Hyoung-Tae Park, and Hong-Gyu Song, "Degradation of Phenanthrene by *Trametes versicolor* and Its Laccase," *Journal of Microbiology* 42, no. 2 (June 2004): 94–98, https://koreascience.kr/article/JAKO 200411922358106.page.

191. Negin Yasrebi et al., "In Vivo and In Vitro Evaluation of the Wound Healing Properties of Chitosan Extracted from *Trametes versicolor*," *Journal of Polymer Research* 28 (September

2021): 399, https://doi.org/10.1007/s10965
-021-02773-x.

192. Seyedeh Kiana Teymoorian, Hoda Nouri, and
Hamid Moghimi, "In-Vivo and In-Vitro
Wound Healing and Tissue Repair Effect
of *Trametes versicolor* Polysaccharide Extract,"
Scientific Reports 14 (February 2024): 3796,
https://doi.org/10.1038/s41598-024-54565-0.

193. Zhuo-Teng Yu et al., "*Trametes versicolor* Extract
Modifies Human Fecal Microbiota

Composition *In Vitro*," *Plant Foods for Human
Nutrition* 68 (June 2013): 107–112, https://
doi.org/10.1007/s11130-013-0342-4.

194. Haiwei Lou et al, "Optimizing the Degradation
of Aflatoxin B_1 in Corn by *Trametes versicolor* and Improving the Nutritional
Composition of Corn," *Journal of the Science
of Food and Agriculture* 104, no. 2 (January
2024): 655–63, https://doi.org/10.1002
/jsfa.12956.

Index

Note: Page numbers in *italics* indicate photographs and illustrations. Page numbers followed by *t* indicate tables.

INDEX

INDEX

About the Authors

The Forest Farmacy: A School of Applied Eco-Mycology is a land-based learning community rooted in the Blue Ridge Mountains of North Carolina. Founded by Christopher and Katherine Parker, The Forest Farmacy teaches mushroom growing, forest co-tending, and spiritual connection to the land as practical, embodied pathways toward personal and ecosystem healing.

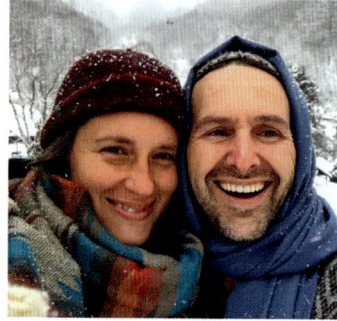

CHRISTOPHER PARKER

Christopher Parker is a self-taught mycologist and member of the Eastern Band of Cherokee Indians grounded in the Southern Appalachian Mountains. He began cultivating mushrooms at age 15, and he brings over three decades of experience, and deep ancestral knowing, in mushroom growing, wild harvesting, forest ecology, and traditional Cherokee foodways. Christopher is known for his hands-on teaching style, humor, and ability to make complex systems accessible and sacred.

Katherine Parker holds a PhD in psychology and has spent her career at the intersection of mental health, ancestral healing, and nature connection. She is certified in Eco-Therapy, Professional Transformational Coaching, and Wilderness Rites of Passage. Katherine creates transformational experiences that blend storytelling, contemplative practice, and nature connection to help people uncover their inner wisdom and access relational consciousness.

Together, Christopher and Katherine guide students—from beginner growers and wild foragers to future mushroom farmers and wild co-tending forest guides—through immersive in-person classes, online courses, and two certification tracks in applied eco-mycology. Their promise is simple and profound:

We teach people to come into right relationship with the forest—through growing food and medicine, tending the land, and deep spiritual connection.